MANUAL OF NEPHROLOGY

MANUAL OF NEPHROLOGY

Editors

Pranaw Kumar Jha
MD (Internal Medicine) DNB (Nephrology)
Consultant
Division of Nephrology and Transplant Medicine
Medanta Kidney and Urology Institute
Medanta—The Medicity
Gurgaon, Haryana, India

Vijay Kher
MD (Internal Medicine) DM (Nephrology) FAMS FRCPE
Chairman
Division of Nephrology and Transplant Medicine
Medanta Kidney and Urology Institute
Medanta—The Medicity
Gurgaon, Haryana, India

JAYPEE

JAYPEE BROTHERS MEDICAL PUBLISHERS

The Health Sciences Publisher

New Delhi | London

Jaypee Brothers Medical Publishers (P) Ltd.

Headquarters
EMCA House
23/23-B, Ansari Road, Daryaganj
New Delhi 110 002, India
Landline: +91-11-23272143, +91-11-23272703
+91-11-23282021, +91-11-23245672
E-mail: jaypee@jaypeebrothers.com

Corporate Office
Jaypee Brothers Medical Publishers (P) Ltd.
4838/24, Ansari Road, Daryaganj
New Delhi 110 002, India
Phone: +91-11-43574357
Fax: +91-11-43574314
E-mail: jaypee@jaypeebrothers.com

Overseas Office
JP Medical Ltd.
83, Victoria Street, London
SW1H 0HW (UK)
Phone: +44-20 3170 8910
E-mail: info@jpmedpub.com

EU GPSR Authorised Representative
Logos Europe, 9 rue Nicolas Poussin
17000, La Rochelle, France
Phone: +33 (0) 6 67 93 73 78
E-mail: Contact@logoseurope.eu

Website: www.jaypeebrothers.com
Website: www.jaypeedigital.com

Manual of Nephrology

First Edition: **2016,** Reprint: 2026
ISBN: 978-93-5250-162-5
Printed in India

Dedicated to

My parents, Mr US Jha and Mrs Neelam Jha—for motivating me to become a doctor and helping me achieve whatever I could in life
My wife, Dr Neha—for her unconditional patience and selfless support
To my teachers—for all the knowledge and guidance
My patients—for being the motivation to pursue medicine

Pranaw Kumar Jha

My parents Late Mrs Lalita and Mr PN Kher for inculcating the idea to become a doctor, Professor Chugh for his excellent mentoring and to all my patients for improving my skills to be a better doctor.

Vijay Kher

Contributors

Amit Gupta MD DNB FRCP
Professor
Department of Nephrology
Sanjay Gandhi Postgraduate Institute of Medical Sciences
Lucknow, Uttar Pradesh, India

Anita Saxena MD (AM) PhD PhD (Cambridge)
Additional Professor
Department of Nephrology
Sanjay Gandhi Postgraduate Institute of Medical Sciences
Lucknow, Uttar Pradesh, India

Arun Kumar Reddy Gorla MD
Senior Resident
Department of Nuclear Medicine
Postgraduate Institute of Medical Education and Research (PGIMER)
Chandigarh, India

Ashish Nandwani MD (Internal Medicine) DNB (Nephro) MNAMS
Consultant
Division of Nephrology and Transplant Medicine
Medanta Kidney and Urology Institute
Medanta—The Medicity
Gurgaon, Haryana, India

Bhagwant Rai Mittal MD DNB
Professor and Head
Department of Nuclear Medicine
Postgraduate Institute of Medical Education and Research (PGIMER)
Chandigarh, India

Georgi Abraham MD FRCP
Consultant Nephrologist
Pondicherry Institute of Medical Sciences
Puducherry, India
Madras Medical Mission
Chennai, Tamil Nadu, India

Gokulnath BSc MD (Med) DM DNB (Nephro) FISN FRCP (Lond)
Senior Consultant and Director
Nephrology Services
Apollo Group of Hospitals
Bengaluru, Karnataka, India

H Sudarshan Ballal MD FRCP (UK)
Board Certified in Internal Medicine
Nephrology and Critical Care (USA)
Chairman, Manipal Health Enterprises Private Ltd
Director
Manipal Institute of Nephrology and Urology Institute
Bengaluru, Karnataka, India

Harbir Singh Kohli MD DM
Professor
Department of Nephrology
Postgraduate Institute of Medical Education and Research (PGIMER)
Chandigarh, India

Indranil Ghosh DM (Nephro)
Classified Specialist (Medicine) and Nephrologist
Command Hospital (WC), Chandimandir
Panchkula, Haryana, India

KC Prakash MD (Int Med) DNB (Nephro)
Senior Consultant and Head
Department of Nephrology
Apollo Hospital
Chennai, Tamil Nadu, India

Kiran Chandra Patro DNB (Med) DNB (Nephro)
Senior Consultant Nephrologist
NU Hospital
Bengaluru, Karnataka, India

Manish Sahay MD (Paeds) DNB (Nephro) MAMS
Professor and Head
Department of Nephrology
Osmania Medical College
Osmania General Hospital
Hyderabad, Telangana, India
Member of Young Nephrologist Committee–International Society of Nephrology
Executive Committee Member–Indian Society of Nephrology and Southern Chapter of Indian Society of Nephrology

Mysore Keshavmurthy Phanish
MBBS MD FRCP CCST (Nephro) PhD
(Renal Cell Biology)
Consultant Nephrologist
St Helier Hospital, Epsom and St Helier
University Hospitals NHS Trust
Surrey, UK, Senior Research Fellow
SW Thames Institute for Renal Research
St Helier Hospital
Honorary Senior Lecturer
St George's University of London, UK

Pranaw Kumar Jha MD (Internal
Medicine) DNB (Nephro)
Consultant
Division of Nephrology and Transplant
Medicine, Medanta Kidney and Urology
Institute Medanta—The Medicity
Gurgaon, Haryana, India

R Kasi Viswesaran MD DM FRCP (Edin)
Senior Consultant in Nephrology
Ananthapuri Hospitals and Research
Institute
Thiruvananthapuram, Kerala, India

Rajan Duggal MD DNB (Pathology)
PDCC (Renal and Transplant Pathology)
ISN-ANIO (Nephropathology) ASH-VTP
(Lymph Node Pathology)
Senior Consultant, Pathology
Medanta—The Medicity
Gurgaon, Haryana, India

Rajesh Ahlawat MS MNAMS MCh
Urology (AIIMS)
Chairman
Division of Urology and Renal
Transplantation, Medanta—The Medicity
Gurgaon, Haryana, India

Ram R MD DM (Nephro)
Associate Professor
Department of Nephrology
Sri Venkateswara Institute of Medical
Sciences (SVIMS)
Tirupati, Chennai, India

Ratan Jha MD DM (Nephro) DNB
(Nephro) DTCD FISN (India)
Senior Consultant Nephrologist
Department of Nephrology
Medwin Hospital
Hyderabad, Telangana, India

Ritambhra Nada MD (Path)
Professor
Department of Histopathology
Postgraduate Institute of Medical
Education and Research
Chandigarh, India

Rohan Augustine MD (Int Med)
DNB (Nephro)
Consultant
Department of Nephrology
Manipal Health Enterprises Pvt Ltd
Bengaluru, Karnataka, India

Satish D MD DNB (Med) DNB (Nephro)
Consultant Nephrology
Apollo Hospitals
Bengaluru, Karnataka, India

Sishir Gang MD DM DNB (Nephro)
Chief
Division of Nephrology
Muljibhai Patel Urological Hospital
Nadiad, Gujarat, India

Sohrab Arora MS MCh Urology and Renal
Transplant (SGPGIMS)
Senior Fellow
Minimally Invasive Urology
Medanta—The Medicity
Gurgaon, Haryana, India

Tarun K George MD (Internal Medicine)
Assistant Professor
Department of Medicine
Christian Medical College
Vellore, Chennai, India

V Ramasubramanian MD FRCP (Glas)
DTM and H (Lon) DGUM (Lon)
Director, Immune Boosters
Adult Immunization and Travel Clinic
Consultant Infectious Diseases and
Tropical Medicine, Apollo Hospitals
Chennai, Tamil Nadu, India
Adjunct Professor
Infectious Diseases
Sri Ramachandra Medical College
Chennai, Tamil Nadu, India
Adjunct Professor, Infectious Diseases
MGR Medical University, Adjunct
Associate Professor, Infectious Diseases
University of Queensland

Vijay Kher MD (Internal Medicine) DM (Nephro) FAMS FRCPE
Chairman
Division of Nephrology and Transplant Medicine
Medanta Kidney and Urology Institute
Medanta—The Medicity
Gurgaon, Haryana, India

Vinay Sakhuja DM (Nephro) FAMS FRCP
Director
Nephrology and Transplant Medicine
Max Superspeciality Hospital
Mohali, Punjab, India

Vinod Kumar K MD DNB (Nephro)
Consultant Nephrologist
Aster Medicity
Kochi, Kerala, India

Vishwanath S DNB (Pediatrics) DNB (Nephro) MNAMSPDCC (Nephro)
Head of Department and Consultant
Department of Nephrology
Manipal Health Enterprises Pvt Ltd
Bengaluru, Karnataka, India

Vivekanand Jha MD DM FRCP FAMS
Professor
Department of Nephrology
Postgraduate Institute of Medical Education and Research
Chandigarh, India
Secretary
Indian Society of Nephrology
Councillor
International Society of Nephrology
Councillor
The Transplantation Society

Preface

During graduation and postgraduation, a medical student usually gets inadequately exposed to nephrology as a subspecialty. But the patients they deal with, more often than not, have one or the other renal issue. This includes acid-base imbalance, electrolyte disorders, acute kidney injury, chronic kidney disease, and renal stones to name a few. India is the world's capital for type II diabetes and the chronic kidney disease burden is thus going to be ever increasing. The number of such patients, a physician sees in his or her day-to-day clinical practice is increasing rapidly. Hence, a good knowledge of these diseases is imperative. The first edition of this manual is an attempt in this direction. This will act as a quick-reference guide to deal with day-to-day renal problems in the patients. It is replete with informative tables, flow charts for quick glance, self-explanatory figures, recent guidelines and concise text for maximum understanding of the subject in a simple yet effective way.

This book will benefit medical interns, postgraduate students, practicing physicians, nephrology fellows and clinicians.

We thankfully appreciate the hard work put by all the authors, who are excellent academicians and teachers, to contribute the chapters for the book. We request you all to let us know the shortcomings in the present edition and the improvements you would like to see. This will go a long way in shaping future editions of the manual. We hope you will find this manual informative, helpful and useful in your routine clinical practice to attain the common goal of improving management of your patients.

Pranaw Kumar Jha
Vijay Kher

Acknowledgments

We would like to thank almighty for giving us the strength and guidance to complete this manual.

We acknowledge and thank all the authors who took time out of their busy schedule and helped to complete the manual in time.

We are indebted to our family members who supported and helped us to realize this dream.

Sincere thanks to all our past and present students who have constantly inspired us to write this manual.

We would like to express our gratitude to one and all who were directly or indirectly involved in completion of this manual.

Special thanks to Dr Vivek Sharma and Dr Rajiv Yadav for helping us with the radiology images.

Last but not least, we would like to acknowledge all our patients who have been constant source of knowledge and motivation. Without them, the book would not have been published.

Contents

CHAPTER

1

Renal Anatomy and Physiology: A Clinical Perspective

Pranaw Kumar Jha, Vijay Kher

SECTION A: RENAL ANATOMY

INTRODUCTION

Kidneys, also known as *"renes"* in Latin, are bean shaped organs located in our body. They function to regulate the acid base balance, maintenance of homeostasis, vitamin D3 and hemoglobin. They remove the waste products of metabolism by filtering the blood passing through. Acute or chronic derangement of kidney function can give rise to various signs and symptoms due to accumulation of these waste products and altered acid-base, electrolytes and fluid homeostasis. This chapter reviews the anatomy of kidneys and describes the physiology of urine formation, which is important to understand the basis of clinic-pathological features of renal dysfunction.

Gross Anatomy

Kidneys are retroperitoneal organs located between D12 and L3 vertebra. The right kidney is slightly lower than the left due to the presence of liver. It is also nearer to median plane when compared to the left.

Each kidney measures about 11 cm in length, 6 cm in width and 3 cm in thickness. It weighs between 125 to 170 grams in adult males and 115 to 155 grams in adult females.

Concave side of each kidney is indented by hilum through which renal artery, vein and ureter enters the kidney. Suprarenal (adrenal) gland is related to the upper pole of kidney.

Each kidney is surrounded by:
- Renal fascia of Gerota—it has two layers
  - Anterior layer—fascia of *Toldt*
  - Posterior layer—fascia of *Zuckerkandl*
- Perirenal fat in the space of Gerota
- Renal capsule around kidney which can be easily stripped off.

Cross-section of each kidney **(Fig. 1.1)** reveals:
- *Cortex*: This is the outer portion between the capsule and medulla. It has number of projections (cortical columns of *Bertini*) extending between the pyramids. It contains renal corpuscles and tubules.

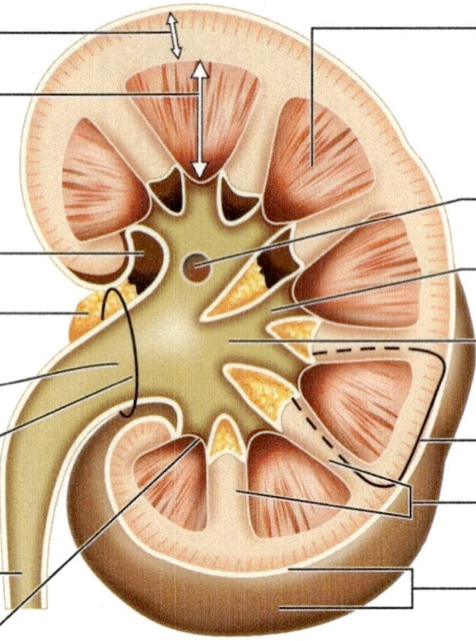

Figure 1.1 Cross-section of kidney

- *Medulla*: This is the innermost part that consists of renal pyramids. This is further divided into:
  - Inner medulla
  - Outer medulla
- *Renal papilla*: It drains urine from medullary pyramids into minor calyx.
- *Renal sinus*: This is a space extending from renal hilum containing branches of renal artery and vein and renal pelvis
- *Renal pelvis*: A funnel shaped dilated upper part of ureter. It divides into 2–3 major calyces which further divides into 7–13 minor calyces.

Blood Supply

Blood supply of the kidney is derived from renal arteries. It arises from aorta at the level of L1-L2 intervertebral disc. **Figure 1.2** shows the blood supply of a kidney.

Flow of blood in arterial side is as follows:
Segmental arteries → Lobar arteries → Interlobar arteries → Arcuate arteries → Interlobular artery (also known as cortical radiate arteries) → Afferent arterioles → Glomerulus.

Venous blood flows in following direction:
Glomerulus → Efferent arterioles → Interlobular vein → Arcuate vein → Interlobar vein → Renal vein.

Nerve Supply

Nerve supply to kidneys is through the renal plexus. Its fibers course along the renal arteries to reach the kidneys.

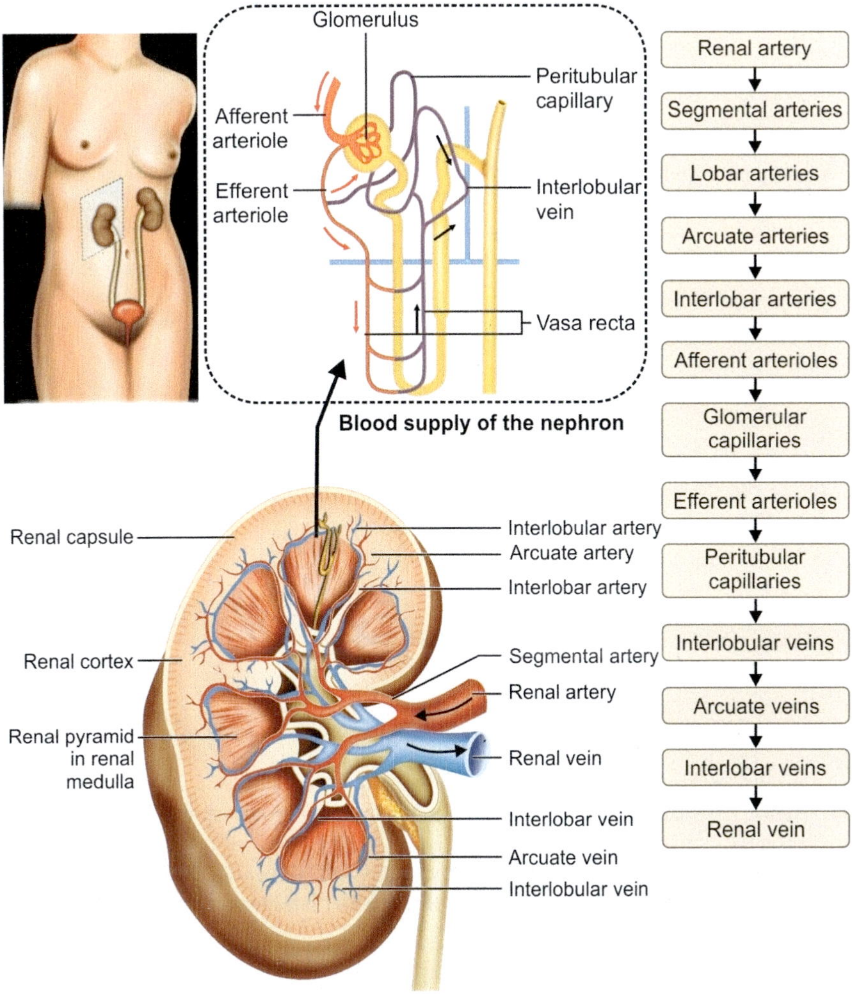

Figure 1.2 Renal blood supply

- *Sympathetic input*: Causes vasoconstriction thereby reducing renal blood flow
- *Parasympathetic input*: Through renal branches of vagus nerve
- *Sensory input*: Travels to spinal cord level T10-11.

MICROSCOPIC ANATOMY: THE NEPHRON

This is the basic functioning and structural unit of a kidney. It derives its name from Greek word *nephros* meaning kidneys. There are about 1.2 million nephrons in each kidney.

Nephrons form urine by process of filtration, secretion and reabsorption. It also functions to control blood pressure, red blood cell production and active vitamin D (calcitriol) synthesis.

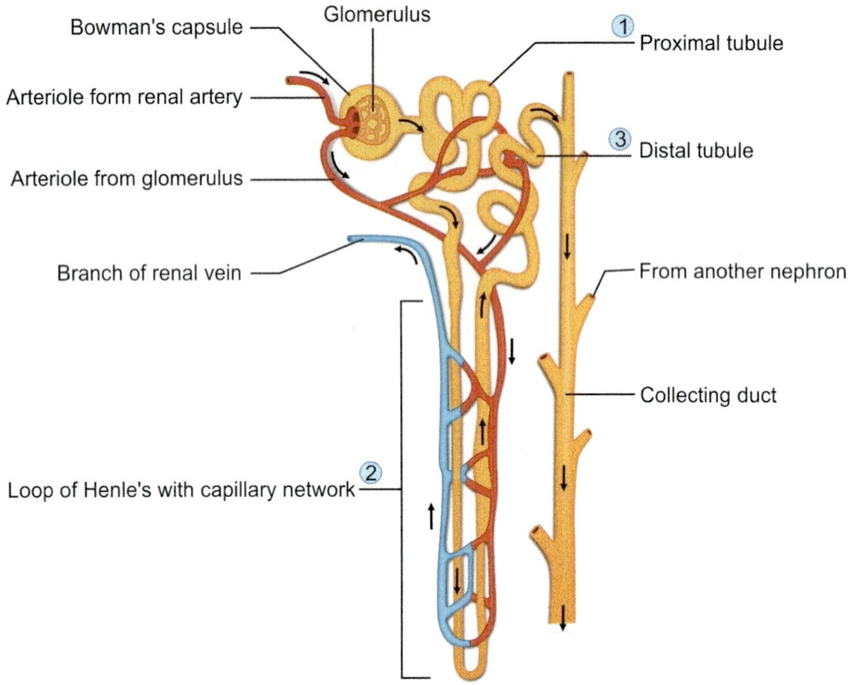

Figure 1.3 Nephron

As shown in **Figure 1.3**, each nephron is composed of:

- *Renal corpuscle (the filtering unit)*: Formed by glomerulus and Bowman's capsule
- *Renal tubule*: Comprising of proximal convoluted tubule (PCT), loop of Henle with its ascending and descending limbs and distal convoluted tubule (DCT).

There are two types of nephrons:

1. *Cortical*: Renal corpuscle of these nephrons are in cortex and loop of Henle located near corticomedullary junction.
2. *Juxtamedullary*: Renal corpuscle of these nephrons are located in cortical part nearing medulla and loop of Henle is located deep in medulla.

Renal Corpuscle

It consists of glomerulus, which is surrounded by Bowman's capsule **(Fig. 1.4)**. Bowman's capsule transfers the filtrate of glomerulus to the PCT. Bowman's capsule has an outer parietal layer, which continues onto the glomerular capillaries to form the inner visceral layer. Visceral layer is composed of visceral epithelial cells also known as podocytes, which covers the extensive capillary network, by its extension known as pedicles. Pedicles interdigitate to form sieve like filtration. The endothelium of glomerular capillaries, the glomerular basement membrane and the podocytes form the filtration barrier.

Most substance less than 8 nm and all the substances less than 4 nm can pass through the filtration barrier. Apart from this size barrier other factor determining

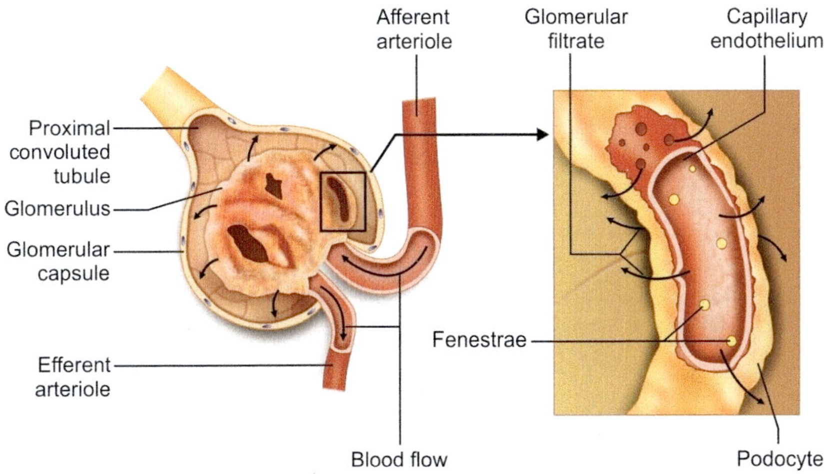

Figure 1.4 Renal corpuscle and filtration barrier

the filtration across the filtration barrier is charge of a particular substance. The negatively charged proteins associated with the pore repel, and thereby reduce, the filtration of negatively charged substance.

Mesangium is a thin membrane that supports the capillary loops. It is surrounded by capillaries. Mesangial cells are phagocytic cells located between the capillaries. These cells also contract to regulate the filtration rate.

Juxtaglomerular Apparatus

The juxtaglomerular (JG) apparatus lies just outside the glomerulus and Bowman's capsule as seen in **Figure 1.5**. It consists of:

- *Macula densa*: The initial part of DCT comes into contact with arterioles near the vascular pole of glomerulus. The wall of DCT at this point is formed by a specialized cluster of cuboidal epithelial cells known as macula densa, which monitors the composition of fluid passing through the DCT. These cells sense the changes in sodium chloride levels in distal tubule of kidney and release paracrine signals to regulate the flow.
- *Juxtaglomerular cells*: These are modified smooth muscle cells that line the media of afferent arterioles. The ATP or adenosine secreted by macula densa leads to contraction or relaxation of these cells, thereby regulating the glomerular blood flow. It also releases *renin* in response to various stimuli such as decreased NaCl concentration at macula densa, stimulation of beta1 adrenergic receptor and decreased renal perfusion pressure.
- *Extraglomerular mesangial cells*: The JG apparatus plays an important role in regulation of fluid balance of the body and helps in autoregulation.

Renal Tubules

Proximal Convoluted Tubule

It is the longest part of the renal tubule and the first one to receive the fluid filtered by Bowman's capsule. It is lined by simple tall cuboidal epithelium. There

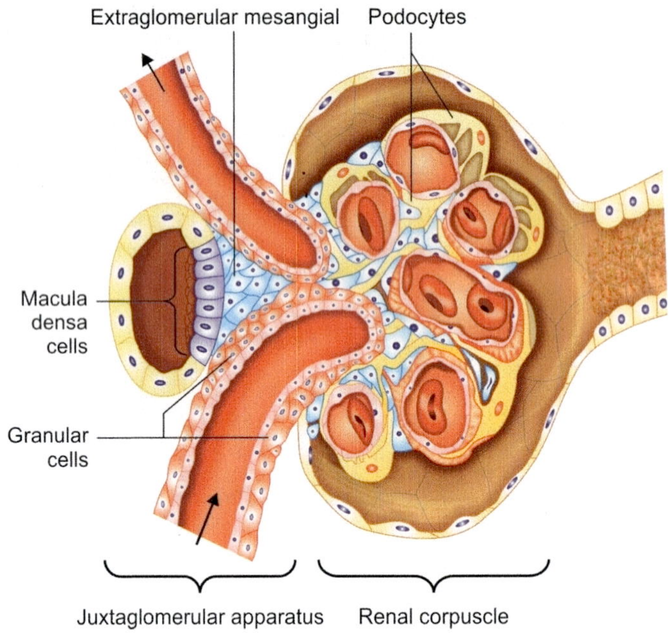

Figure 1.5 Juxtaglomerular and renal apparatus

are numerous microvilli on the apical surface of these cells, which considerably increase the surface area for reabsorption and secretion; two important functions of PCT. PCT cells contain numerous mitochondria due to high-energy requirements.

Henle's Loop

PCT continues as Henle's loop. It has following parts:

- Descending limb—this consists of:
  - *Initial short thick portion (pars recta)*: It has simple cuboidal epithelium like PCT
  - *Long thin portion*: This has simple squamous epithelium
- Hairpin turn
- Ascending limb—this consists of:
  - *Short thin portion*: Containing simple squamous epithelium
  - *Long thick portion*: It has simple cuboidal epithelium like DCT.

They have different water and solute permeabilities, which play role in diluting and concentrating the urine by countercurrent mechanisms, which will be described later in section on physiology.

Distal Convoluted Tubule

It is tortuous like PCT and contain similar simple cuboidal cells but with fewer microvilli on the apical surface. It contains lesser number of mitochondria compared to PCT.

Collecting Duct System

Technically speaking this is not a part of the nephron. Each collecting duct drains several nephrons. Collecting duct can be divided into cortical and medullary part, while the medullary part is further divided into inner and outer segments. Medullary collecting ducts end at renal papilla. It has both cuboidal and columnar epithelium (near the papilla). There are two types of cells in collecting ducts – the intercalated and principal cells, which will be described in detail in section on physiology.

The squamous epithelium of collecting duct has receptors for anti-diuretic hormone (ADH). On stimulation of these receptors by ADH, aquaporins (the water channels) get inserted into the cell membrane and allow water to pass from lumen into the interstitial space. In the absence of ADH, dilute high volume urine is formed.

SECTION B: RENAL PHYSIOLOGY AND URINE FORMATION

INTRODUCTION

Having gone through the anatomical details of the kidneys, it's the time to proceed to the physiology of urine formation.

Kidney uses three key steps in urine formation:

1. *Filtration*: This happens in the renal corpuscles where a filtrate is formed out of the blood passing through the glomerulus. This filtrate passes through the tubular system where its composition is altered by reabsorption or secretion leading to eventual formation of urine.
2. *Reabsorption*: This involves transport of water, important ions and minerals (such as glucose, amino acids, sodium, potassium, magnesium, etc.) from the filtrate in the tubular lumen back into the blood surrounding the renal tubules.
3. *Secretion*: This is a process by which various substance are transported into the tubular filtrate from the blood surrounding the tubules.

GLOMERULAR FILTRATION RATE AND PRESSURE

Kidney receives about one fifth of the blood pumped by the heart every minute (cardiac output). This blood is filtered to form about 125 ± 15 mL of filtrate every minute in men and about 110 ± 15 mL/min in women. Hence, a normal functioning kidney has a glomerular filtration rate (GFR) of about 180 L/day in men and 150 L/day in women.

The pressure that drives the filtrate out of the glomerular capillaries into the tubular lumen is known as the glomerular filtration pressure or *net filtration pressure*. This is determined by the forces favoring (hydrostatic pressure in glomerular capillaries i.e. *PG*) and opposing (hydrostatic pressure in Bowman's capsule i.e. *PB* and oncotic pressure exerted by plasma in glomerular capillaries i.e. *OG*) the flow. The oncotic pressure in Bowman's capsule is negligible.

Net filtration pressure $= PG - (PB + OG)$
$= 55 - (15 + 30)$
$= 10$ mm Hg

Clearance of any substance is defined as volume of plasma, which gets completely cleared off of a substance per unit time.

Determination of GFR is an important step in assessment of renal function. There are various methods of GFR estimation. The gold standard is inulin clearance. *Inulin* is a polysaccharide that is neither reabsorbed nor secreted by the kidneys. Assessment of GFR by inulin requires intravenous administration of this drug. Method of inulin clearance is cumbersome; hence, an endogenous molecule serum creatinine is used to assess GFR in day-to-day clinical practice.

TRANSPORT MECHANISMS

There are various mechanisms by which substances are transported across membranes. These include:

- *Active transport*: This involves movement of molecules from lower to higher concentration across a cell membrane. As the movement is against the concentration gradient, this requires energy, which is usually derived form adenosine tri-phosphate (ATP)
- *Diffusion*: Simple diffusion involves movement of molecules down the concentration gradient, i.e. from higher to lower concentration.
- *Facilitated diffusion*: Here the molecules move from higher to lower concentration but require specific transmembrane proteins.
- *Secondary active transport*: Here the substance is moved in energetically unfavorable direction against the gradient facilitated by co-transport of another molecule down the gradient. These are of two types
  - *Symport*: Two or more substances move in same direction.
  - *Antiport*: Substances move in opposite direction across the cell membrane.
- *Osmosis*: This involves movement of solvent from the region of lower solute concentration to higher solute concentration across a semi-permeable membrane.

These mechanisms are involved in the process of reabsorption and secretion in renal tubules leading to the formation of urine.

TUBULAR TRANSPORTS

Proximal Convoluted Tubule

PCT is an important site for reabsorption of most of the water, electrolytes such as sodium, potassium etc. and organic solutes such as glucose and amino acids **(Table 1.1)**. There are many channels present in the cells of PCT to facilitate the movement of various substances across the cell membrane. The Na^+K^+ ATPase pump present in the basolateral membrane actively transports Na out of the cell creating a gradient across the cell membrane leading to sodium reabsorption. This is an energy driven process. Reabsorption of Na is coupled with the movement of various substances either in the same (*symport*) or the opposite (*antiport*) direction **(Fig. 1.6)**. **Table 1.2** shows substances transported across the apical and basolateral membrane of PCT.

Table 1.1 Reabsorption of various substances across PCT

Substance	*Reabsorption*
Salt and water	67%
Glucose	100%
Amino acid	100%
Urea	50%
Phosphate	80%
Magnesium	20–30%
Potassium	65%
Citrate	70–90 %

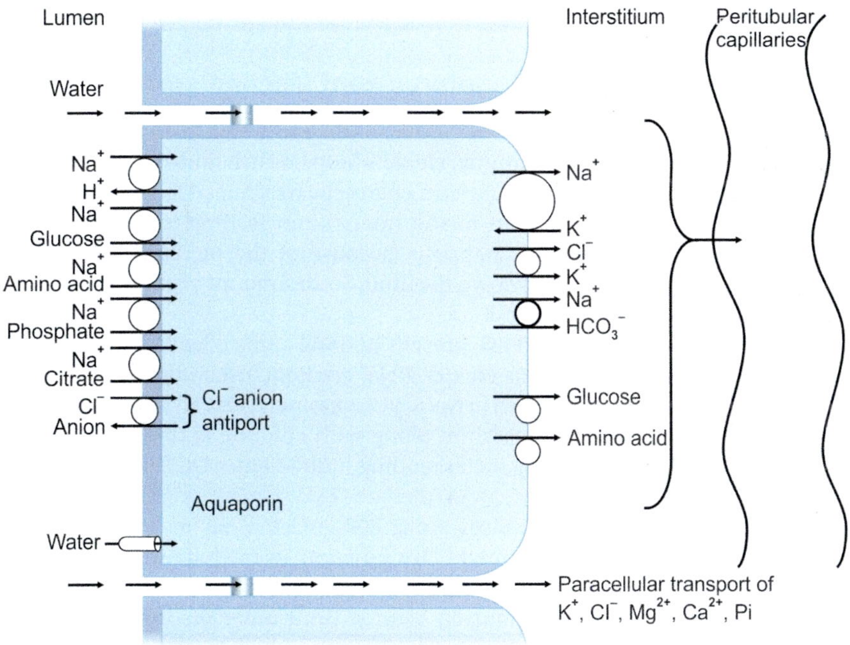

Figure 1.6 Proximal convoluted tubular cells and channels

Carbonic anhydrase (CA) is an important enzyme located inside the PCT cells. It is also present on the cell surface in small amount. In the tubular lumen, HCO_3^- combines with H^+ to form H_2O and CO_2 in presence of CA. CO_2 diffuses into the cell. Here the reverse reaction occurs, in presence of CA, leading to the formation of HCO_3^- and H^+. HCO_3^- is cotransported with Na across basolateral membrane and apical Na/H antiporter secretes H^+ back in the lumen. This process recovers the bicarbonate.

Table 1.2 Substances transported across the membranes of PCT	
Across apical membrane	
Symport with Na	K, Cl, HCO_3, Mg, Ca, amino acid, glucose, galactose, fructose, lactate, succinate, citrate
Antiport with Na	H^+ ion
Transcellular diffusion	K, Mg, Ca
Across basolateral membrane	
Active	Na (exchanged for K)
Facilitated diffusion	Ca, K, Cl, HCO_3, glucose, fructose, galactose, citrate, succinate

There are few substances secreted in PCT. Most of the drugs are secreted here. These include furosemide, indomethacin, penicillin, and probenecid to name a few. Apart from this PCT is the site for formation of most of the ammonia secreted in urine.

Loop of Henle and the Countercurrent Mechanism

The Henle's loop functions to reclaim the solute and water from the filtrate. As discussed in the section on anatomy, Henle's loop has two limbs:

1. *Descending limb*: This has aquaporin channels, which lead to free movement of water from tubular lumen to the interstitium leading to about 15–20% reabsorption of water. This happens because of the increasing interstitial osmolarity as one descends down the limb. Some amount of urea, sodium and other ions are also reabsorbed.
2. *Ascending limb*: Na+K+ ATPase present in basal surface leads to extrusion of sodium outside the cell. This creates a Na^+ gradient. Ascending limb cells are impermeable to water but rich in $Na^+K^+2Cl^-$ channels **(Fig. 1.7)**. Sodium moves down the gradient and potassium along with chloride is transported along with it. tubular fluid leaving the ascending limb to enter DCT is hypoosmotic (100 mOsm/kg).

Interstitial osmolarity increases from 300 mOsmol/kg to 1200 mOsmol/kg as one moves from corticomedullary junction to medulla. Apart from the sodium reclaimed by ascending tubule by $Na^+K^+2Cl^-$ channels and Na^+K^+ ATPase described above, facilitated diffusion of urea from inner medullary collecting ducts into the medullary interstitium add to produce high medullary osmolarity. This happens due to the countercurrent multiplier mechanism. The name countercurrent multiplier exchange is derived from *countercurrent arrangement* of the two limbs of Henle's loop leading to flow of tubular filtrate in opposite directions **(Fig. 1.8)**.

Due to the above arrangement the medullary interstitium becomes hyperosmotic (almost 1200 mOsm/kg at the tip). This facilitates the water movement across the descending limb as described leading to concentration of tubular filtrate.

Further, the presence of vasa recta serves as a countercurrent exchangers to prevent the solute washout from the hyperosmotic interstitium. This is also helped by the low medullary blood flow (<5% of total renal blood flow).

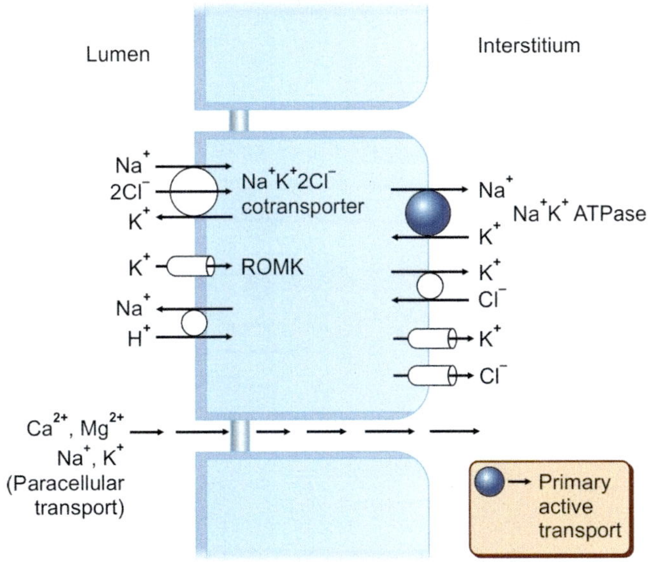

Figure 1.7 Thick ascending limb of Henle's loop cell
Abbreviation: ROMK, renal outer medullary K-channel

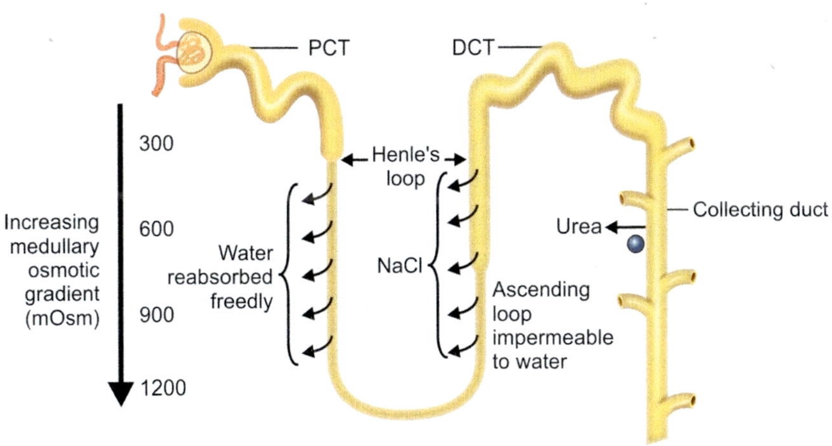

Figure 1.8 Countercurrent system

Distal Convoluted Tubule

The DCT functions to recover water and various solutes from the hypotonic fluid reaching it. Various channels of DCT play significant role in this **(Fig. 1.9)**.

- The basal Na^+K^+ ATPase channel of DCT moves Na out of the cell creating gradient for
  - Na to be absorbed from the apical Na/Cl symporter
  - Ca reclamation by Na/Ca antiporter in basolateral membrane
  - Up to 10–15% of total filtered water reabsorption

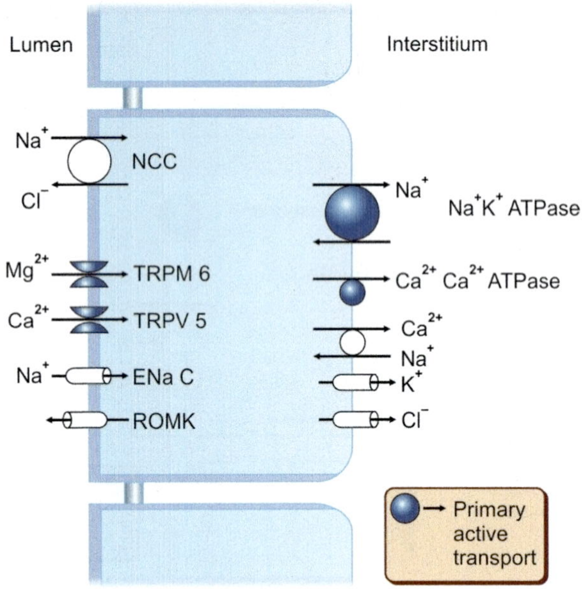

Figure 1.9 Distal convoluted cell and channels

Abbreviations: ROMK, renal outer medullary K^+ channel; ENaC, epithelial sodium channel; TRPV, transient receptor potential vanilloid; TRPM, transient receptor potential melastatin; NCC, Na^+–Cl^--cotransporter

- About 7–10% of filtered calcium is reabsorbed via transcellular route by TRPV5 channel
- Basal transport of calcium also occurs via calcium ATPase
- Magnesium is reabsorbed by TRPM6 apical channel
- Regulation of sodium and potassium levels by apical ENaC (sodium reabsorption) and ROMK (potassium excretion) channels.

Collecting Duct

Collecting duct drains urine from the DCTs. It serves an important function in formation of diluted or concentrated urine. It also helps in sodium, potassium and acid-base regulation.

- *Urine volume and osmolarity regulation*: Antidiuretic hormone (ADH) (vasopressin) is the hormone responsible for regulation of urine volume and osmolarity. It leads to insertion of aquaporin channels into the apical membrane of principal cells lining the collecting duct. Water is reabsorbed through these aquaporin channels because of the increasing interstitial osmolarity as the collecting duct traverses the medulla. In case blood becomes hyperosmotic, more water is reabsorbed by above-mentioned ADH action. In case blood is hypoosmotic, opposite occurs, leading to formation of dilute urine.

- *Sodium and potassium homeostasis by principal cells*: An important hormone, aldosterone, stimulates luminal Na and K channel formation as well as the activity of basal Na/K ATPase pump **(Fig. 1.10A)**. In case of increase in serum aldosterone, more sodium is reabsorbed and potassium is lost in urine. Water is reabsorbed as well.
- *Acid-base balance by intercalated cells*: There are two types of intercalated cells which are mirror images of each other **(Figs 1.10B and C)**
  - α *intercalated cells*: Secretes H+ ion and reabsorbs bicarbonate
  - β *intercalated cells*: Secretes bicarbonate ion and reabsorbs H+

  Damage to these cells can lead to renal tubular acidosis.

AUTOREGULATION

Renal blood flow remains relatively stable to maintain a normal GFR over a wide range of blood pressure (mean arterial pressure of 70–160 mm Hg). This is known as autoregulation and has two important components:

1. *Myogenic response*: The afferent arteriole wall smooth muscle cells are stretched when BP increases. It contracts in response to this, leading to little change in blood flow. The opposite happens when BP drops.
2. *Tubuloglomerular feedback (TGF)*: Important components of TGF are juxtaglomerular apparatus (JGA) and a paracrine signaling mechanism. Macula densa cells of DCT respond to the flow of tubular filtrate as well as sodium and chloride concentration of the filtrate. Increasing GFR leads to increase in tubular flow. Macula densa detects it and releases ATP and adenosine. These lead to contraction of the juxtaglomerular (JG) cells of afferent arterioles thereby reducing GFR. Drop in GFR has the opposite effect.

Other important mechanisms involved in controlling the effective circulatory volume include sympathetic nervous system and renin-angiotensin-aldosterone system (RAAS).

SYMPATHETIC NERVOUS SYSTEM

Kidneys receive the sympathetic supply from the celiac plexus and the splanchnic nerves. Reduced effective circulatory volume results in reflex increase in sympathetic nerve discharge leading to vasoconstriction and reduced glomerular flow and filtration. This also leads to stimulation of renin secretion. Renin further leads to circulatory volume augmentation as described below.

RENIN-ANGIOTENSIN-ALDOSTERONE SYSTEM (RAAS)

Decrease in renal perfusion leads to secretion of renin by granular cells of afferent arteriole at the JGA. It converts angiotensinogen derived from liver to angiotensin I. This is further converted by angiotensin converting enzyme (ACE) to angiotensin II. This enzyme is produced in lungs and binds to endothelial cells of afferent arteriole and glomerulus **(Fig. 1.11)**.

Angiotensin II has multiple effects by which it tries to maintain blood volume and pressure such as:

- Increased sympathetic activity leading to afferent and efferent vasoconstriction and preservation of blood volume.

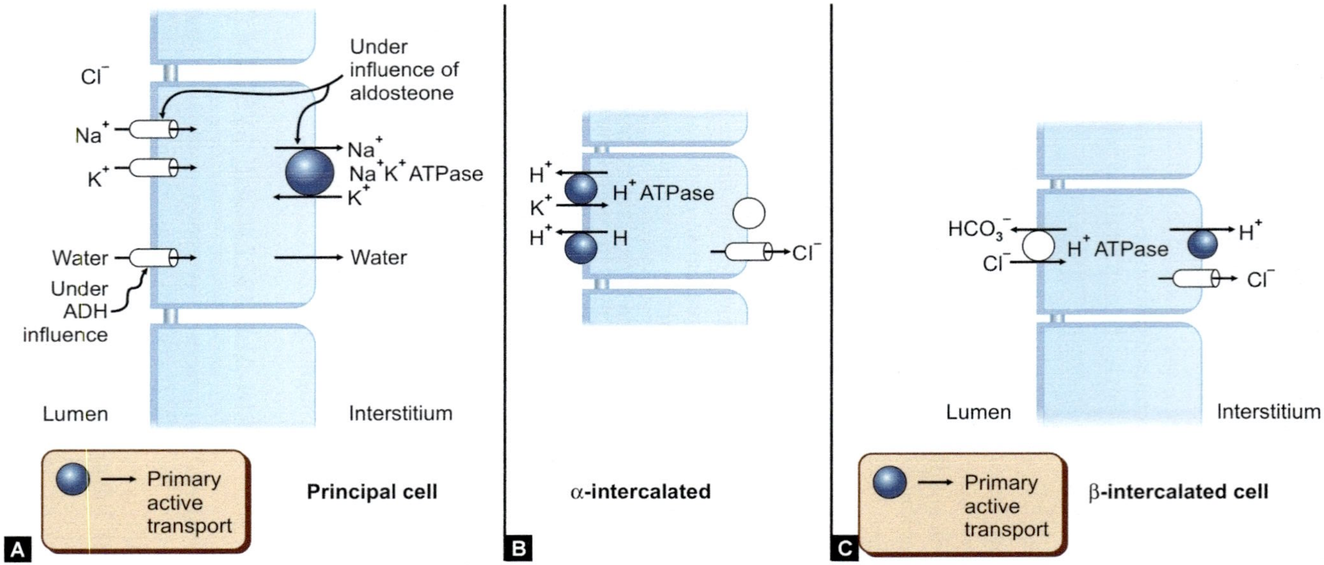

Figures 1.10A to C Principal and intercalated cells

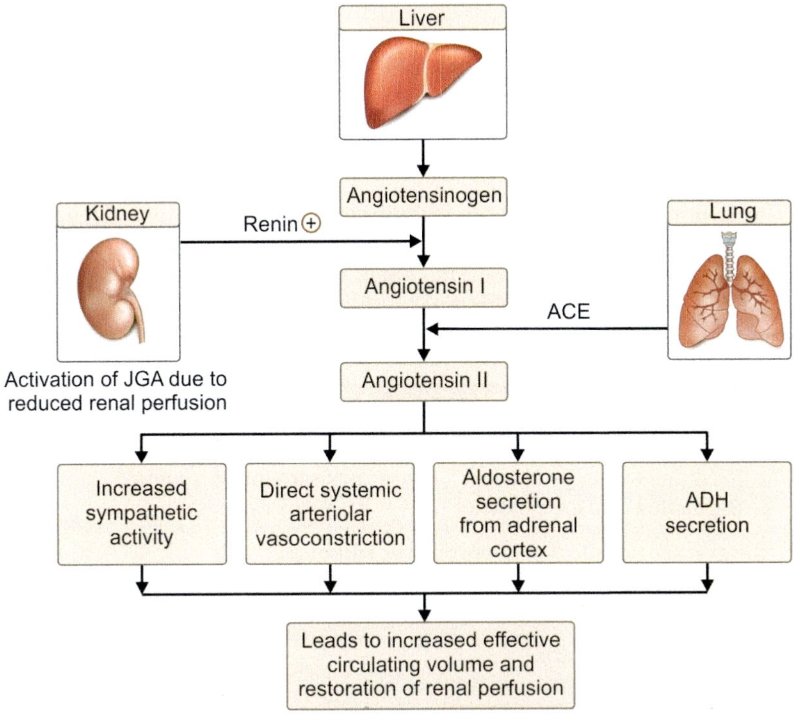

Figure 1.11 Renin-angiotensin-aldosterone system (RAAS)
Abbreviations: JGA, juxtaglomerular apparatus; ACE, angiotensin-converting enzyme; ADH, antidiuretic hormone

- Direct systemic arteriolar vasoconstriction leading to increased blood pressure
- Promotes secretion of aldosterone from adrenal cortex. This leads to sodium reabsorption and potassium excretion. This also leads to reabsorption of water along with sodium.
- Secretion of ADH leading to fluid retention.

ENDOCRINE FUNCTION OF KIDNEYS

Apart from its role in RAAS and ADH mediated fluid regulation there are few other important endocrine functions of kidney worth mentioning here:

- *Erythropoiesis*: Kidney secretes erythropoietin hormones in response to hypoxia. It is secreted by renal cortical interstitial cells near the base of PCT. Kidneys account for about 85% secretion of EPO. In chronic kidney disease, deficiencies of these hormones lead to anemia requiring EPO supplementation.
- *Active vitamin D (calcitriol) synthesis*: Active form of vitamin D i.e. 1,25-dihydrocholecalciferol also known as calcitriol is synthesized in the renal PCT. The enzyme 1-alpha-hydroxylase acts on its substrate 25-hydroxycholecalciferol leading to the formation of active vitamin D.

SUMMARY

- Kidney performs important function of maintaining fluid, electrolytes and acid-base balance in the body.
- It also secretes important hormones such as active vitamin D3 and erythropoietin and has an important role to play in the regulation of blood pressure.
- Compromise of these functions leads to various manifestations of renal failure, which may be fatal.
- Understanding of the basic renal anatomy and physiology is important for management of patients with renal dysfunction.

Multiple Choice Questions

1. Kidney has following function:
a. Excreting waster product
b. Secreting hormones
c. Regulating acid base balance
d. All of the these

2. The average numbers of nephrons per kidney is:
a. 1.2 lakh
b. 1.2 million
c. 2.4 million
d. 12 million

3. Macula densa cells are:
a. Extraglomerular mesangial cells
b. Cluster of cuboidal epithelial cells forming wall of DCT where it comes in contact with the arterioles
c. Modified smooth muscle cells lining media of afferent arterioles
d. None of the above

4. Which one of the following about flow of renal blood supply is correct?
a. Lobar arteries → Segmental arteries → Interlobar arteries → Arcuate arteries → Afferent arterioles
b. Segmental arteries → Arcuate arteries → Lobar arteries → Interlobar arteries → Afferent arterioles
c. Segmental arteries → Lobar arteries → Interlobar arteries → Arcuate arteries → Afferent arterioles
d. None of the above

5. Filtration barrier is formed by:
a. Endothelium of glomerular capillaries
b. Glomerular basement membrane
c. Podocytes
d. All of the above

6. Average net filtration pressure is:
a. 5 mm Hg
b. 10 mm Hg
c. 25 mm Hg
d. 100 mm Hg

7. Gold standard for GFR determination is:
a. DTPA renal scan
b. eGFR by Cockcroft Gault formula
c. Inulin clearance
d. eGFR by MDRD formula

8. Glucose is absorbed completely in:
a. Distal convoluted tubule
b. Proximal convoluted tubule
c. Loop of Henle
d. Collecting duct

9. Angiotensin converting enzyme is synthesized in:
a. Liver
b. Lungs
c. Kidneys
d. All of these

10. Collecting duct functions to:
a. Maintain urine volume and osmolarity
b. Sodium and potassium homeostasis
c. Acid-base balance
d. All of the above

Answers

1. d	2. b	3. b	4. c	5. d	6. b	7. c	8. b
9. b	10. d						

SUGGESTED READING

1. Bailey MA, Shirley DG, Unwin RJ, Renal physiology. In: Johnson RJ, Feehally J, Floege J (Eds). Comprehensive Clinical Nephrology, 5th edn. Philadelphia, PA: Elsevier/Saunders. 2015. pp.14-27.
2. Barajas L. Anatomy of the juxtaglomerular apparatus. Am J Physiol. 1979:237(5): F333-43.
3. Barrett KE, Barman SM, Boittano S, Brooks HL, Renal physiology. In: Barrett KE, Barman SM, Boittano S, Brooks HL (Eds). Ganong's Review of Medical Physiology, 23rd edn. New York,: McGraw-Hill Medical. 2010. pp. 639-86.
4. Blaine J, Chonchol M, Levi M. Renal control of calcium, phosphate, and magnesium homeostasis. Clin J Am Soc Nephrol. 2015:10(7):1257-72.
5. Danziger J, Zeidel. Osmotic homeostasis. Clin J Am Soc Nephrol. 2015:10(5): 852-62.
6. Healy JC. Urogenital system. In: Standring S (Ed). Gray's Anatomy: The Anatomical Basis of Clinical Practice, 41st edn. Philadelphia: Elsevier. 2015 .pp. 74-8.
7. Kriz W, Elger M. Renal anatomy. In: Johnson RJ, Feehally J, Floege J (Eds). Comprehensive Clinical Nephrology, 5th edn. Philadelphia, PA: Elsevier/ Saunders. 2015. pp. 2-13.
8. Subramanya AR, Ellison DH. Distal convoluted tubule. Clin J Am Soc Nephrol. 2014;9(12):2147-63.

CHAPTER

2

Basics of Renal Histopathology

Ritambhra Nada, Rajan Duggal

INTRODUCTION

The renal biopsy is a safe medical procedure and should be undertaken only after consideration of possible morbidity and rare mortality that can occur with this invasive procedure.

The renal biopsy sample needs to be examined with optimal methods for a complete evaluation, including light microscopy (LM), immunofluorescence (IF), immunohistochemistry (wherever required) and electron microscopy (EM). The correct diagnosis requires a well-trained nephropathologist with thorough knowledge of not only renal pathology but also clinical nephrology in order to correlate intricate tissue derived information with clinical data in order to provide the best possible clinicopathologic diagnosis.

RENAL BIOPSY FIXATION AND PROCESSING

The renal biopsy tissue delivered to histopathology laboratory should be accompanied by adequate clinical information to enable proper interpretation of findings. Majority of the laboratories provide a special clinical information form to the physician to ease the recording of the overall renal syndrome, symptoms and laboratory data. Although this does not replace direct communication with the submitting nephrologist/physician. This basic medical information provides a good initial background for overall interpretation of the renal biopsy tissue. The use of a dissecting microscope can be of help in assessing sample adequacy.

Another option is the use of a standard light microscope. The renal tissue is placed on a glass slide with normal saline and examined with or without a coverslip producing a wet mount. Knowledge of the glomerular content of the sample can help in correct division of tissue for the various histologic modalities. If no glomerulus is visualized then the standard protocol for dividing the tissue obtained at each 'pass' should be used to avoid inadequate glomerular sampling for LM, IF or EM **(Fig. 2.1)**. The standard approach is to first procure tissue for electron microscopy from each core by removing 1 mm cubes from the ends and placing them in glutaraldehyde or other fixative suitable for EM. Some clinicians prefer that the pathology laboratory obtain tissue for EM from the ends of the formalin fixed tissue. Electron microscopic examination can also be performed on formalin fixed paraffin embedded tissue, however fresh tissue is always preferred.

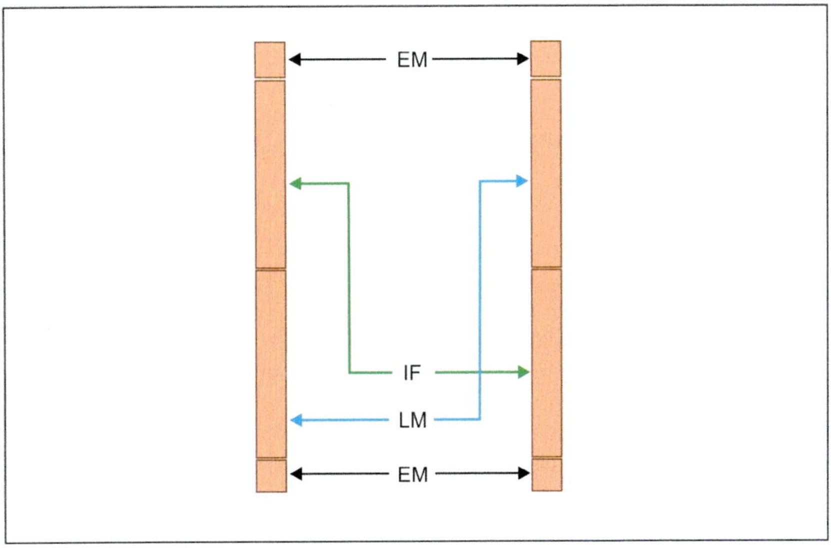

Figure 2.1 Division of renal biopsy cores in the absence of a dissecting microscope for laboratories using immunofluorescence (IF). The ends from all cores are taken for electron microscopy (EM) with the remainder divided for light microscopy (LM) and IF.
Source: Modern Pathology. 2004;17:1555-63.

SPECIMEN ADEQUACY

How much renal biopsy tissue is necessary for a definite pathologic diagnosis is a difficult question, and the answer depends on the indication for biopsy. If the differential diagnosis includes renal diseases defined by electron microscopy or immunohistology, then tissue must be processed for these studies as well as for light microscopy. A single glomerulus may be sufficient for the diagnosis of diffusely distributed glomerular diseases, such as amyloidosis or membranous glomerulopathy. In many cases, specimen adequacy is a statistical consideration of the number of glomeruli required to definitely exclude a focal pathology and to know what proportion of the glomeruli is involved.

LIGHT MICROSCOPIC EXAMINATION OF RENAL BIOPSY

The complex microscopic anatomy of the kidney requires an examination of all the histologic elements (glomeruli, tubules, interstitium, and blood vessels) in multiple serial sections to avoid missing pathologic lesions.

When confronted with a renal biopsy specimen, an initial task is to decide what renal compartment is the primary or initial site of injury, i.e. glomeruli, tubules, and interstitium, or extraglomerular vessels. In some instances, multiple compartments will be affected simultaneously by the primary pathogenic process, for example, glomeruli and vessels in certain form of vasculitis, and tubules and interstitium in tubulointerstitial nephritis. Once a particular renal compartment is injured, secondary injury often develops in other compartments, especially if there is chronic progression of renal disease. For example, primary glomerular injury results in secondary interstitial, tubular and vascular disease through multiple mechanisms. As chronic renal disease approaches end stage, injury to all compartments may be so severe that the primary site of disease is completely obscured.

Evaluation of Glomerular Compartment

Primary glomerular diseases have many patterns of injury, including but not limited to glomerular inflammation, necrosis, thrombosis, scarring (sclerosis), capillary wall thickening by light microscopy (LM), immune deposits by electron microscopy (EM) or immunofluorescence (IF), and glomerular basement membrane abnormalities by EM. Soon after the onset of glomerular diseases, secondary tubulointerstitial changes appear, such as interstitial edema or fibrosis, interstitial inflammation, and tubular simplification or atrophy.

Table 2.1 lists some of the terms that are used to describe the pathologic features that characterize glomerular injury. The presence and sometimes the absence of these features are used to resolve the differential diagnosis and to describe the glomerular injury in the renal biopsy report. **Table 2.2** and **Figs 2.2A and B** lists some general patterns of glomerular lesions seen by light microscopy and the diseases that most often cause them alongwith their clinical manifestations. **Figures 2.3A to D** illustrate several LM patterns of glomerular injury.

Some glomerular diseases that have overt clinical manifestations and unequivocal lesions by EM or IF may have no detectable abnormalities by LM, such as minimal change glomerulopathy, thin basement membrane nephropathy, early immune complex disease (e.g. class I lupus nephritis, mild IgA nephropathy, stage I membranous glomerulopathy). The thickness and texture of glomerular capillary walls must be assessed. Special stains, such as periodic acid-Schiff (PAS), Jones silver and Masson trichrome stains, are helpful in determining whether capillary wall thickening is most consistent with membranous glomerulopathy, thrombotic microangiopathy, or some infiltrative process such as fibrillary glomerulonephritis or amyloidosis. However, EM and/or IF are helpful in the diagnosis of most glomerular diseases both by ruling in and ruling out disease and are essential for the pathologic diagnosis of some glomerular diseases. For example, immunofluorescence (IF) is required for a definite pathologic diagnosis of anti-GBM disease, IgA nephropathy, C1q nephropathy, and monoclonal immunoglobulin deposition disease; and EM is required for a definite pathologic diagnosis of thin basement membrane nephropathy, dense deposit disease, fibrillary glomerulonephritis, and immunotactoid glomerulonephritis. In addition, there are many early or mild expressions of disease that cannot be detected or will be overlooked by LM that are readily apparent by EM, such as early or mild Fabry's disease, early hereditary nephritis, mild or resolving TMA or eclampsia, and many others.

Electron Microscopic Evaluation of Glomeruli

Renal pathology is the only anatomic pathology subspeciality that uses transmission electron microscopy for routine evaluation of tissue specimens. EM allows detailed evaluation of the cellular and extracellular contents of each glomerular compartment and definite assessment of thickness, contour,

Table 2.1 Terms used to describe histologic lesions in glomeruli

Term	*Definition*
Focal	Involving less than 50% of glomeruli
Diffuse	Involving all or almost all glomeruli (≥ 50% of glomeruli)
Segmental	Involving portions of individual glomeruli
Global	Involving all of a glomerular tuft
Mesangial hypercellularity **(Figure 2.3)**	Four or more nuclei in the contiguous matrix of a peripheral mesangial segment
Endocapillary hypercellularity **(Figure 2.3)**	Increased cellularity internal to the glomerular basement membrane (GBM) composed of leukocytes, endothelial cells and mesangial cells
Lobular **(Figure 2.3)**	Consolidated expansion of the glomerular segments representing major anatomic subunits (lobules) of the glomerular tuft formed by dichotomous branching of the afferent arteriole (hypersegmentation of the glomerular tuft)
Extracapillary hypercellularity **(Figure 2.3)**	Increased cellularity in Bowman space or more than one layer of parietal or visceral epithelial cells
Crescent	Extracapillary hypercellularity other than the epithelial hyperplasia of the collapsing variant of focal segmental glomerulosclerosis (FSGS), often accompanied by fibrin extravasation into Bowman space
Fibrinoid necrosis	Lytic destruction of cells and matrix with deposition of acidophilic fibrin-rich material and often accompanied by GBM rupture and apoptosis of infiltrating leukocytes
Mesangiolysis	Detachment of the paramesangial GBM from the mesangial matrix resulting in a capillary aneurysm, or lytic dissolution of the mesangial matrix
Sclerosis	Increased collagenous extracellular matrix that is expanding the mesangium, obliterating capillary lumens, or forming adhesions to Bowman capsule. The sclerotic areas stain positively with periodic acid-Schiff (PAS), Masson's trichrome, and periodic acid-silver methenamine (PASM)
Hyaline	Glassy acidophilic extracellular material. Acellular material that stains red with eosin and PAS but is unstained by PASM. Contents include serum proteins, other glycoproteins and lipids.

and integrity of the glomerular basement membrane and mesangial matrix. Abnormal deposits (such as electron-dense immune deposits or organized fibrillary or microtubular deposits), can be detected in subepithelial, intramembranous, subendothelial and mesangial locations. Diagnostically informative ultrastructural abnormalities in the GBMs include thickening, thinning, lamellation, mesangial cell interposition and subendothelial electron-lucent expansion. Glomerular deposits with an organized substructure are pathognomic of some renal/systemic conditions or at least narrow the differential diagnosis substantially. Abnormalities in cells (podocytes/visceral epithelial cells

Table 2.2 Patterns of glomerular injury observed by light microscopy and some but not all diseases that can cause each pattern of injury

No abnormality by light microscopy
No glomerular disease
Glomerular disease with no light microscopic changes (e.g. minimal change disease, thin basement membrane nephropathy)
Mild or early glomerular disease (e.g. lupus nephritis, IgA nephropathy, C1q nephropathy, membranous glomerulonephritis, amyloidosis, Alport syndrome, etc.)
Thick capillary walls without hypercellularity or mesangial expansion
Membranous glomerulonephritis (primary or secondary) with thick GBM
Thrombotic microangiopathy with expanded subendothelial zone
Pre-eclampsia/eclampsia with endothelial swelling
Fibrillary glomerulonephritis with predominance of capillary wall deposits
Thick capillary walls with mesangial expansion but little or no hypercellularity
Diabetic glomerulosclerosis with diffuse rather than nodular sclerosis
Secondary membranous glomerulonephritis with mesangial immune deposits
Amyloidosis
Monoclonal immunoglobulin deposition disease
Fibrillary glomerulonephritis
Dense-deposit disease
C3 glomerulonephritis
Focal segmental glomerular sclerosis without hypercellularity
Focal segmental glomerulosclerosis
Chronic sclerotic phase of focal glomerulonephritis
Hereditary nephritis (Alport syndrome)
Mesangial or endocapillary hypercellularity
Focal or diffuse mesangioproliferative glomerulonephritis
Focal or diffuse (endocapillary) proliferative glomerulonephritis
Acute diffuse proliferative postinfectious glomerulonephritis
Membranoproliferative glomerulonephritis
Dense-deposit disease
Extracapillary hypercellularity
ANCA crescentic glomerulonephritis (paucity of immunoglobulin by IFM)
Anti-GBM crescentic glomerulonephritis (linear immunoglobulin by IFM)
Immune complex and C3 glomerulopathy crescentic glomerulonephritis (granular immunoglobulin and/ or complement by IFM)
Collapsing variant of FSGS (including HIV nephropathy)
Membranoproliferative, lobular, or nodular pattern
Membranoproliferative glomerulonephritis
Dense-deposit disease
C3 glomerulonephritis
Diabetic glomerulosclerosis with nodular mesangial expansion (KW nodules)
Monoclonal immunoglobulin deposition disease with nodular sclerosis
Thrombotic microangiopathy
Fibrillary glomerulonephritis
Immunotactoid glomerulopathy
Advanced diffuse global glomerular sclerosis
End-stage glomerular disease
End-stage vascular disease
End-stage tubulointerstitial disease

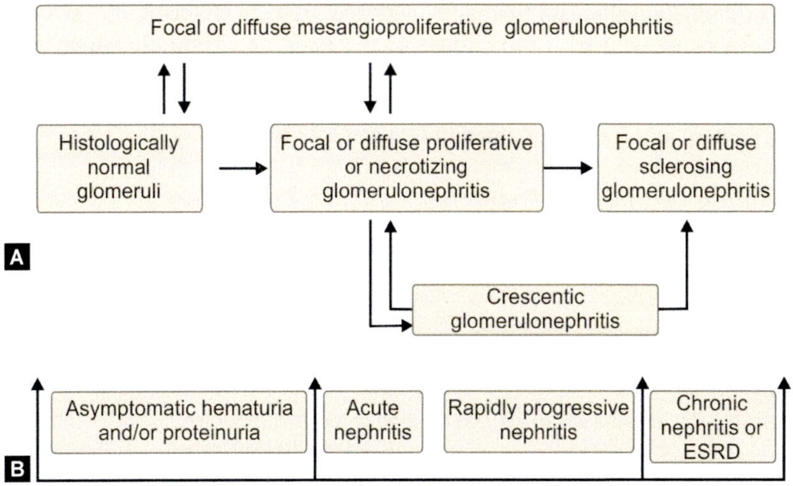

Figures 2.2A and B Correlation of various histopathologic patterns of glomerular response to injury correlated with the usual clinical manifestations of renal injury: (A) Spectrum of light microscopic morphology; (B) Spectrum of clinical manifestations
Source: Med Clin North Am. 1997;81:653.

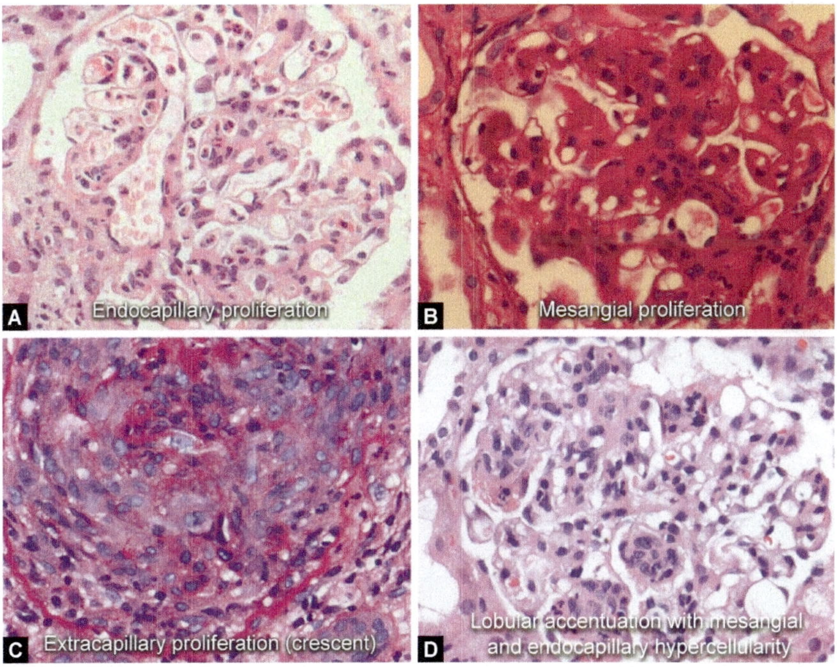

Figures 2.3A to D (A) Panel of photomicrographs show endocapillary proliferation as highlighted by glomerular capillary loops filled with polymorphs; (B) Mesangial proliferation as highlighted by mesangial matrix expansion with presence of 4 and/or more nuclei in the mesangial compartment; (C) Extracapillary proliferation with compressed glomerular tuft; (D) Lobular appearance of glomerulus as highlighted by mild mesangial and segmental endocapillary proliferation with nonuniform thickening of the capillary basement membrane (classical of MPGN)

and endothelial cells) can be readily detected, such as effacement of podocytic foot processes seen with proteinuria or the swelling of endothelial cells seen with eclampsia/pre-eclampsia and the thrombotic microangiopathies. **Table 2.3** illustrates varied location of immune-complex deposits in electron microscopic examination and is demonstrated in **Figures 2.4A to D**.

Common Glomerular Diseases

Minimal change disease (MCD): Light microscopy of this disease shows no or minimal glomerular abnormality. The glomerular capillaries are patent, with

Table 2.3 Terms related to location of immune-complex deposits

Term	*Definition*
Subepithelial or epimembranous	Located between the glomerular basement membrane and the podocytes
Intramembranous	Within the basement membrane
Subendothelial	Between the glomerular basement membrane and the endothelium
Mesangial	Within the mesangium

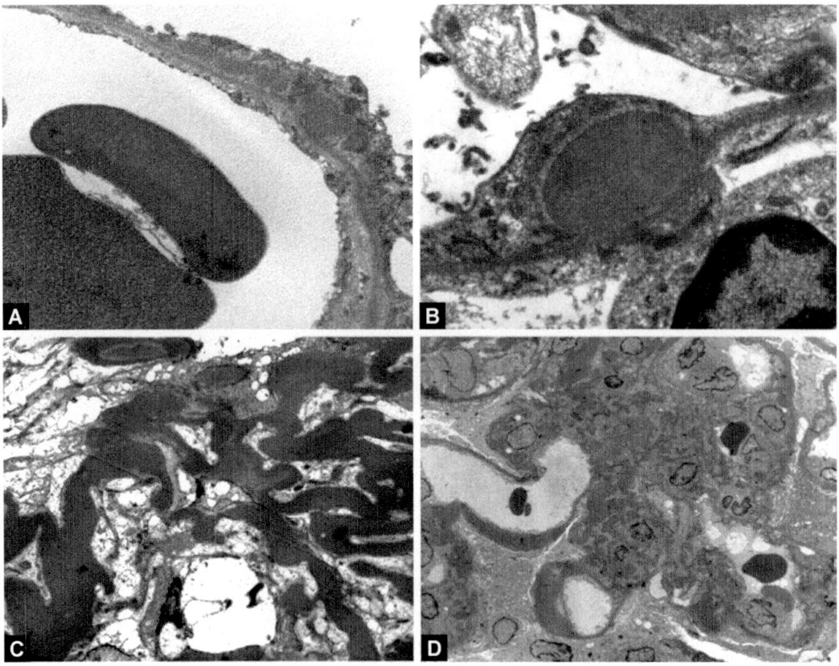

Figures 2.4A to D Panel of electron microscopic photomicrographs show varied location of immune-complex deposits: (A) Uniform sized subepithelial immune-complex like electron dense deposits (classical of Membranous GN); (B) Subepithelial hump (classical of postinfectious GN. Also seen in C3 GN); (C) Dense osmiophilic intramembranous deposits (classical of dense deposit disease); (D) Dominant mesangial deposits (classical of IgA nephropathy)

neither thickening nor irregularity of the capillary wall. Some specimens show a slight increase in the mesangial matrix or cellularity, the presence of focal segmental glomerular collapse or scarring, endocapillary proliferation, or adhesions is not supportive of the diagnosis of MCD. Immunofluorescence show no staining for immunoglobulins in most cases except for minimal trace staining for IgM and C3. Presence of significant immune deposits excludes a diagnosis of MCD. Electron microscopy show diffuse effacement of podocytic foot processes **(Fig. 2.5)**.

Focal segmental glomerulosclerosis (FSGS): The "classic" lesion of FSGS consists of segmental solidification of the glomerular capillary tuft by an acellular extracellular matrix that is eosinophilic, periodic acid-Schiff (PAS) reactive, and argyrophilic. This may be accompanied by hyalinosis. FSGS lesions are often associated with adhesion to the Bowman capsule and the smallest lesions may consist of a simple synechial attachment, without prominent matrix accumulation in the underlying glomerular tuft. Immunofluorescence show nonspecific trapping for IgM and C3 in areas of segmental sclerosis. Electron microscopy show diffuse effacement of foot processes in primary FSGS and show very focal effacement in secondary FSGS **(Figs 2.6 and 2.7)**. The lack of standardized approach to definition and classification has hindered study of various morphological variants of FSGS (collapsing variant, tip variant, cellular variant, perihilar variant and FSGS NOS) **(Fig. 2.8)**. Collapsing variant is also known as collapsing glomerulopathy is characterized by capillary collapse with accompanied prominent epithelial cell

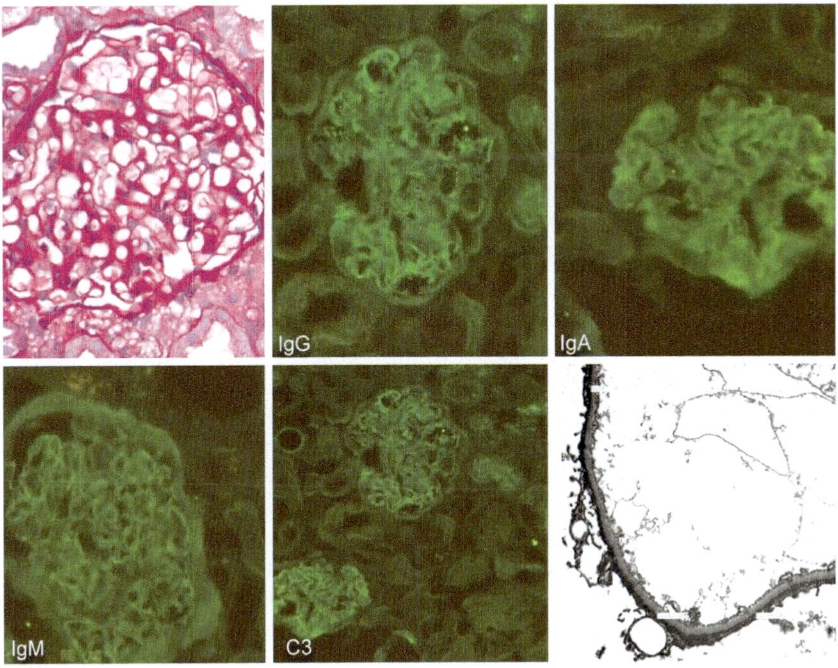

Figure 2.5 Panel of photomicrographs show normal glomerular morphology with completely negative immunofluorescence with diffuse foot process effacement in electron microscopy consistent with minimal change disease

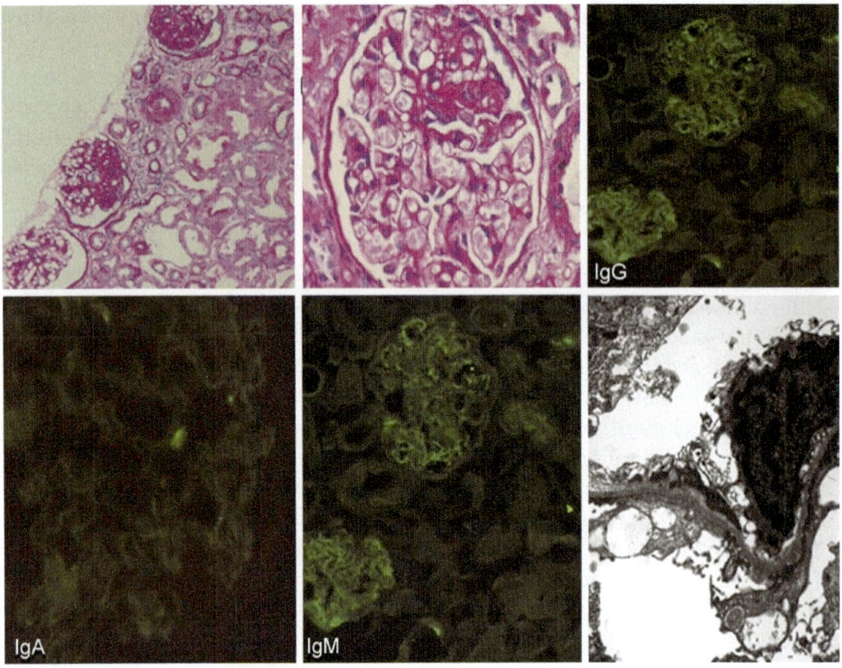

Figure 2.6 Panel of photomicrographs show a lesion of segmental sclerosis with synechiae formation, completely negative immunofluorescence with diffuse foot process effacement in electron microscopy consistent with primary focal segmental glomerulosclerosis

hypertrophy and hyperplasia within Bowman space. The epithelial cells typically line the external surface of the glomerular tuft but may fill the Bowman space, forming a "pseudocrescent". Collapsing FSGS usually presents with severe nephrotic syndrome and renal insufficiency and could be primary or secondary to viruses (HIV), drugs (pamidronate, interferon), and vaso-occlusive disease.

Membranous glomerulonephritis (MGN): The light microscopic findings in MGN may be subtle, especially in early cases, diagnostic changes may not be obvious by light microscopy alone. In these cases, IF and EM readily establish the diagnosis. In later stages there is marked global thickening of the glomerular basement membrane with vacuolization of the GBM. Immunofluorescence show granular deposition of IgG for C3 along capillary wall. Membranous lupus nephritis (secondary MGN) is a close light microscopy differential diagnosis for primary MGN, however secondary membranous lupus nephritis show intense IgA, C3 and C1q staining alongwith IgG in immunofluorescence. Fortunately, staining for the PLA2R has emerged as a far more effective strategy to differentiate primary and secondary forms of disease (PLA2R will be positive in primary MGN and negative in membranous lupus nephritis) **(Figs 2.9 and 2.10)**.

Primary IgA nephropathy: Light microscopy show varied glomerular histopathology in form of mesangial proliferation, segmental sclerosis, necrotizing lesion, endocapillary proliferation and extracapillary proliferation.

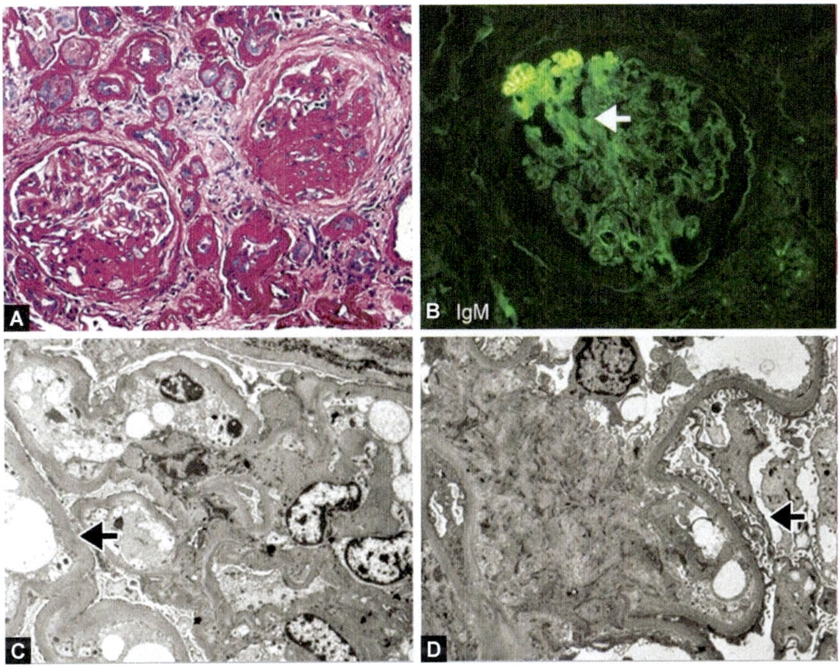

Figures 2.7A to D Panel of photomicrographs show segmental sclerosis with significant tubular atrophy and immunofluorescence show nonspecific segmental IgM trapping in area of sclerosis. The electron microscopy show preserved foot processes in the first EM image, however the second EM image show very focal foot process effacement (as highlighted by arrow head) and GBM thickening (related to underlying diabetic nephropathy) consistent secondary FSGS

Because of highly diverse histologic presentation of IgA nephropathy, a number of histologic classification systems have been devised and tested for their value in predicting clinical outcome. Recently Oxford MEST classification and scoring system has come in which includes four histologic parameters, M, E, S, and T:

- M0 or M1, indicating mesangial hypercellularity in ≤50% versus >50% of glomeruli
- E0 or E1, indicating endocapillary hypercellularity in zero versus one or more glomeruli
- S0 or S1, indicating segmental sclerosis in zero versus one or more glomeruli
- T0, T1, or T2, indicating TA/IF in ≤ 25%, 26% to 50%, or > 50% of renal cortex, respectively.

Immunofluorescence show dominant IgA deposits predominantly in the mesangium and very focally along capillary loops. Electron microscopy confirm electron dense deposits in mesangium **(Figs 2.11A and B)**.

Lupus nephritis: Renal biopsy plays a significant role in the management of patients with SLE. In some patients, it is instrumental in establishing a diagnosis of SLE. This is especially common early in disease and applies most frequently to patients with mesangial proliferative or membranous patterns who lack serologic markers of SLE and may present months or even years before the American

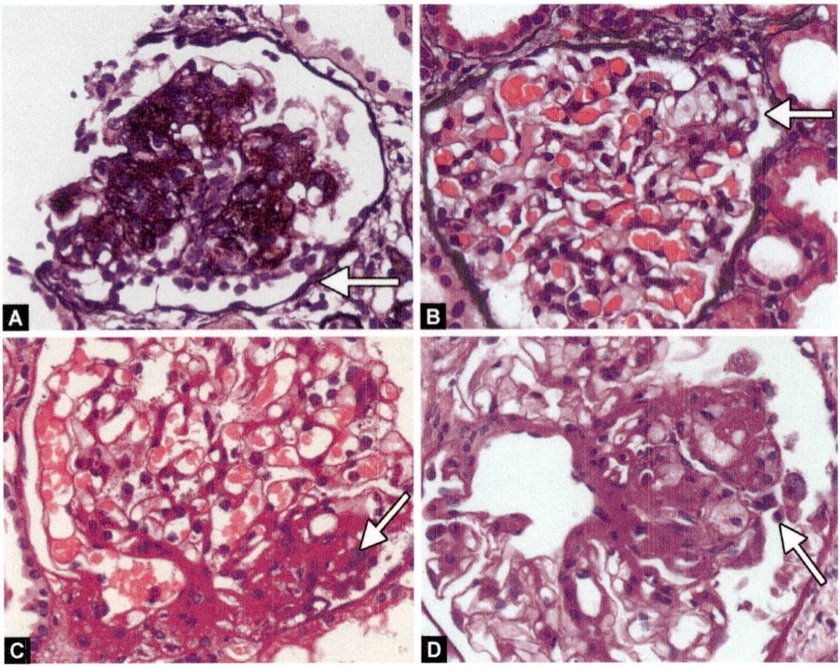

Figures 2.8A to D (A) Panel of photomicrographs show collapse of the glomerular tuft with proliferation of overlying podocytes appearing as crown over collapsed glomerular tuft (collapsing pattern of FSGS; (B) Other image show endocapillary foam cells projecting into the tubular pole (FSGS, tip variant; (C) Segmental sclerosis in perihilar location (FSGS, perihilar variant); (D) A glomerulus with segmental endocapillary hypercellularity occluding lumina, with or without foam cells and karyorrhexis (FSGS, cellular variant)

College of Rheumatology (ACR) criteria for SLE have been met. In cases in which diagnosis of SLE has already been made prior to renal biopsy, the biopsy provide information about the class, severity, activity, and chronicity of the lupus nephritis that cannot be accurately predicted on the basis of clinical manifestations. The major histologic abnormalities of the glomerulus include immune deposits, glomerular proliferation, influx of leukocytes, glomerular necrosis, and scarring. Glomerular proliferation may be mesangial, endocapillary, and extracapillary. Immunofluorescence show full house IF pattern with strong staining of the glomerulus for all immunoglobulins (IgG, IgA, IgM) and complements (C3, C1q). Electron microscopic examination reveals massive immune-complex deposits in subendothelial, subepithelial and mesangial location **(Figs 2.12A and B)**.

Crescentic glomerulonephritis: Light microscopic morphological recognition of crescentic glomerulonephritis is only the beginning of an adequate nephropathologic analysis. A pathologic diagnosis of crescentic glomerulonephritis is incomplete unless the disease is further categorized, which usually requires immunofluorescence and electron microscopy, serology, or both. Accurate and definite categorization of crescentic glomerulonephritis is critical for optimal patient clinical outcome, because one of the major positive

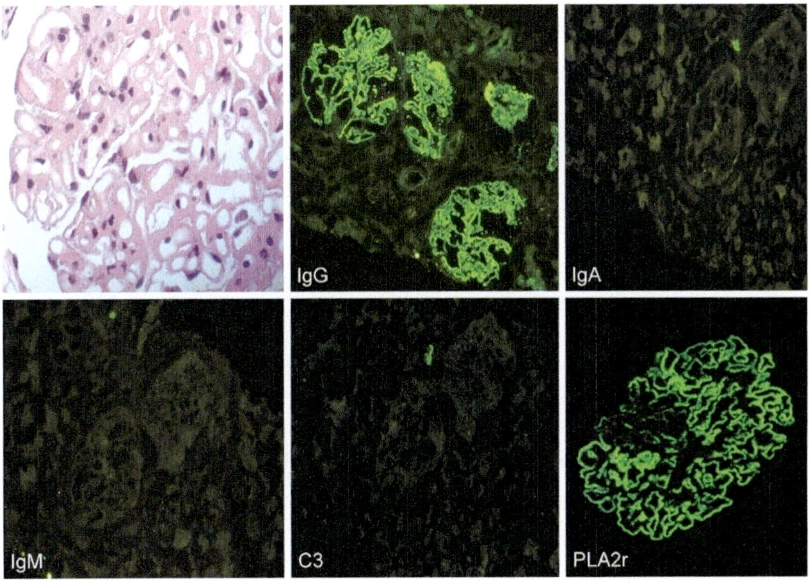

Figure 2.9 Panel of photomicrographs show diffuse thickening of the glomerular capillary wall along with granular deposition of IgG along capillary wall. Other immunoglobulins (IgA, IgM) and complements (C3,C1q) are negative. This immunofluorescence pattern is classical of primary idiopathic membranous glomerulonephritis. In addition, PLA2r staining is seen confirming idiopathic/primary membranous nephropathy

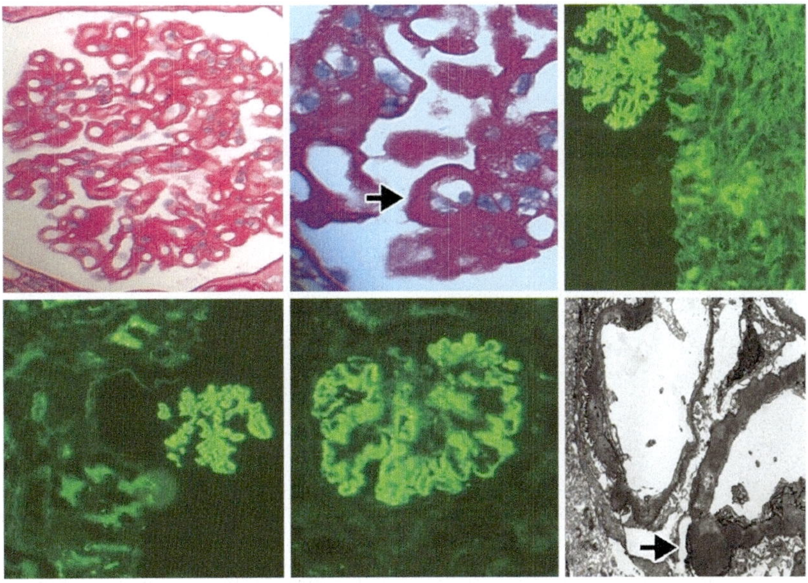

Figure 2.10 Panel of photomicrographs show diffuse thickening of the glomerular capillary wall along with granular deposition of IgG, C3 and C1q consistent with secondary membranous glomerulonephritis (Class V Lupus). In addition, the arrow heads point wire-loop like lesion in light microscopy and electron microscopy reveal immune-complex like electron dense deposits

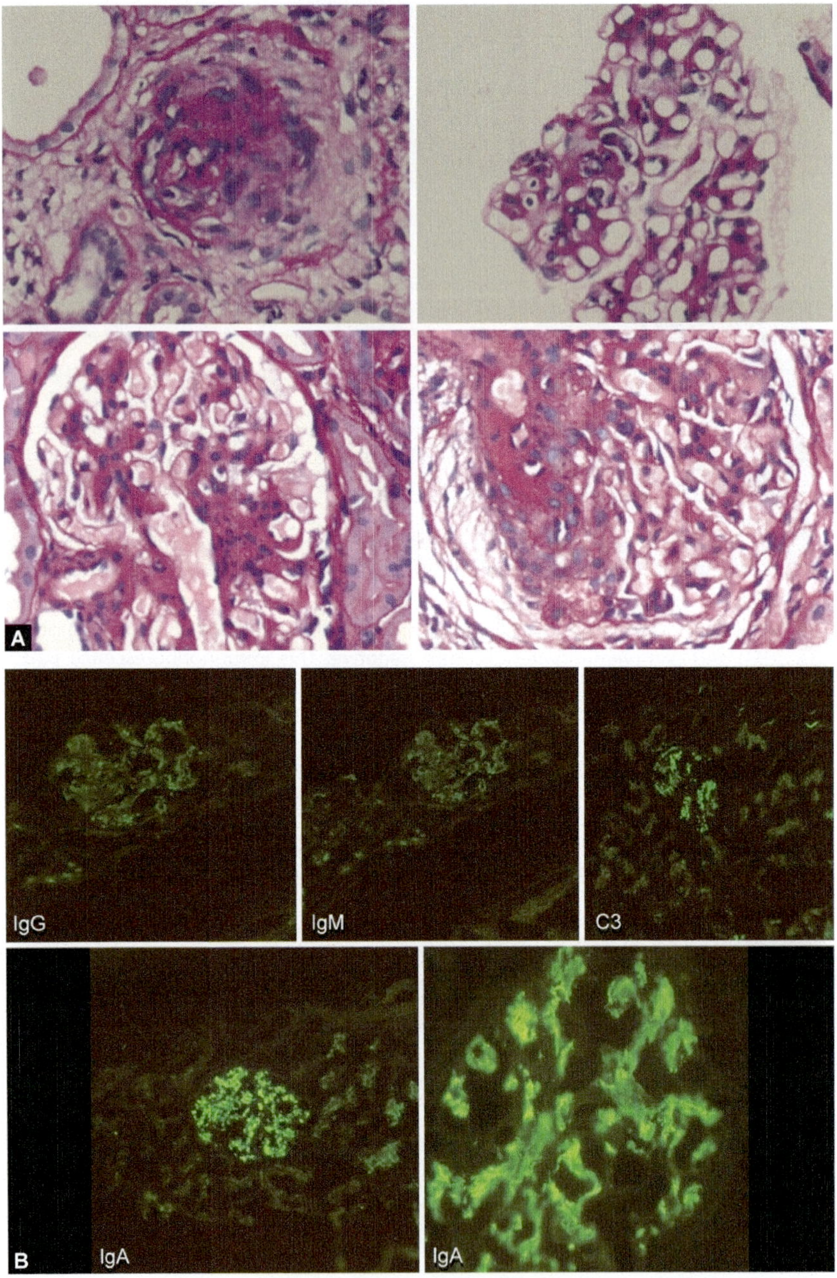

Figures 2.11A and B (A) Panel of photomicrographs show variable glomerular morphology in form of occasional glomerulus with fibrocellular crescent, occasional one with segmental endocapillary proliferation, occasional one with mesangial matrix expansion with mesangial hypercellularity and occasional one with segmental sclerosis. Variable glomerular morphology is commonly seen in IgA nephropathy; (B) Panel of immunofluorescence photomicrographs show dominant granular deposition of IgA in mesangium along with minimal staining for C3. IgG and IgM are negative. This immunofluorescence pattern is classical of IgA nephropathy

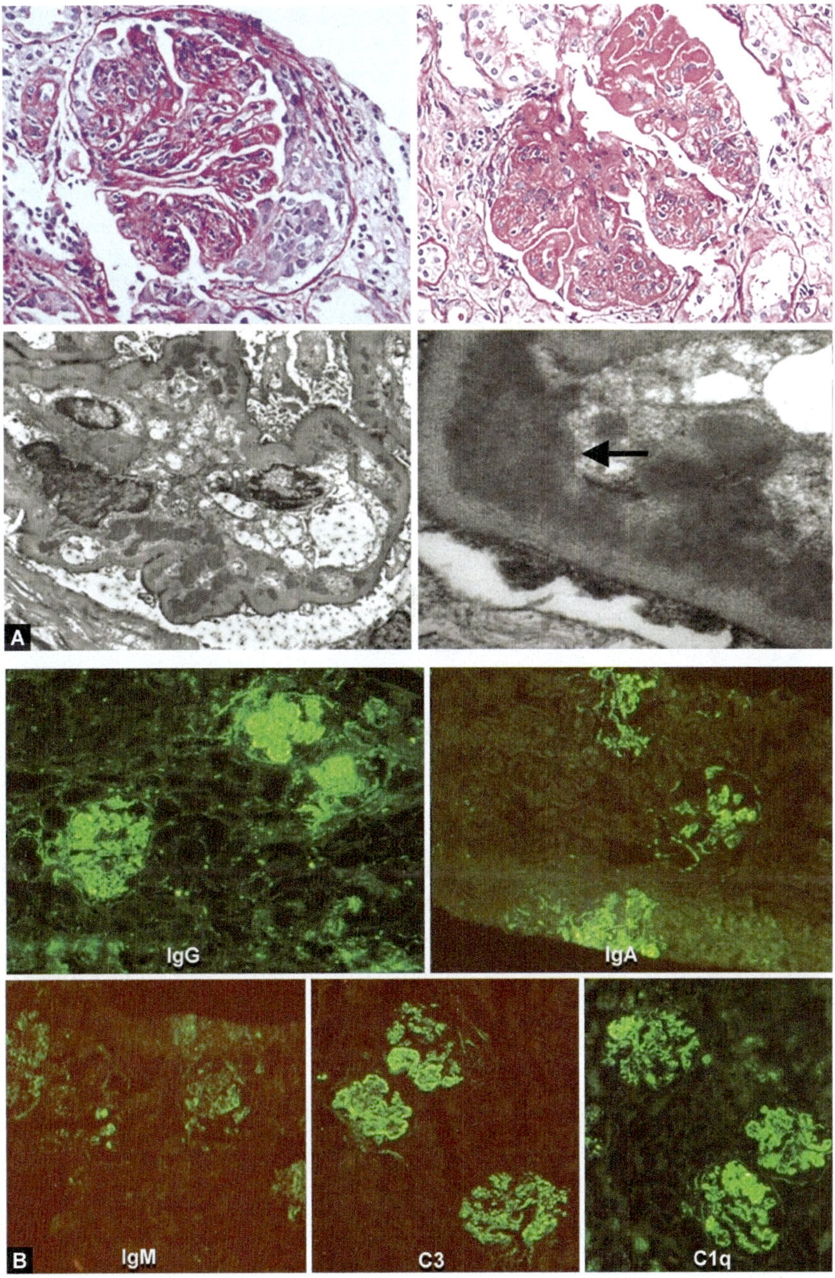

Figures 2.12A and B (A) Panel of photomicrographs show variable glomerular morphology in form of segmental endocapillary proliferation, small cellular crescent and wire-loop lesion with few hyaline thrombi. Electron microscopic photograph show massive immune-complex like electron dense deposits in the subendothelial location. Higher magnification of the immune-complex deposits show finger print impression (shown by an arrow); (B) Panel of immunofluorescence photomicrographs show full house IF pattern seen in diffuse proliferative lupus nephritis (Class IV)

prognostic factors in the most aggressive forms of crescentic glomerulonephritis is rapid institution of immunosuppressive therapy.

Crescentic glomerulonephritis is categorized by immunofluorescence into *anti-GBM* crescentic glomerulonephritis with linear GBM staining for immunoglobulin IgG, *immune complex* crescentic glomerulonephritis with granular staining of glomeruli for immunoglobulin (IgG, IgA, IgM) or complement (C3, C1q), or crescentic glomerulonephritis with little or no glomerular staining for immunoglobulin (i.e. *pauci-immune* crescentic glomerulonephritis) (**Figs 2.13A to D**). Varying ages of crescent (from cellular to fibrocellular and fibrous crescents) are more commonly seen in pauci-immune GN and in anti-GBM GN crescents are mostly of the same age **(Fig. 2.14)**.

Proliferative glomerulonephritis with isolated C3 deposits in immunofluorescence: Light microscopic morphology of diffuse or focal proliferative GN (with endocapillary, extracapillary or mesangial proliferation) with isolated or dominant C3 deposits is characteristically seen in *postinfectious GN* and

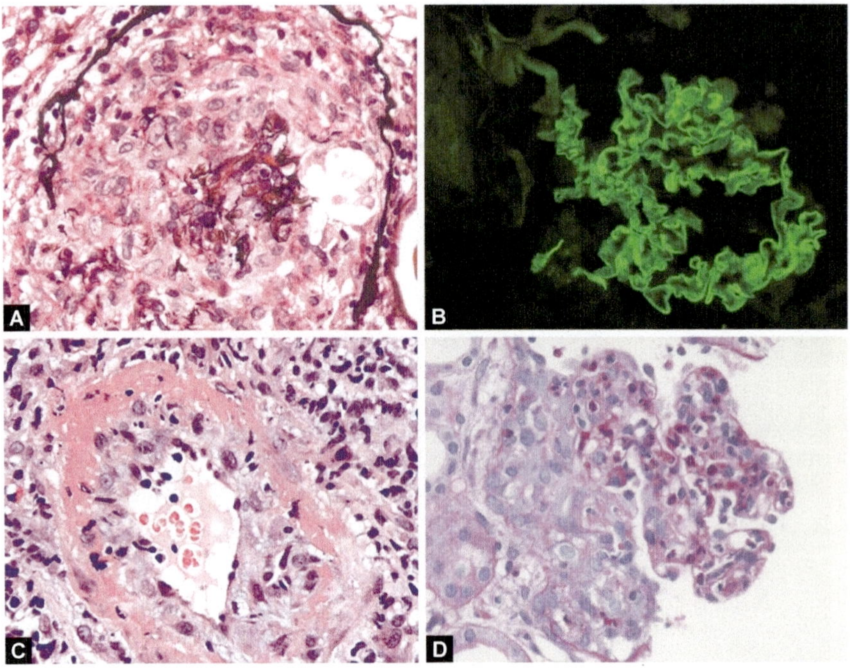

Figures 2.13A to D (A) Highlight presence of global circumferential cellular crescent with compressed underlying glomerular tuft. The present morphology is classical of anti-GBM disease or pauci-immune glomerulonephritis. Presence of linear staining along glomerular basement membrane confirm the diagnosis of anti-GBM disease (B) and its absence along with absence or very minimal staining for other immunoglobulins confirm the diagnosis of pauci-immune glomerulonephritis. In addition, pauci-immune GN biopsy show evidence of vasculitis in form of transmural arteritis or fibrinoid necrosis of the vessel wall (C); (D) small cellular crescent with endocapillary proliferation in the underlying glomerular tuft, feature of immune-complex/compliment mediated glomerulonephritis. The immunofluorescence show presence of dominant C3 deposits (not shown)

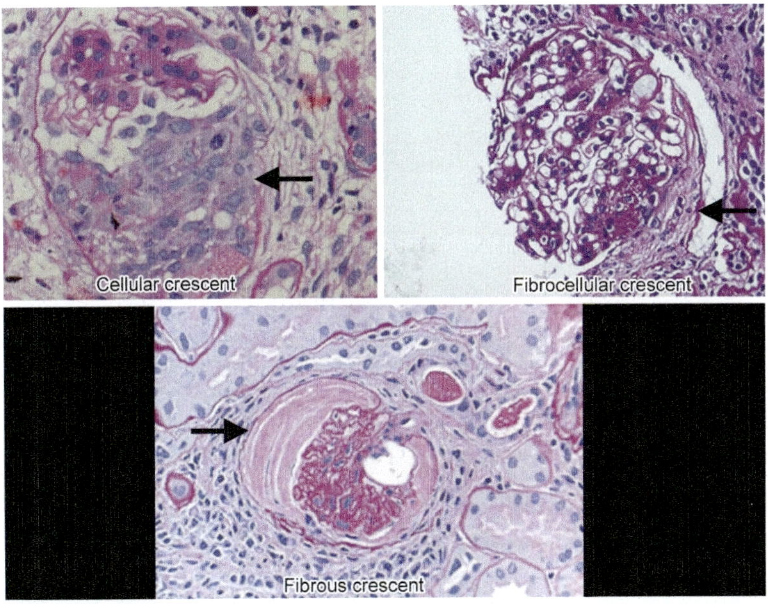

Figure 2.14 Panel of light microscopic photomicrographs show crescents of varying ages ranging from cellular to fibrocellular to fibrous crescent (highlighted by arrow)

C3 glomerulopathy (which includes C3 GN and dense deposit disease). The characteristic features of postinfectious glomerulonephritis on kidney biopsy are a proliferative glomerulonephritis on light microscopy, bright C3 staining with or without immunoglobulins on immunofluorescence microscopy, and subepithelial deposits called 'humps' on electron microscopy **(Figs 2.15A to D)**. In some cases, the diagnosis of postinfectious glomerulonephritis is made on the basis of these biopsy findings even in the absence of any clinical, bacterial, or serological evidence of a preceding infection. If there is persistent low C3 levels along with persistent hematuria/proteinuria then these patients should be evaluated for alternate complement pathway defects and possibility of C3 glomerulopathy remains a strong possibility. Definite categorization of C3 glomerulopathy into *C3 glomerulonephritis* and *dense deposit disease (DDD)* requires electron microscopy as dense deposit disease will show dense osmiophilic intramembranous deposits whereas C3 GN show pale deposits in mesangium, subendothelial, occasionally subepithelial and intramembranous location.

Membranoproliferative glomerulonephritis (MPGN): The definite diagnosis of MPGN is based on renal biopsy. Renal histological features include mesangial widening due to an increase in matrix and cells, and diffuse capillary wall thickening resulting from the presence of subendothelial and/or intramembranous immune deposits and mesangial cell interposition.

Historically, the MPGN was subclassified into MPGN type I (the most common form), type II (dense deposit disease), and type III based on combined features of light, immunofluorescence, and electron microscopy. In recent years, there have been great advances in our understanding of the pathogenesis of

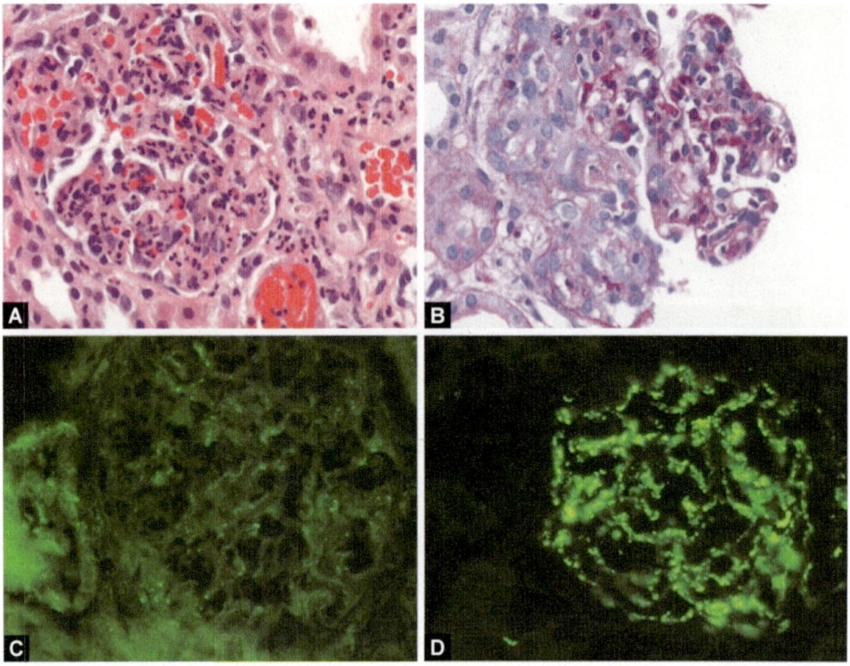

Figures 2.15A to D (A and B) Highlight presence of global endocapillary proliferation rich in polymorphs. An occasional glomerulus show a small cellular crescent and underlying glomerular tuft show endocapillary proliferation. Immunofluorescence show absent to trace IgG staining (C) and strong 3+ coarse granular staining for C3 (D). In view of isolated C3 deposits and diffuse endocapillary proliferation rich in neutrophils and a recent history of infection, case was reported as diffuse proliferative GN consistent with postinfectious GN

MPGN, particularly in the area of complement-mediated C3 glomerulonephritis, including DDD and C3 glomerulonephritis. The current classification recognizes the importance of IF in further subdividing MPGN into immune-complex mediated MPGN with glomerular immunoglobulins and complement deposition and MPGN with abnormalities in alternate complement pathway regulation resulting in isolated C3 deposits with little or no immunoglobulins by IF. MPGN type II is currently designated as DDD and is recognized as a variant of C3 glomerulopathy.

MPGN type I is commonly associated with infections, autoimmune diseases and dysproteinemic state **(Figs 2.16A and B)**.

Diagnostic criteria for C3 glomerulopathy **(*Figs 2.17A to D*)**:

- Membranoproliferative glomerulonephritis (MPGN) pattern on light microscopy
- C3-predominant staining with staining ≥2 + (on a 0–3 + scale)
- Electron-dense deposits by electron microscopy that are of the immune complex type.

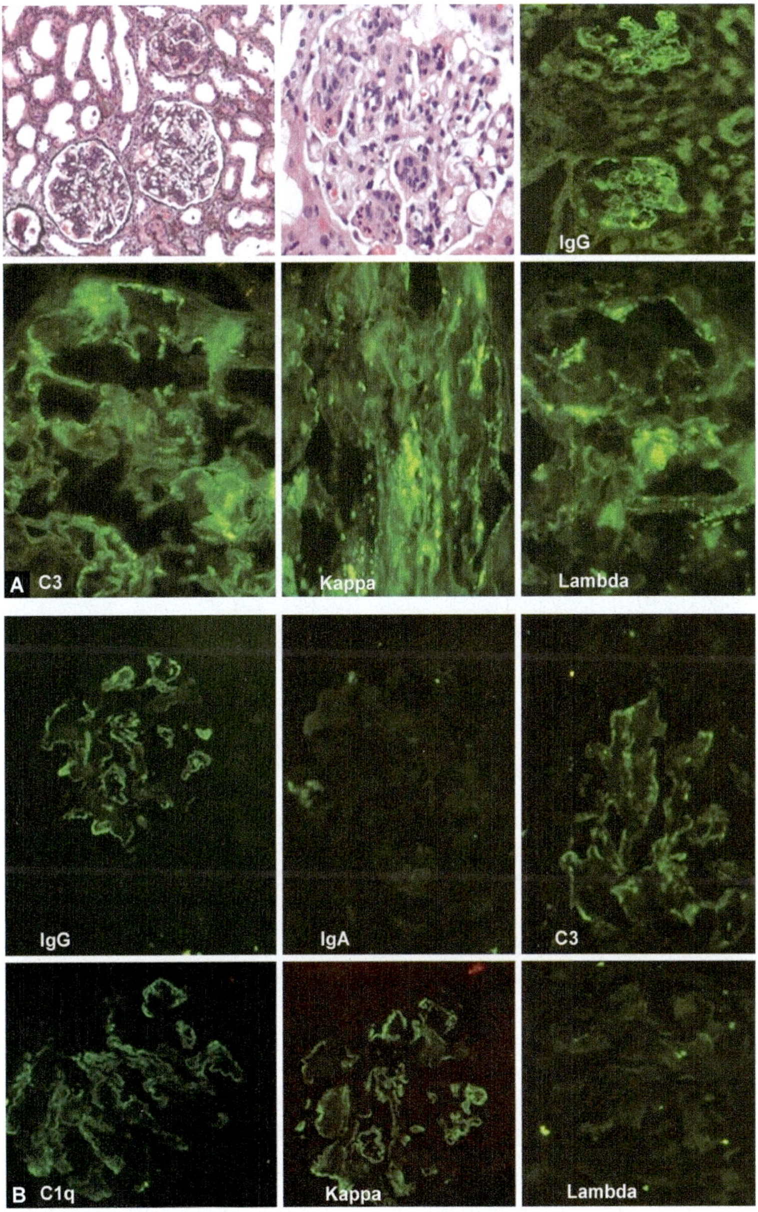

Figures 2.16A and B (A) Photomicrograph panel show lobular accentuation of the glomerulus due to mesangial and segmental endocapillary proliferation (classical of MPGN). Immunofluorescence show both IgG and C3 deposits. Both kappa and lambda show positivity, thereby excluding any monoclonal restriction or a dysproteinemic state. This case was reported as Immune-complex mediated MPGN; (B) Photomicrograph panel show immunofluorescence images in a case of MPGN. IF images show granular deposition of immunoglobulin (IgG) and complements (c3, c1q), however kappa is positive and lambda is negative. The case was reported as MPGN IgG kappa (MPGN with dysproteinemia)

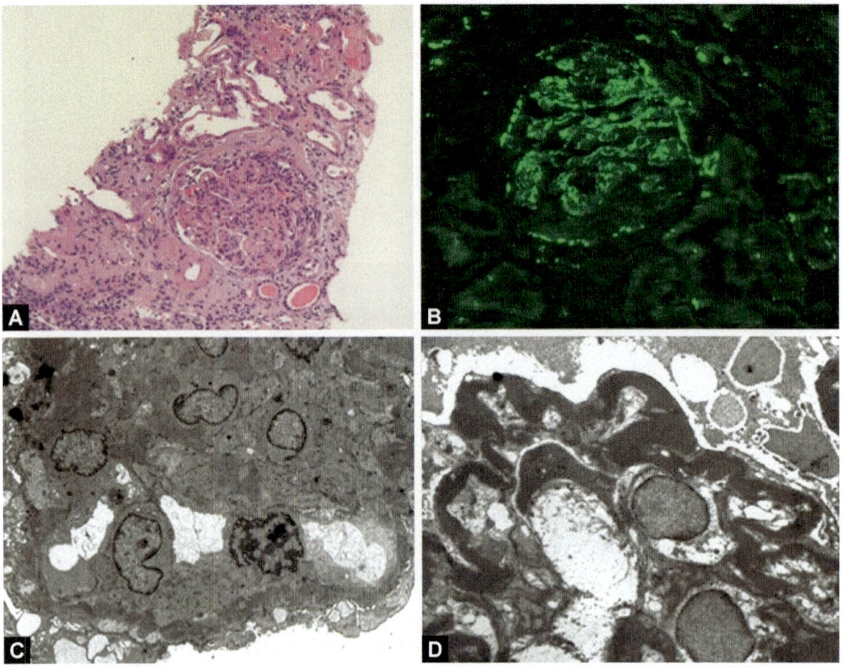

Figures 2.17A to D (A) Photomicrograph panel show immunofluorescence images in a case of C3 glomerulopathy. Light microscopy show lobular accentuation; (B) IF image show granular deposition of C3 only; (C) Immunoglobulins are negative (not shown). Based on light microscopy and isolated C3 deposits, diagnosis is C3 glomerulopathy. If electron microscopy show predominantly less osmiophilic or less electron dense deposits predominantly in the mesangial and subendothelial location than diagnosis of C3 glomerulonephritis is given; (D) However, if there are more dense osmiophilic intramembranous deposits than it is diagnosed as DDD

Diagnostic criteria for C3 glomerulonephritis:

- MPGN pattern (most common); less common patterns include mesangial proliferative, diffuse proliferative, crescentic, or sclerosing.
- C3-dominant staining ≥ 2 + (on a 0–3 + scale), ± Ig trace to 1+.
- Electron-dense deposits, often large mesangial and subendothelial, ± intramembranous and subepithelial deposits. The only C3 deposits appear different from immune deposits as they are lobular, paler, waxy, smooth and not as sharp.

Amyloidosis: The light microscopic features of amyloidosis are always the same, regardless of the type of amyloid. In hematoxylin and eosin-stained sections, amyloid appear as eosinophilic, amorphous, "hyaline" material. In a PAS stain, amyloid is usually weakly positive and in silver stain amyloid is silver negative. A definite diagnosis of amyloid requires examination under polarized light, with the demonstration of apple green birefringence. If there is either of the light chain restriction then amyloid is likely primary in nature, however if no light chain restriction is demonstrated and serum amyloid associated protein is positive in areas of amyloid deposition then it is secondary amyloidosis **(Figs 2.18 and 2.19)**.

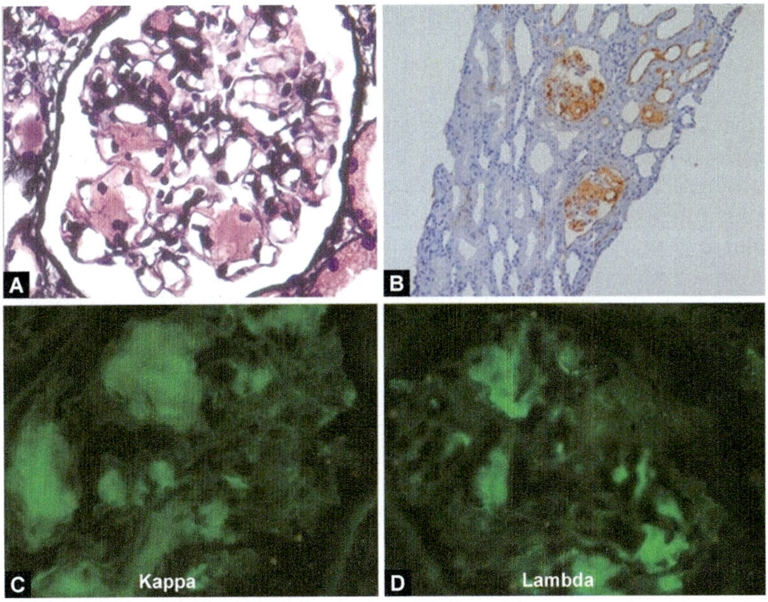

Figures 2.18A to D Photomicrograph panel show images in a case of secondary amyloidosis. Light microscopy show mesangial expansion by silver negative material (A) which show strong staining for serum amyloid associated protein [SAA immunohistochemistry, (B)]. Kappa and lambda immunofluorescence show no monoclonal restriction, thereby excluding primary amyloidosis (C and D)

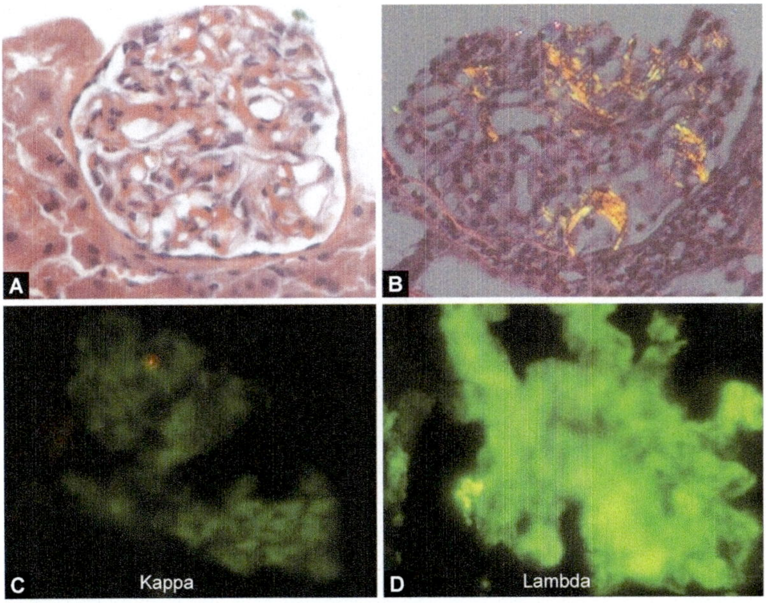

Figures 2.19A to D Photomicrograph panel show images in a case of primary amyloidosis. Light microscopy show mesangial expansion by congophilic material (A) which show apple-green birefringence thereby confirming amyloid deposition (B). Kappa and lambda immunofluorescence show lambda light chain restriction, thereby confirming primary amyloidosis (C and D)

Evaluation of Tubular Compartment

Diseases primarily affecting the renal tubules can be divided histologically into following headings: acute tubular epithelial injury (including acute tubular necrosis), tubulointerstitial inflammation, tubular casts, tubulitis, and chronic changes (tubular atrophy).

In normal renal cortex, tubules are arranged in back to back manner, virtually without interstitium. The histologic differential diagnosis between primary acute tubular injury (ATI) with secondary interstitial inflammation versus primary acute tubulointerstitial nephritis (TIN) is critical but often difficult. Since most inflammatory diseases affecting the tubules also involve the interstitium and because interstitial inflammation may be accompanied by tubulitis, the term acute or chronic tubulointerstitial nephritis is more appropriate than interstitial nephritis. **Table 2.4** illustrates terms used to describe histopathology lesions in tubules. Light chain (myeloma) cast nephropathy show tubular casts commonly in distal nephrons. In fact, most casts are located in the collecting ducts, and if medulla is not included in the renal biopsy specimen, the diagnosis may be missed **(Figs 2.20A to D)**.

Table 2.4 Terms used to describe histologic lesions of the tubules

Term	*Definition*
Acute tubular injury	Acute simplification with loss of brush border and flattening of cells without necrosis
Acute tubular necrosis	Coagulative necrosis of the tubular epithelium, usually secondary to toxins and/or ischemia
Tubulitis	Presence of lymphocytes/other inflammatory cells infiltrating the tubular epithelium
Tubular atrophy	Wasting of tubules as a result of ischemia, obstruction, or severe cellular injury. The tubular cells are usually simplified, reduced in size, or dilated and filled with casts. The tubular basement membranes are often thickened and wrinkled
Tubular casts	Various coagulated proteins and formed elements in the tubular lumens (e.g. RBC casts, WBC casts, hyaline or pigmented casts).
Myeloma fractured tubular casts	Distal nephron casts with brittle consistency, resuting in fracture planes and associated multinucleated giant cell reaction around cast
Hydropic change	Fine regular vacuolization of the proximal tubules
Hyaline droplet formation	PAS/silver-positive resorption droplets in the proximal tubular epithelium, betraying glomerular permeability to proteins
Hypokalemic changes	Irregular-sized, course vacuoles occupying the renal epithelium
Intranuclear inclusions	Dense inclusions in the nuclei often indicative of viral infection. Need to rule out lead nephropathy, tubular epithelial cell regeneration following ATN

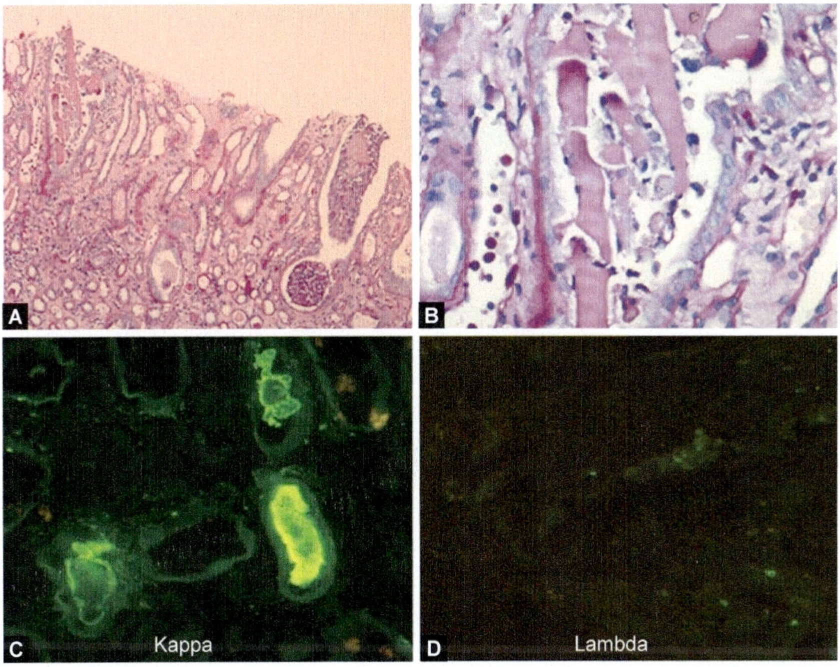

Figures 2.20A to D Photomicrograph panel show images in a case of cast nephropathy. Light microscopy show fractured PAS negative fractured casts with surrounding tubular epithelial cell reaction (A and B). Kappa and lambda immunofluorescence show kappa light chain restriction (C and D)

Evaluation of Interstitial Compartment

The interstitium is that part of renal parenchyma not occupied by glomeruli, tubules, and vessels. It occupies <5% of the cortex and outer medulla but occupies a greater percentage of the inner medulla where the tubules are more widely spaced. Increased interstitial volume due to fibrosis correlates with impaired renal function and is a negative prognostic indicator in diseases of the interstitium as well as in diseases involving the other renal compartments. **Table 2.5** highlights terms used to describe interstitial pathology. **Table 2.6** focuses on the terms that describe vascular disease in renal biopsy and their major features.

Evaluation of Vascular Compartment

Vessels may be damaged by hypertension, inflammation, deposition of material, toxins, and hypercoagulable states. Each of these mechanisms of injury results in different forms of damage that may aid in determination of the cause of injury. Vasculitis has mural infiltration by leukocytes, often with leukocytoclasia. Materials such as amyloid or monoclonal light chain may be deposited in the wall of the vessel, interfering with its normal function.

Table 2.5 Terms used to describe histologic findings in interstitial disease

Term	*Definition*
Interstitium	Space between the glomeruli, tubules, and blood vessels
Edema	Interstitial expansion by protein—poor, aqueous fluid
Interstitial foam cells	Interstitial macrophages with cytoplasmic lipid-containing vacuoles
Fibrosis	Interstitial expansion by collagen-rich matrix and increased fibroblasts
Granuloma	Inflammatory reaction characterized by coalescence of epithelioid macrophages with or without surrounding lymphocytes, fibroblasts, and giant cells
Primary interstitial disease	Renal injury with primary pathology in the interstitium
Secondary interstitial disease	Secondary pathologic changes in the interstitium caused by primary injury to the glomeruli, tubules, or blood vessels
Tubulointerstitial nephritis	Inflammation of the interstitium and tubules
Acute TIN, pathologic	Interstitial leukocyte infiltrates with or without edema and tubulitis in the absence of interstitial fibrosis and tubular atrophy
Chronic TIN, pathologic	Interstitial inflammation with fibrosis and tubular atrophy
Acute pyelonephritis	Acute TIN caused by bacterial infection of the kidney
Chronic pyelonephritis	Chronic TIN caused by bacterial infection of the kidney

Table 2.6 Terms used to describe vascular disease in renal biopsy and their major pathologic features

Term	*Major pathologic features*
Arterionephrosclerosis, including chronic hypertensive nephrosclerosis and age-related arterionephrosclerosis	Arterial fibrotic intimal thickening, arteriolar hyalinosis, regional (often subcapsular) global glomerular sclerosis with adjacent tubular atrophy, interstitial fibrosis, and chronic inflammation
Malignant hypertensive nephropathy and thrombotic microangiopathies	Arterial edematous and myxoid intimal thickening, arteriolar fibrinoid necrosis, glomerular subendothelial and acute ischemic tubular epithelial injury
Renal artery stenosis with chronic ischemic nephropathy	Renal artery stenosis (e.g. caused by atherosclerosis, arteriosclerosis, arteritis, fibromuscular dysplasia, vasculitis, retroperitoneal fibrosis, etc.), tubular "endocrine" atrophy, and glomerular crowding
Renal atheroembolization (cholesterol crystal embolization)	Cholesterol clefts in vascular lumens with or without adjacent atheromatous debrosi, thrombosis, leukocytes or fibrosis

CONCLUSION

Renal diagnosis requires a more sophisticated integeration of histology with immunopathology, ultrastructure, clinical information, and laboratory data.

Multiple Choice Questions

1. **PLA2r immunofluorescence is positive in:**
   a. Primary membranous glomerulonephritis
   b. Class V lupus nephritis
   c. MPGN
   d. Secondary membranous glomerulonephritis

2. **Subepithelial hump are seen in:**
   a. Postinfectious glomerulonephritis
   b. C3 glomerulonephritis
   c. Dense deposit disease
   d. Postinfectious and C3 glomerulonephritis

3. **Dense deposit disease show dominant:**
   a. Subepithelial deposits
   b. Subendothelial deposits
   c. Intramembranous deposits
   d. Mesangial deposits

4. **Mesangioproliferative pattern is commonly seen in:**
   a. IgA nephropathy
   b. Membranous GN
   c. Postinfectious GN, resolving phase
   d. IgA nephropathy and resolving phase of postinfectious GN

5. **Dominant C3 deposits are seen in:**
   a. C3 glomerulonephritis
   b. Dense deposit disease
   c. Postinfectious GN
   d. All the above

6. **Myeloma cast nephropathy show one of the following features:**
   a. Tubular hyaline casts
   b. Fractured cast with associated epithelial reaction
   c. More commonly lambda restriction
   d. Always associated with light chain deposition disease

7. **Linear staining along glomerular capillary wall for IgG is seen in:**
   a. Membranous glomerulonephritis
   b. Membranoproliferative glomerulonephritis
   c. Anti-GBM disease
   d. Pauci-immune GN

8. **Pauci-immune GN is characterized by:**
   a. Normal glomerular morphology
   b. Absence of crescents
   c. Absent or trace immunoglobulin staining in immunofluorescence
   d. Massive immunoglobulin deposition in immunofluorescence

9. C3 glomerulopathy include following entities:
a. Postinfectious GN
b. Pauci-immune GN
c. C3 GN and dense deposit disease
d. Only dense deposit disease

10. Following comment is correct about FSGS:
a. Primary FSGS is characterized by diffuse foot process effacement
b. Secondary FSGS is characterized by diffuse foot process effacement
c. FSGS show massive immune-complex deposits
d. FSGS show true crescents

Answers

1. a 2. d 3. c 4. d 5. d 6. b 7. c 8. c
9. c 10. a

SUGGESTED READING

1. Cattran DC, Coppo R, Cook HT, Feehally J, Roberts IS, Troyanov S, et al. Working Group of the International IgA Nephropathy Network and the Renal Pathology Society: The Oxford classification of IgA nephropathy: Rationale, clinicopathological correlations, and classification. Kidney Int. 2009;76:534-45.
2. Chang A, Gibson IW, Cohen AH, Weening JW, Jennette JC, Fogo AB. Renal Pathology Society: A position paper on standardizing the nonneoplastic kidney biopsy report. Hum Pathol. 2012;43:1192-6.
3. Falk RJ, Nachman PH, Hogan SL, Jennette JC. ANCA glomerulonephritis and vasculitis: A Chapel Hill perspective. Semin Nephrol. 2000;20:233-43.
4. Jennette JC, Olson JL, Silva FG, D' Agati VD. Heptinstall's pathology of the kidney, 7th edn. Wolter Kluwer; 2015.
5. Larsen CP, Walker PD. Redefining C3 glomerulopathy: 'C3 only' is a bridge too far. Kidney International. 2013;83:331-3.
6. Sethi S, Fervenza FC. Membranoproliferative glomerulonephritis—a new look at an old entity. N Engl J Med. 2012;366:1119-31.
7. Weening JJ, D'Agati VD, Schwartz MM, Seshan SV, Alpers CE, Appel GB, et al. The classification of glomerulonephritis in systemic lupus erythematosus revisited. J Am Soc Nephrol. 2004;15:241-50.
8. Zand L, Fervenza FC, Nasr SH, Sethi S. Membranoproliferative glomerulonephritis associated with autoimmune diseases. J Nephrol. 2014;27:165-71.

CHAPTER 3

An Approach to Patient with Kidney Disease

Vijay Kher

INTRODUCTION

Patients with kidney disease may have a variety of clinical presentations. Some have symptoms directly related to the kidney (gross hematuria, flank pain) while others may have extra-renal symptoms (edema, hypertension, signs of uremia). However, many patients are asymptomatic and are noted on routine examination to have an elevated plasma creatinine concentration or an abnormal urinalysis. Each of these groups requires a step-wise approach so, as to arrive at a definitive diagnosis.

Over the last few years, there have been certain changes in the terminology of kidney disease. Acute renal failure (ARF) is now termed as acute kidney injury (AKI) to reflect the entire spectrum of severity of ARF. Similarly chronic renal failure (CRF) is now termed as chronic kidney disease (CKD). The term renal has been replaced by kidney to make it more patient friendly. The term failure has been replaced by disease as like AKI, CKD has a spectrum of severity as well as failure seemed to connote a helplessness on part of the nephrologists in managing patients with kidney disease. The term end stage renal disease (ESRD) has also been changed to chronic kidney disease stage V [glomerular filtration rate (GFR) less than 15 mL/min], as most of these patients can be given many years of good quality life with kidney transplantation or maintenance dialysis and cannot be considered as end stage.

The diagnosis of kidney disease is based on the evaluation of signs, symptoms and a series of investigations. The diagnosis is complicated by the fact that most of the signs and symptoms are nonspecific and also appear fairly late in the course of the disease. A simple approach to a patient with kidney disease is to match the patient's clinical features into one of the following syndromes:

- Asymptomatic urinary abnormality
- Urinary tract infection (UTI)
- Hypertension
- Acute kidney injury
- Rapidly progressive renal failure (RPRF)
- Acute nephritic syndrome
- Nephrotic syndrome (NS)
- Chronic kidney disease
- Urinary tract obstruction
- Tubule function defects
- Congenital/genetic syndromes.

SIGNS AND SYMPTOMS OF KIDNEY DISEASE

The first step in evaluating a patient for kidney disease is to look for clinical features suggestive of kidney disease. These could be a change in urine output like polyuria or nocturia, which relates to loss of the concentrating ability of the kidney or oliguria (<400 mL urine in 24 hours) or anuria (<50 mL urine in 24 hours) which may be symptoms of AKI; whereas dysuria, frequency, urgency could suggest urinary tract infection (UTI), or a pathology in bladder, prostate or urethra. Edema around eyes, hematuria, proteinuria and hypertension are suggestive of glomerular disease. Flank pain, hematuria and graveluria may suggest stone disease.

The window to kidney disease is the examination of the urine, for specific gravity, glycosuria, proteinuria and microscopic examination for red blood cells (RBCs), white blood cells (WBCs) and casts or any other cells. The urinary specific gravity and osmolality may be relatively fixed around 1010 and 290 mOsmol/L respectively, signifying the inability of the kidneys to concentrate or dilute the urine. Presence of RBCs casts with proteinuria suggests glomerulonephritis; WBCs casts in a patient with fever, chills and flank pain suggest acute pyelonephritis; eosinophiluria and eosinophilia in a patient with AKI suggests drug-induced interstitial nephritis; broad casts suggest CKD. An ultrasound is mandatory for evaluation of any patient with kidney disease as it provides information on the size and echogenicity of the kidneys as well as the morphology of the ureters, urinary bladder, urethra, and prostate.

ASYMPTOMATIC URINARY ABNORMALITY

Asymptomatic patients are most commonly detected to have kidney disease following routine investigations, such as urine analysis, blood pressure measurement, and biochemical analyses or as part of a health-screening programme. In some patients, kidney disease is detected during clinical examination for health insurance, occupational purposes, or during pregnancy. Asymptomatic patients may be detected as a result of investigation of family members following the diagnosis of a familial renal disease. Asymptomatic patients may have either abnormal urinary excretion of protein, microscopic hematuria, abnormal imaging of kidney or urinary tract or a combination of these.

Technetium 99mm mercaptoacetyltriglycine diethylene-triamine-penta-acetic acid (DTPA) or MAG3 scan provides an excellent evaluation of function and GFR assessment of each kidney and can be used for the diagnosis and follow-up of patients with obstructive uropathy and renovascular hypertension. ^{99}Tc DMSA is useful in detecting scars in the renal parenchyma.

Routine ultrasound screening during pregnancy has resulted in prenatal detection of urological disorders. Neonatal ultrasound scanning has led to a predictable increase in the detection of urinary tract abnormalities, the most common of which is hydronephrosis.

Mild, asymptomatic proteinuria can be divided into three categories: transient, orthostatic, and persistent. Transient proteinuria is by far the most common, occurring in 4% of men and 7% of women on a single examination, with resolution on subsequent examinations. A transient increase in protein excretion may be seen with fever and exercise, as well as with symptomatic UTI. Orthostatic proteinuria primarily occurs in adolescents; it is characterized by increased protein excretion in the upright position, but normal protein excretion when the patient is supine. Both transient and orthostatic proteinurias are benign conditions requiring no further evaluation or specific therapy. Persistent proteinuria, in comparison, is more likely to reflect some underlying renal or systemic disorder. There are three types of persistent proteinuria: glomerular, tubular, and overflow.

- *Glomerular proteinuria* implies proteinuria as a result of increased glomerular permeability and usually consists of excretion of albumin.
- *Tubular proteinuria* implies increased excretion of proteins due to non-absorption of low molecular weight proteins, which are filtered through a normal glomerular filter as in tubulo interstitial disease.
- *Overflow proteinuria* is excretion of proteins, which are increased in the plasma as in multiple myeloma and light chain proteinuria.

The evaluation of the patient with mild proteinuria should begin by testing the urine on at least two occasions. The urine sediment should also be examined. If the proteinuria persists, a renal ultrasonogram should be performed looking for a structural lesion, such as chronic pyelonephritis or polycystic kidney disease. A renal biopsy is generally performed if there is some sign of progressive disease, such as increasing protein excretion or a rise in the plasma creatinine concentration.

Hematuria may be grossly visible or microscopic. Gross hematuria is suspected because of the presence of red or brown urine. The color change does not necessarily reflect the degree of blood loss, since as little as 1 mL of blood per liter of urine can induce a visible color change. In addition, the intermittent excretion of red to brown urine can be seen in a variety of clinical conditions (myoglobinuria or porphyria) other than bleeding into the urinary tract. Thus, the initial step in the evaluation of such patients is centrifugation of the specimen to see if the red color is in the urine sediment (RBCs) or the supernatant (pigments like myoglobin as in myoglobinuria, hemoglobin in urine as in intravascular hemolysis). Although hematuria is commonly defined as the presence of more than 2 RBCs per high power field in spun urine sediment, there is no 'safe' lower limit below which significant disease can be excluded. The causes vary with age with the most common being inflammation or infection of the prostate or bladder, stones, and in older patients, malignancy. The investigations should be done as per the **(Flow chart 3.1)**. If no diagnosis is apparent from the history, urinalysis, radiologic tests, or cystoscopy, then the most likely causes of persistent isolated hematuria are a mild glomerulopathy or a predisposition to stone disease, particularly in young and middle-aged patients. If hematuria is associated with nephrotic range proteinuria, it almost always suggests glomerular disease. Microscopic hematuria in itself cannot cause heavy proteinuria.

URINARY TRACT INFECTION

Infections of the urinary tract are common, distressing, and can occasionally be life-threatening. The clinical features, diagnosis, treatment, complications, and

Flow chart 3.1 An approach to a patient with chronic kidney disease

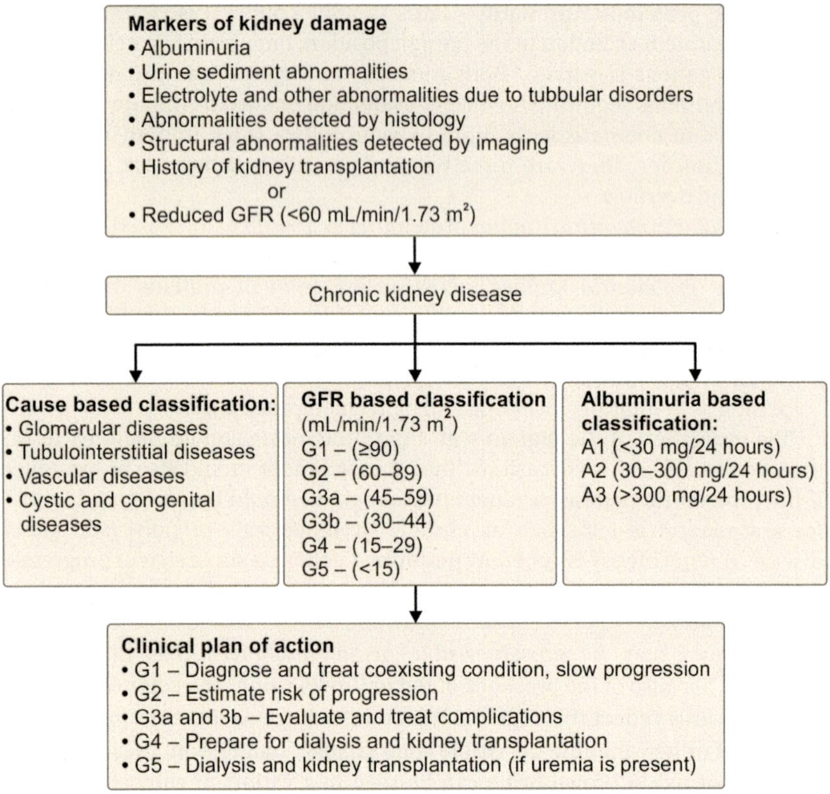

long-term significance of infection vary, depending on the site of infection and the presence or absence of structural or functional abnormality within the urinary tract. Diagnosis requires demonstration of bacteriuria and/or pyuria. In children, UTI may cause significant long-term morbidity, particularly, renal scarring, hypertension and renal impairment, which may not be evident clinically until adult life. Hence, in children even the first episode of UTI mandates a detailed work-up and evaluation.

HYPERTENSION

Hypertension is defined as an elevation of blood pressure ≥140/90 mm Hg. This may be the first sign of an underlying kidney disease, especially in patients <35 years of age. In referral centers, 2-5% of hypertensive patients have renovascular hypertension. Renal ultrasound may reveal a unilateral contracted kidney suggesting an underlying renovascular etiology and/or renal parenchymal etiology. Another important cause of renal hypertension is reflux nephropathy, which leads to scarring of the kidneys.

ACUTE KIDNEY INJURY

Acute kidney injury is a sudden and reversible loss of kidney function usually preceded by loss of blood or fluid, kidney ischemia, hypotension or caused by drugs. AKI is now categorized and defined by acute kidney injury network (AKIN) criteria. Details are in chapter on AKI. It mostly recovers in 4–12 weeks time. The incidence of AKI is very high in hospitalized patients. An incidence of 15–30% has been reported among patients admitted to intensive care units, whereas among all hospitalized patients, rates of 2–5% have been reported. The two major causes of AKI are acute tubular necrosis (ATN, due to ischemia or the administration of a nephrotoxin) and prerenal disease (due to heart failure, true volume depletion, or sepsis).

RAPIDLY PROGRESSIVE RENAL FAILURE

Rapidly progressive renal failure (RPRF) is described as insidious onset (*versus* abrupt onset in AKI) deterioration (over days to weeks) in renal function. The most important cause of RPRF is rapidly progressive glomerulonephritis (RPGN). This is characterized morphologically by extensive crescent formation and clinically by progression to end-stage renal disease in most untreated patients within a period of weeks to months. The severity of the disease is in part related to the degree of crescent formation: patients with circumferential crescents in more than 80% of the glomeruli tend to present with advanced renal failure that may not respond well to therapy. Patients should undergo early renal biopsy, which should include immunofluorescence and light microscopy and appropriate serologic assays. These include antineutrophil cytoplasmic antibodies (ANCA), anti-GBM antibodies, antinuclear antibodies and complement levels. The other important causes of RPRF are acute interstitial nephritis (which could be drug-induced or due to acute pyelonephritis), malignant hypertension, hemolytic uremic syndrome and obstructive uropathy.

ACUTE NEPHRITIC SYNDROME

Acute nephritic syndrome is characterized by hematuria, proteinuria, edema and hypertension. The prototype of this disease is acute poststreptococcal glomerulonephritis. However, it can occur as a result of many bacterial or viral infections. This occurs 10–20 days following infection. Some of these patients may present with severe hypertension, edema and renal failure. Most of these patients resolve completely with time. The other important renal diseases mimicking this syndrome are immunoglobulin (Ig) A nephropathy and mesangiocapillary glomerulonephritis.

NEPHROTIC SYNDROME

The nephrotic syndrome is caused by renal diseases that increase the permeability across the glomerular filtration barrier. It is classically characterized by four clinical features, but the last two may not be seen in all patients: (i) nephrotic range proteinuria—urinary protein excretion greater than 50 mg/kg per day or urine protein-to-creatinine ratio >2, (ii) hypoalbuminemia—serum albumin concentration <3 g/dL (30 g/L), (iii) edema, and (iv) hyperlipidemia. Although, edema is generally the presenting sign of nephrotic syndrome, the diagnosis is confirmed by the presence of nephrotic range proteinuria and hypoalbuminemia.

Primary nephrotic syndrome refers to nephrotic syndrome in the absence of an identifiable systemic disease. Within this category are patients who have usually a bland sediment and no glomerular inflammation on renal biopsy, i.e. minimal change disease (MCD), focal glomerulosclerosis and membranous nephropathy. Patients with primary glomerulonephritis, who have an active sediment and glomerular inflammation on renal biopsy have mesangiocapillary glomerulonephritis or mesangioproliferative glomerulonephritis. Secondary nephrotic syndrome refers to nephrotic syndrome in the presence of an identifiable systemic disease, e.g. lupus nephritis.

In children corticosteroid therapy can be initiated in patients with a high probability of having MCD without confirmation of the diagnosis by renal biopsy. In adults, a kidney biopsy is considered mandatory prior to starting any kind of immunosuppressive therapy. Children with idiopathic nephrotic syndrome treated with empirical steroid therapy can be further classified based upon their response to corticosteroid therapy: (a) steroid-responsive nephrotic syndrome—majority of the children with idiopathic nephrotic syndrome are steroid responsive. In these patients, the most likely histologic lesion is MCD, although some patients with focal segmental glomerulosclerosis (FSGS) will also respond to corticosteroid therapy. Patients who are steroid responsive have a favorable long-term outcome; and (b) steroid-resistant nephrotic syndrome—approximately 25% of all children with nephrotic syndrome will not respond to corticosteroids. The response rate is better in younger children, who are much more likely to have MCD. Some children with steroid-resistant nephrotic syndrome have genetic mutations of podocyte proteins.

Chronic Kidney Disease

Chronic kidney disease (CKD) is a syndrome that results from progressive and irreversible destruction of nephrons resulting from a number of causes. It is defined as kidney damage for ≥3 months, as defined by structural or functional abnormalities of the kidney, with or without decreased GFR, manifest by either: (i) pathological abnormalities or the presence of markers of kidney damage, including abnormalities in the composition of the blood or urine, or abnormalities in imaging studies or (ii) GFR <60 mL/min/1.73 m^2 for 3 months, with or without kidney damage. This is usually progressive in nature. In most of the cases, demonstration of bilateral contracted kidneys, along with the clinical features of uremia serve as the distinguishing features of chronicity. However, in CKD due to diabetes, amyloidosis and polycystic kidney disease, the kidney size may be normal or even bigger. Recent Kidney Disease: Improving Global Outcomes (KDIGO) guidelines have classified CKD based on cause, GFR category and albuminuria category (collectively referred to as CGA) **(Tables 3.1 and 3.2)**.

Once a patient has been diagnosed to have kidney disease, the next step is to assess his level of renal function. Routinely a physician diagnoses kidney disease when serum creatinine and blood urea are elevated. However, the patient is said to have renal dysfunction once the GFR declines below normal.

Table 3.1 Glomerular filtration rate categories in chronic kidney disease

GFR category	*GFR (mL/min/1.73 m²)*	*Terms*
G1	≥ 90	Normal or high
G2	60–89	Mildly decreased
G3a	45–59	Mildly to moderately decreased
G3b	30–44	Moderately to severely decreased
G4	15–29	Severely decreased
G5	<15	Kidney failure

Table 3.2 Albuminuria categories in chronic kidney disease

Category	*AER (mg/24 hours)*	*ACR (approximate equivalent) mg/mmol*	*ACR (approximate equivalent) mg/g*	*Terms*
A1	<30	<3	<30	Normal to mildly increased
A2	30–300	3–30	30–300	Moderately increased
A3	>300	>30	>300	Severely increased

Normal GFR in an adult varies from 100–130 mL/min. There is an age-related decline in GFR of 1 mL/min/year after the age of 30 years. The relationship of serum creatinine and urea to GFR is curvilinear and not linear, where serum creatinine and urea does not rise till the GFR declines to about 50%. Most of the patients are usually asymptomatic or mildly symptomatic at that stage. This is because of functional and structural adaptations that take place in the surviving nephrons, which compensate by increasing their functional capability. GFR can be assessed by either 24 hours urinary creatinine clearance or estimating GFR from serum creatinine by either modification of diet in renal disease (MDRD) formula or Cockcroft-Gault formula. Recently a new CKD-EPI equation has been developed in 2009 for estimation of eGFR. This was shown to have lesser bias and more accuracy compared to other formulae, especially when GFR > 60 mL/min/1.73 m^2 **(Table 3.3)**. But when applied to a wide population based study in India, it performed similar to MDRD.

Serum cystatin C is an alternative endogenous filtration marker used to calculate eGFR. It has been shown that serum cystatin C based equations to calculate GFR are more accurate than serum creatinine based equations in individuals with malnutrition and reduced muscle mass. But this test is not widely available and standardization is another major issue associated with it. For most clinical circumstances serum creatinine based eGFR are good enough. Serum cystatin C based eGFR estimation may be useful in specific circumstances such as confirming a diagnosis of CKD, determining suitability for kidney donation and dose adjustment of few drugs excreted by kidneys.

Once the diagnosis of CKD is established, it is important to make an attempt to find out the specific disease that caused the kidney failure. According to the recent United States Renal Data System (USRDS) data, diabetes mellitus is

Table 3.3 Formula for estimation of glomerular filtration rate

Cockcroft-Gault formula eGFR in men : $\frac{(140 - \text{age}) \times \text{weight}}{72 \times \text{P. creatinine}}$ eGFR in women : 0.85 × value from above [Where age in years, weight in kilograms and P. creatinine in mg/dL]
Abbreviated modification of diet in renal disease (MDRD) study equation eGFR (mL/min/1.73 m^2) = 186 × [Pcr]$^{-1.154}$ × [age]$^{-0.203}$ × [0.742 if patient is female] × [1.210 if patient is black] -exp (5.228 – 1.154 × ln (Scr) – 0.203 × IN (Age) – 0.299 if female) + (0.192 if African – American)
CKD-EPI equation eGFR = 141 × min (Scr /κ, 1)$^{\alpha}$ × max (S_{Cr} /κ, 1)$^{-1.209}$ × 0.993^{Age} × 1.018 [if female] × 1.159 [if black] Where: • Scr is serum creatinine in mg/dL • κ is 0.7 for females and 0.9 for males • α is –0.329 for females and –0.411 for males • min indicates the minimum of Scr/κ or 1, and • max indicates the maximum of Scr/κ or 1

regarded as the leading cause of kidney failure. In India, most of the data has been generated from single center experiences. Of late, CKD registry of India and SEEK (Screening and Early Evaluation of Kidney disease) study have included multiple centers from different regions and provided data from a wider population base. Chronic glomerulonephritis and diabetic nephropathy are leading causes of CKD. In order to establish the underlying cause, one must look for appropriate clinical features and use suitable laboratory tests. If the kidney size is preserved then one should attempt a kidney biopsy to find out the cause but if kidneys are shrunken then the cause of kidney disease may be difficult to detect. It is important to identify factors, which may have aggravated the degree of kidney failure, as once these factors are corrected, kidney function may improve at least partially **(Table 3.4)**. An appropriate plan of action for a patient of CKD is detailed in **Flow chart 3.1**.

CONGENITAL/GENETIC SYNDROMES

This includes a varied spectrum of diseases like autosomal dominant and recessive polycystic kidney disease, congenital nephrotic syndrome (Finnish type), Alport's syndrome, Fabry's disease and juvenile nephronopthisis. The diagnosis of these entities is suspected on a positive family history, characteristic clinical features and requires a high index of suspicion. Genetic counseling is an integral part of the management of these diseases.

SUMMARY

- Kidney diseases have varied presentation. Loss of renal function may be reversible leading to AKI or there may be irreversible damage as in CKD.
- Early diagnosis is important to improve the outcome and reduce the associated morbidity and mortality. A thorough evaluation, which sometimes

Table 3.4 Common reversible factors in chronic kidney disease

Volume depletion
Vomiting, diarrhea, excessive diuresis, congestive heart failure
Urinary tract obstruction
Nephrolithiasis, papillary necrosis, bladder outlet obstruction
Infection
Renal or extra-renal
Vascular disease
Uncontrolled or accelerated hypertension
Nephrotoxic drugs
Aminoglycosides, cephalosporins, tetracycline, amphotericin, radiocontrast agents, Nonsteroidal anti-inflammatory drugs (NSAIDs), diuretics
Electrolyte and metabolic disorders
Hyperphosphatemia, hyperuricemia, acidosis
Catabolic states
Surgery, burns, gastrointestinal bleed, steroids, chemotherapy
Vasculitis
Systemic lupus erythematosus, Wegener's granulomatosis, microscopic polyarteritis
Pregnancy
Pre-eclampsia, eclampsia

may include a renal biopsy, is warranted to establish the type of renal disease and to look for any reversible factor.

- Accurate estimation of GFR is needed to establish the stage and progression of CKD so that appropriate action is taken at right time.
- Traditional and nontraditional risk factors play important role in development of cardiovascular disease in patients with CKD.
- High index of suspicion, appropriate genetic testing and counseling is required in patients with familial kidney disease.

*The source of above chapter is "*Kidney Disease: A Clinical Approach* —Vijay Kher, Pranaw Kumar Jha" in "API Textbook of Medicine —YP Munjal" 10th edition

Multiple Choice Questions

1. **Age related decline in renal function after 30 years of age is at the rate of:**
   a. 1 mL/min/year
   b. 3 mL/min/year
   c. 5 mL/min/year
   d. 10 mL/min/year

2. **Type of proteinuria in multiple myeloma:**
   a. Glomerular proteinuria
   b. Overflow proteinuria
   c. Tubular proteinuria
   d. All of the above

3. **Not characteristic of nephrotic syndrome:**
   a. Urinary protein excretion greater than 50 mg/kg/day
   b. Edema
   c. Hypoalbuminemia
   d. Active urine sediments

4. CKD is defined as presence of functional or structural abnormalities in kidneys with or without reduced GFR for duration of more than:

a. 2 months
b. 3 months
c. 4 months
d. 5 months

5. Recent CKD classification is based on:

a. Cause
b. Glomerular filtration rate
c. Albuminuria
d. All of the above

6. Nuclear imaging method used to look for renal scar is:

a. Tc-99m-DTPA
b. Tc-99m-DMSA
c. Tc-99m-MAG-3
d. All of the above

7. A 24-year-old gentleman presented with history of passing cola colored urine, edema and hypertension ten days after an episode of cough and sore throat. Urine examination showed active sediments and RBC casts. The clinical picture is consistent with:

a. Acute nephritic syndrome
b. Nephrotic syndrome
c. Rapidly progressive glomerulonephritis
d. None of the above

8. A 7-year-old boy presented with history of anasarca since 10 days. On evaluation, urine showed 3+ proteinuria but no active sediments, 24 hour urinary protein excretion of 4 gm, serum albumin of 2 g/dL and total cholesterol 300 mg/dL. The clinical picture is consistent with:

a. Acute nephritic syndrome
b. Nephrotic syndrome
c. Rapidly progressive glomerulonephritis
d. None of the above

9. Most probable cause of nephrotic syndrome in above patient is:

a. Focal segmental glomerulosclerosis
b. Membranous nephropathy
c. Minimal change disease
d. Membranoproliferative glomerulonephritis

10. A 67-year-old male who is a chronic smoker with history of COPD and claudication pain in both legs presented with accelerated hypertension. On examination, he had bilateral carotid bruit and renal bruit with absent popliteal and, posterior tibial and dorsalis pedis pulse. On evaluation, his serum creatinine was 2.3 mg/dL, urine routine showed 1+ proteinuria and ultrasound abdomen showed bilaterally small sized kidneys. Most probable cause of hypertension in this case is:

a. Essential hypertension
b. Renovascular hypertension
c. Pheochromocytoma
d. All of the above

Answers

1. a 2. b 3. d 4. b 5. d 6. b 7. a 8. b
9. c 10. b

SUGGESTED READING

1. Davison AM, Grunfeld JP, Fitzpatrick M. History and clinical examination of the patient with renal disease. In: Ponticelli C, Ritz E, Winearls CG, van Ypersele CC, (Eds). New York, Oxford Textbook of Nephrology. Oxford University Press. 2005. pp.3-22.
2. Fogazzi GB. Urinalysis and microscopy. In: Ponticelli C, Ritz E, Winearls CG, van Ypersele CC, (Eds). New York: Oxford Textbook of Nephrology. Oxford University Press. 2005.pp.23-46.
3. Kidney Disease Improving Global Outcome (KDIGO) CKD Work Group: KDIGO 2012 Clinical Practice Guideline for the Evaluation and Management of Chronic Kidney Disease. Kidney Int Suppl. 2013;3:1-150.
4. Mehta RL, Kellum JA, Shah SV, Molitoris BA, Ronco C, Warnock DG, et al. Acute Kidney Injury Network: Acute Kidney Injury Network: report of an initiative to improve outcomes in acute kidney injury. Crit Care. 2007;11:R31.
5. Rose BD, Black RM. Boston: Manual of Clinical Problems in Nephrology. Little, Brown and Co. 1988.p.130.

CHAPTER

4 Investigations in Renal Diseases

BIOCHEMICAL INVESTIGATIONS IN RENAL DISEASES

Ratan Jha, Kiran Chandra Patro

INTRODUCTION

In renal diseases, clinical history and examination alone are not enough to diagnose and biochemical analysis (including urine examination, sometime urinary electrolytes and acid/base assessment) is an absolute necessity to classify the disease, prognosticate and to plan therapy. Urine and blood investigations are commonly employed to determine renal disease, but occasionally other samples like urinary stones, kidney biopsy samples, urine cytokines/proteomic analysis and other specialized tests could be employed for biochemical analysis. An accurate history and careful examination will determine the usual sequence and spectrum of clinical investigations to make a diagnosis or decide on prognosis or treatment.

URINE ANALYSIS

Also termed as the non-invasive renal biopsy, is simple and cost effective approach to identify the upstream renal abnormalities.

The complete urine analysis consists of identifying the physical characteristics, chemical analysis and the microscopy. In contrast to the earlier times when various instruments were required for urine examination, a reliable, easy and fairly accurate dip stick method is used now. A detailed urine examination has been discussed elsewhere and hence only urinary tests relevant to renal diseases which will direct us to required blood biochemistry have been tabulated **(Tables 4.1 to 4.4)**.

PROTEINURIA

Normally 30-130 mg/day of protein and 30 mg/day of albumin is lost in urine daily. Tamm-Horsfall protein (protein formed on epithelial surface of the thick ascending limb of the loop of Henle and early distal convoluted tubule), immunoglobulin A (IgA) and urokinase constitute the various proteins in urine.

Table 4.1 Variations and abnormalities on macroscopic examination of urine

Macroscopic appearance	*Diagnosis/Examples*
Amount	Oliguria/Anuria/Polyuria
Color	Straw, light yellow, yellow, dark yellow, amber (hepatitis with increased bilirubin), red/hematuria (cystitis, glomerulonephritis)
Clarity/cloudiness	Frothy urine (heavy proteinuria), precipitates, sediments, pyuria
Milky	Chyluria
Dark/brown	Drugs implicated—Chloroquine, methyldopa, levodopa, quinine, sulphonamides, nitrofurantoin, ferrous salts, metronidazole
Blue/blue green	Drugs implicated—Methylene blue, amitriptyline, triamterene
Pink-orange	Drugs implicated—Rifampicin, chlorzoxazone, heparin, warfarin, sulfasalazine

Table 4.2 Abnormalities of urinary pH

Causes of alkaline urine	*Causes of acidic urine*
• Urinary tract obstruction • Pyloric stenosis • Salicylate intoxication • Renal tubular acidosis • Chronic kidney disease • Respiratory alkalosis	• Metabolic acidosis • Uncontrolled diabetes • Starvation and dehydration • Respiratory diseases—carbon dioxide retention and acidosis

The earliest sign of renal disease is proteinuria and identification of type of proteinuria can help us in identifying the area of damage (glomerular, tubulo-interstitial), help in prognosticating disease and monitor response to therapy **(Tables 4.5 to 4.8)**.

BLOOD AND URINE BIOCHEMISTRY

The kidney participates in a number of essential biochemical processes in the human body to maintain constant extracellular environment for adequate functioning of the cells:

- This is achieved by excretion of the waste products of metabolism (like urea, creatinine, and uric acid) and by adjusting the urinary excretion of water and electrolytes such as sodium, potassium, and hydrogen (that precisely matches net intake and endogenous production). This is achieved by tubular reabsorption or secretion which helps maintain equilibrium in the body fluids.
- Kidney secretes many hormones that participate in the regulation of systemic and renal hemodynamics (renin, prostaglandins, and bradykinin), red blood cell production (erythropoietin), and bone health (1,25-dihydroxyvitamin D3 or calcitriol).

In renal disease, some or all of these functions may be variably diminished or absent leading to altered biochemistry of blood, urine and other fluid

Table 4.3 Urinary dipstick test interpretation

Dipstick urine testing	*Diagnosis/examples*
pH	*Normal:* 5.5–7 (<5.3 may rule out a renal acidification defect)
Specific gravity Hypersthenuria (concentrated) Hyposthenuria (dilute)	*Normal:* 1.003–1.035 Dehydration, diarrhea, emesis, excessive sweating, urinary tract/bladder infection, glycosuria, renal artery stenosis, hepatorenal syndrome, decreased blood flow to the kidney (as a result of heart failure), excess of antidiuretic hormone (SIADH) Renal failure, pyelonephritis, diabetes insipidus, acute tubular necrosis, interstitial nephritis, and excessive fluid intake (e.g., psychogenic polydipsia)
Glycosuria	When serum glucose more than renal threshold of 160–180 mg/dL or in renal glycosuria or in Fanconi's syndrome—reported as trace ,1+, 2+, 3+4+ (equivalent to 100, 250, 500, 1000, 2000 mg% of plasma glucose approximately)
Nitrite and leukocyte esterase	>90% of common urinary pathogens produce nitrite
Blood	Dysmorphic RBCs suggest glomerular hematuria. Blood is also positive in hemoglobinuria or myoglobinuria
Bilirubin and urobilinogen	Suggests jaundice
Protein	Positive only with albuminuria

Table 4.4 Urinary abnormality and clinical correlation

Condition	*Causes*
Hematuria	Glomerulonephritis, kidney stones, infections, tumors and other conditions
Pyuria	Tubulointerstitial nephritis, urinary infections, stone disease
Eosinophiluria	Allergic interstitial nephritis, atheroembolic disease
Red blood cell casts	Glomerulonephritis, vasculitis, or malignant hypertension
White blood cell casts	Acute interstitial nephritis, exudative glomerulonephritis, or severe pyelonephritis
Granular casts	Acute tubular necrosis
Crystalluria	Acute urate nephropathy [(or acute uric acid nephropathy (AUAN)]
Calcium oxalate	Ethylene glycol
Waxy casts	Chronic renal disease

compartments. Biochemical tests should therefore be directed towards assessing the glomerular filtration rate, glomerular function, tubular function, function of divalent ions and assess acid-base abnormalities **(Tables 4.9 to 4.11)**.Overall renal function can be assessed by combining the tests of glomerular function, tubular function and the maximal capacity of tubules.

Table 4.5 Urinary albumin and protein creatinine ratios

Urinary albumin creatinine ratio	Normal (<20 mg/g in men and <30 mg/g in women)
Protein-creatinine ratio (PCR)	Normal <30 mg/g on a spot sample

Table 4.6 Dipstick protein grading

Designation	*Approximate amount*	
	Concentration (mg/dL)	*Per day loss (g/day)*
Trace	5–20	–
1+	30	<0.5
2+	100	0.5–1
3+	300	1–2
4+	>300	>2

Table 4.7 Definition of microalbuminuria

24 hours urine	30–300		Milligram albumin per 24 hours
Time voided urine	20–200		Microgram albumin per minute
Spot urine	30–300		Milligram albumin per liter of urine
Spot urine albumin/creatinine ratio	Women	2.5–25 (or 30)	Milligram albumin per millimole creatinine
		30–400	Microgram albumin per milligram creatinine
	Men	2.5 (or 3.5) to 25 (or 30)	Milligram albumin per millimole creatinine
		30–300	Microgram albumin per milligram creatinine

Table 4.8 Diagnosis and prognosis of proteinuria

- Quantify urine protein excretion—to differentiate glomerular versus tubular proteinuria
- Nephrotic proteinuria (greater than 3 g/24 hours)—indicates glomerular proteinuria
- Selective glomerular proteinuria (Immunoglobulin G (IgG)/albuminuria ratio less than 0.1)—indicates albuminuria
- Tubular proteinuria—heterogeneous—α2-microglobulin being major constituent—low-molecular-weight proteinuria—caused by proximal tubular injury—markers include α-glutathione-*S*-transferase, α_1-macroglobulin, and retinol-binding protein.
- Beta-2 microglobulin is a low molecular weight (11.8-kDa) protein—indicates proximal tubule defects
- Plasma dyscrasias causes overflow proteinuria—Bence-Jones proteinuria is not specific or sensitive—needs M spike on protein electrophoresis/immunofixation to diagnose plasma dyscrasias
- Once proteinuria is diagnosed—follow-up of protein creatinine ratio will help in identifying response to therapy and prognosticate the disease
- Albumin, α2-microglobulin, IgG, α2-macroglobulin, beta 2-microglobulin are used to differentiate between prerenal, renal and postrenal diseases

Table 4.9 Categories of biochemical panel of test

Categories	*Biochemical test*
Screening	eGFR, urinary protein/creatinine ratio
Proximal tubular function	TMP GFR, fractional HCO_3 excretion, measurement of aminoaciduria/glycosuria/urinary β-2-microglobulin and n-acetyl-β-d-glucosaminidase excretion
Distal tubular function	Concentrating ability in polyuria/diluting ability in hyponatremia, acidification of urine in metabolic acidosis (ammonium chloride load test)/dyselectrolytemia (sodium/potassium/calcium disturbance in various tubulopathies
Endocrine functions	PTH/1, 25 (OH) vitamin D/erythropoietin levels, renin/aldosterone/testosterone levels/ TSH/ thyroid hormones
Stone disease	*Blood:* Urea, creatinine, uric acid, sodium, potassium, calcium, magnesium, phosphorus, chloride, inorganic sulfate, alkaline phosphatase, oxalate and bicarbonate. *24-hour urine:* Urea, creatinine, uric acid, sodium, potassium, calcium, magnesium, phosphorus, chloride, oxalate, inorganic sulphate, citrate, pH, ammonia, bicarbonate and titratable acid. *Fasting urine:* Calcium, citrate, creatinine, OH-proline, Brand's test for cystinuria. urinalysis urine culture chemical analysis of available stone fragments/vitamin D/ intact PTH
Infection related tests	Serum procalcitonin in sepsis/leukocyte esterase test/ Griess nitrate test in urinary tract infection/immunocytochemistry for viral infection in tissues like BK virus / CMV in renal transplant/ galactomannan assay in fungal infection/ detection of cryptococcal antigen by latex agglutination test
Specialized biochemical tests for renal tubular acidosis confirmation	Ammonium chloride load test/furosemide/fludrocortisone test, urine pCO_2 after sodium bicarbonate load; fraction excretion of bicarbonate; urinary citrate/acid excretion; urine osmolal gap/urine anion gap/ arterial blood gases/ electrolytes
Tests to help determine the cause and/or guide treatment	Urinalysis with a urine culture/hepatitis B or C testing/ antinuclear antibody (ANA); kidney stone risk panel and kidney stone analysis/complement tests (C3, C4); urine and serum protein electrophoresis
Research tests	Early AKI diagnosis—N-GAL; Pre-eclampsia prediction—sflt1, VEGF, Renal transplantation—tests for antigen/antibody/cytokines/ mRNA expression in renal tissues in renal transplant to diagnose rejection—identification of abnormal genes involved in T/B-cell activation and leukocyte trafficking: DUSP1, PBEF1, PSEN1, MAPK9, and NKTR can discriminate acute rejection from all other non-acute rejection phenotypes. Urinary concentrations of mRNA for CD3ε, perforin, granzyme B, IP-10, and 18s RNA also can add to the diagnosis of acute rejection.

*Corrected calcium levels (mg/dL) = serum calcium (mg/dL) + 0.8 (4 – serum albumin (g/dL))

Table 4.10 Biochemical tests to identify complications or diseases

Condition	*Biochemical assays*
Inflammatory marker	C-reactive protein, IL-6,TNF-α, homocysteine and other CKs, ferritin and platelet count
Nutritional markers	Albumin, transferrin
Anemia	Ferritin, transferrin saturation
Dyslipidemia	Lipid profile
Mineral bone disorder	Calcium, phosphorus, alkaline phosphatase (bone), parathyroid hormone, crossed collagen peptide, serum osteocalcin, 25-hydroxy vitamin D
Coagulation disorder	Serum fibrinogen levels, fibrin degradation products
Pregnancy	sFlt1, VEGF (in pre-eclampsia); complement levels (for hemolytic uremic syndrome/lupus)

Table 4.11 Evaluation of renal failure

BUN and creatinine	Serial levels to indicate worsening renal disease
Calcium and phosphorous	Rising levels indicate worsening renal disease
Serum and urine electrolytes	Na+, K+ (hyperkalaemia—a significant complication of renal failure)
ABG (Bicarbonate level)	Acidosis often accompanies renal failure
Hemoglobin	Marker of decreased erythropoiesis in renal failure
Parathyroid hormone (PTH)	often increased in kidney disease and may be checked to help determine if enough calcium and vitamin D are being taken to prevent bone damage
Erythropoietin	Level may suggest renal failure
Cystatin C	Marker to confirm known or suspected renal disease
Blood and urine β-2 microglobulin (B2M) tests	Useful to evaluate kidney damage and disease, and also to distinguish between disorders that affect glomeruli or renal tubules (blood levels raised in glomerular injury and urinary level raised in tubular injury)—also useful to monitor a kidney transplant to detect early signs of rejection, monitor people who are exposed to high levels of cadmium and mercury (with occupational exposure).

Markers of Glomerular Function

Serum creatinine, urea, cystatin C and β-trace protein are the usual biomarkers of renal function. Cystatin C in particular, is being utilized to assess early renal dysfunction and several studies have confirmed and consolidated the usefulness of this marker. These biomarkers are used to calculate GFR through derived equations or by measurement of its clearance (from blood in urine) by multiple estimations over a timed collection, a cumbersome process as discussed in the following paragraphs.

Glomerular Filtration Rate and Renal Clearance

Glomerular filtration rate (GFR) is the measure of renal clearance of an endogenous (urea, creatinine, or cystatin) or exogenous substance (inulin, radio-pharmaceuticals) that is removed from plasma. Clearance is expressed as weight of the substance removed per volume per time or the volume of plasma that can be completely cleared of the substance in a unit of time.

If there is no extra renal elimination, tubular reabsorption or tubular secretion of the marker, then GFR can be calculated as:

$$GFR = (U \times V) / (P \times T)$$

(U is the urine concentration, V is the urine volume, and P is the average plasma concentration of the marker over the time (T) of the urine collection).

An ideal indicator should have following qualities:
- Constant production
- Safe
- Convenient
- Readily diffusible in extracellular space
- No protein binding and freely filterable
- No tubular reabsorption
- No tubular secretion
- No extra renal elimination or degradation
- Accurate and reproducible assay
- No compounds interfere
- Inexpensive
- No influence on the glomerular filtration rate.

No such ideal substance has yet been identified and the closest substance which fulfils these criteria is an exogenous substance inulin—however, it requires to be infused intravenously at a constant rate so as to measure the GFR and is therefore a cumbersome, expensive and invasive process. It is therefore easier to estimate endogenous substances eliminated by the kidney to assess the renal function.

Plasma Urea and Urea Clearance

Urea was one of the first indicators used to measure GFR. Increased urea or BUN (blood urea nitrogen) (which is derived by dividing urea by 2.14) levels suggest impaired kidney function, although they can also be elevated due to a condition that results in decreased blood flow to the kidneys, such as congestive heart failure, upper gastrointestinal (GI) bleed or shock. Serum urea is considered a poor marker of renal function, because it varies significantly with hydration and diet, is not produced constantly and is reabsorbed by the kidney. Urea clearance varies between 50 mL/min and 80 mL/min based on urine flow rate and is occasionally calculated in calculation of residual renal function in patients on dialysis. The level of this waste product in the blood increases as kidney filtration declines. Despite limitation it should always be done together with creatinine as the high BUN/creatinine ratio (>15:1) could suggest hidden GI bleed, volume contraction, catabolic state and a low value of BUN/creatinine (<10:1) could suggest a muscle disorder (rhabdomyolysis). It is also useful in differential diagnosis of acute renal failure where in a prerenal state presents with increased ratio of blood urea nitrogen–creatinine ratio and the same does not hold true for pure renal dysfunction.

Serum Creatinine

Creatinine, a metabolic product of creatine and phosphocreatine, almost exclusively found in muscle (hence production is proportional to muscle mass) and varies little from day-to-day (though can vary over longer periods of time if there is a change in muscle mass) is now a popular substance estimated to assess renal function. Age, gender, nonvegetarian diet and few drugs (Cimetidine, Trimethoprim, Pyrimethamine and Dapsone) can alter creatinine excretion.

Serum creatinine though for all practical purposes is easy and ideal choice to measure GFR the levels of serum creatinine may remain fairly constant despite a loss of over 50% of renal function (due to tubular excretion or extra renal loss of creatinine). Therefore many are looking at alternatives to detect renal dysfunction at an earlier stage and more accurately.

Alkaline picrate method (Jaffé method), enzymatic method, high-performance liquid chromatography (HPLC), isotope dilution mass spectrometry (IDMS), gas chromatography and liquid chromatograph have been used to measure serum creatinine out of which Jaffé method is the most common.

To overcome fallacies in serum creatinine estimation, an estimated GFR using a serum creatininebased formula have been identified of which Cockcroft and Gault is the most simple bed side formula which can be utilized to assess GFR using serum creatinine value.

Estimated GFR = (140 – age (in years)) × weight (in kg)/72 × serum creatinine

The whole multiplied by 0.85 for women estimates the GFR.

The alternate formulae include the modification of diet in renal disease (MDRD) study formula (most suited for people with renal dysfunction—not standardized for Asians or oriental races) and the chronic kidney disease epidemiology collaboration (CKD-EPI) equation (supposedly more accurate), but require calculator or online software.

MDRD equation:

GFR in $(mL/min/1.73\ m^2) = 175 \times (S_{cr})^{-1.154} \times (Age)^{-0.203} \times (0.742 \text{ if female}) \times (1.212$ if African-American).

CKD-EPI equation:

$GFR = 141 \times \min(S_{cr}/\kappa, 1)^{\alpha} \times \max(S_{cr}/\kappa, 1)^{-1.209} \times 0.993^{Age} \times 1.018$ [if female] $\times$ 1.159 [if black]

where: S_{cr} is serum creatinine in mg/dL, κ is 0.7 for females and 0.9 for males, α is -0.329 for females and -0.411 for males, minimum indicates the minimum of S_{cr}/κ or 1 and maximum indicates the maximum of S_{cr}/κ or 1.

Serum Cystatin C

Though it was used for a few years (1985) now, commercially serum cystatin C has been in vogue only recently. Rise in cystatin C occurs at an earlier stage (when GFR fell to88 mL/min/1.73 m^2) as compared to serum creatinine (increases after a drop to 75 mL/min/1.73 m^2 or lesser). Serum cystatin C estimation can be an useful tool to assess GFR changes early, however cystatin C too is reabsorbed by tubules and needs validation in larger studies.

Inulin

Inulin was once considered the gold standard of exogenously administered markers of GFR; however, need for constant infusion, invasive nature of the test; costs and availability of inulin have limited its utility.

Radionuclide and Radiocontrast Markers of Glomerular Filtration Rate

As of now the practical gold standard to estimate GFR remains the isotope GFR estimation. The most commonly studied isotopes are technetium 125m-radio labelled diethylenetriaminepentaacetic acid (99mTc-DTPA), iodine 125m-radiolabelled iothalamate (125I-iothalamate) and 51Cr-EDTA. Of these the DTPA underestimated the GFR as compared to the other radionuclide agents possibly due to protein binding.

The radioisotope method is invasive and requires intravenous bolus injection followed by estimation using:

$$\text{Clearance} = \frac{V_0\,[\log(2)]}{t_{1/2}}$$

where V_0 is the volume of distribution and $t^{1/2}$ is the half-time for decay in plasma levels. Various computer base equations like GATES method are employed to give GFR and such methods are useful for follow-up and detecting trends after intervention.

An ionic radiocontrast agent, iothalamate sodium acid, has also been studied to measure GFR as it behaves very similar to inulin. However, its long-term effects have not been studied so far.

In clinical practice, tests of GFR are most commonly used for:

- Screening for the presence of kidney disease
- Measuring disease progression to determine prognosis and effects of therapy
- Confirming the need for treatment of end-stage renal disease with dialysis or transplantation
- Estimating renal clearance of drugs to guide dosing, and
- Assessing GFR as a risk factor for cardiovascular disease

Serum creatinine as of now is a practical marker to assess GFR.

Markers of Tubular Function

The tubules reabsorb the electrolytes, especially sodium, chloride, calcium, phosphorus, magnesium, bicarbonate, water, amino acids and glucose and the proximal tubules account for nearly 75% of absorption. The loop of Henle is involved in absorption of sodium, chloride and excretion of potassium leading to dilute urine reaching the thick ascending loop of Henle. The distal tubules later secrete hydrogen ions, further absorb sodium and water (with the help of aquaporins under the influence of antidiuretic hormone) and thus concentrated urine is excreted. Hence, tubular function tests involve evaluation of functions of the proximal tubule (i.e. tubular handling of sodium, glucose, phosphate, calcium, bicarbonate and amino acids) and distal tubule (urinary acidification and concentration).

Proximal Tubular Function Tests

Ninty-nine percent of amino acids excreted into the filtrate are reabsorbed by the proximal tubule. Any defect in proximal tubule will therefore affect acidification and can lead to aminoaciduria. Glycosuria too can occur due to proximal tubular defect or if the renal threshold of glucose (200 mg/dL plasma glucose) is exceeded as in diabetes. Ammonia formation and secretion helps in acidification of urine and occurs in the proximal tubule. Excess bicarbonate loss (fractional excretion 15%) indicates proximal tubule damage.

Phosphaturia is also an indicator of proximal tubule damage and is indirectly measured as the maximal tubular reabsorption capacity phosphate (T_mP GFR). Analysis of excretion of the following substances can assist in the diagnosis of proximal tubular disorders:

- *Glucose:* The maximum reabsorption rate for glucose (T_mG) in the proximal tubule can be determined following infusion of 20% dextrose and is normally about 15 mmol/liter (T_mG/GFR)
- *Phosphate:* The theoretical maximum tubular threshold of phosphate (T_mP/GFR) can be estimated by formula from the plasma and urinary phosphate and creatinine concentrations, or can be measured directly following infusion of phosphate
- *Amino acids excretion:* Five types of renal aminoaciduria are distinguished: dibasic amino acids, neutral amino acids (monoamino monocarboxylic acids), glycine and imino acids, dicarboxylic amino acids, and generalized amino aciduria (Fanconi's syndrome). Of all tests TmP/GFR is the commonest test done in nephrological practice.
- Tubular reabsorption of phosphorus (TRP)
  1. = $1-\{C^*_{PO4}/C_{Cr}\}$ * C = Clearance
  2. = 1-[serum creatinine × urine phosphate]/[serum phosphate × urine creatinine]

TmP/GFR—calculated by nomogram **(Fig. 4.1)** by plotting TRP and serum phosphate: If serum phosphate is low—TmP/GFR should be high (if low suggests renal phosphate wasting).

Distal Tubular Function Tests

Distal tubules absorb water through aquaporins only under the influence of antidiuretic hormone (ADH) action and any defect in ADH action (either central or renal) leads to diuresis or excess urine loss or diabetes insipidus. If ADH action occurs inappropriately then too much water is retained in the body leading to hyponatremia (syndrome of inappropriate ADH secretion/SIADH).

Water deprivation test is done in polyuric states to differentiate between primary or secondary nephrogenic diabetes insipidus or central (or neurologic) diabetes insipidus from primary polydipsia. Serum and urine osmolality, serum sodium levels pre- and postwater deprivation helps in identifying concentration

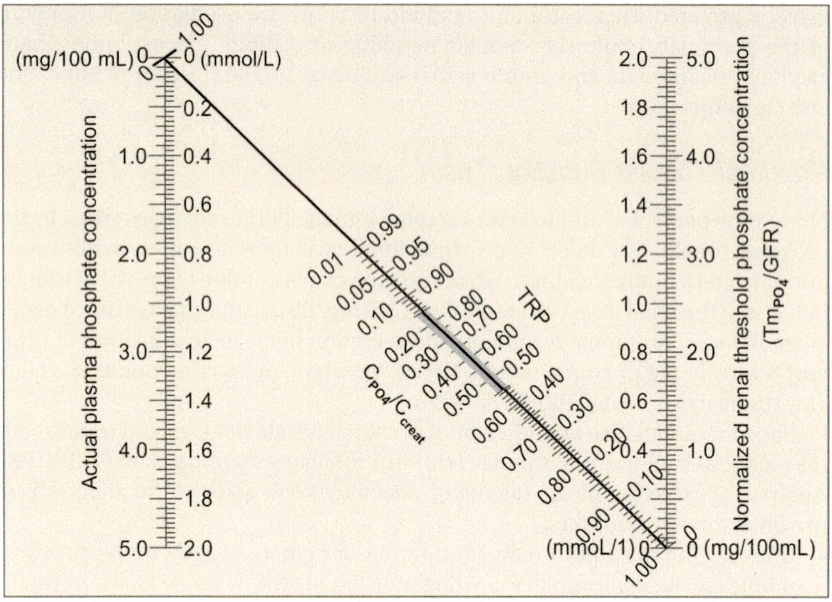

Figure 4.1 TmP/GFR calculation by nomogram by plotting TRP and serum phosphate
Source: Nat Clin Pract Oncol © 2006 Nature Publishing Group (www.medscape.com)

defects. It is done in 2 stages—overnight supervised water deprivation for nearly 12 hours followed by checking body weight, serum and urine osmolality. If urine remains hypotonic or remains dilute (not concentrated) Desmopressin is administered to assess the response. If response is noted it indicates central cause and if no response it indicates renal cause.

WATER LOAD TEST (15 mL/kg water load orally) is done in hyponatremia to assess the diluting capacity of tubules. Normally 80% of the water is excreted in 4 hours. This should not be carried out in presence of renal dysfunction, fluid overload state or in poor cardiac function.

Distal tubules also help in acidification of urine by excreting hydrogen and potassium and hence any defect in distal tubules can lead to metabolic acidosis, hypokalemia or hyperkalemia. If first voided urine pH is less than 5.5, then distal renal tubular acidosis is ruled out. However, if pH is more than 6 then ammonium chloride loading test (0.1 g/kg ammonium chloride (in empty capsules) given orally and urine samples collected at 2, 4 and 6 hours are tested for pH and serum sample taken at 4 hours for bicarbonate levels) or furosemide challenge test (single oral dose of 2 mg/kg body weight furosemide) are utilized to look for drop in urine pH over 4 to 6 hours. If the urine pH does not drop to 5.5 or less it indicates distal tubular acidosis.

Other Tubular Function Tests

Employed to aid diagnosis are—fractional excretion of bicarbonate ($FeHCO_3$); urine anion gap and urine osmolal gap **(Table 4.12)** and transtubular potassium gradient (TTKG).

Table 4.12 Diagnosis of renal tubular acidosis (RTA)

Type of RTA	*UAG/UOG*	*Urine pH*	*Plasma potassium*	*$FeHCO_3$*
Proximal (HCO_3 wasting)	Negative/low	< 5.5	Normal/low	>15%
Distal (Classical)	Positive/high	>5.5	Low	<5%
Hyperkalemic distal RTA (dRTA)	Positive/high	>5.5	High	<5%
Rate limiting dRTA	Positive/high	N/<5.5	Normal	<5%
Type 4 RTA	Positive	<5.5	High	<10%

- Fe-HCO_3 = (urinary bicarbonate × serum creatinine)/(serum bicarbonate × urine creatinine) (helps identify bicarbonate loss either proximal or distal tubular loss)
- Urine anion gap (UAG) can be estimated to assess ammonium excretion. A positive urine anion gap indicates distal renal tubular acidosis (dRTA). Similarly a low urinary osmolal gap (<100) indicates distal renal tubular acidosis. These urinary gaps are calculated as follows:
  - UAG = Urinary ($Na^+ + K^+ - Cl^-$)
  - Urine Osmolal gap (UOG) (measured – calculated*)
  - Urine osmolality calculated* = Na + K + Cl + urea + glucose + 90 mosm/L
- Estimation of transtubular potassium gradient (TTKG) is advocated by some as useful in analysis of disorders of potassium = (urinary potassium × serum osmolality/serum potassium × urinary osmolality).

TTKG below 4 is considered abnormal in hyperkalemia and above 2 in hypokalemia.

Renal Calculi and Divalent Ions

In renal stone disease abnormalities of calcium (corrected to serum albumin levels*), phosphorus and uric acid identifies primary cause of renal calculi such as hyperuricemia or hyperparathyroidism which are treatable conditions. If calcium, phosphorus and uric acid are normal then metabolic work-up by collecting 24 hours urine to estimate oxalate, cysteine, sulphate and citric acid is to be undertaken to identify the underlying cause which can sometimes be elusive. The renal stones are usually radio-opaque due to presence of calcium and phosphorus, however radiolucent stones made-up of predominantly uric acid or cysteine too can be noted. And urine examination could be the clue of the type of stone.

Identification of monohydrate calcium oxalate stones requires identification of abnormal functioning of vitamin B_6-dependent liver-specific peroxisomal enzyme alanine: glyoxylate aminotransferase (AGT) or mutation in AGXT gene, or dysfunction of the enzyme glyoxylate/hydroxypyruvate reductase (GRHPR) and mutation in GRHPR gene if the patient presents with renal failure at young age with bilateral stone.

Other Biochemical Tests in Specific Situations

In cases of glomerulonephritis, to assess the etiology of the glomerulonephritis, antinuclear antibody titres, antineutrophil cytoplasmic antibodies (ANCA)-

cANCA or proteinase 3 and pANCA or myeloperoxidase antibody titres, complement 3 (C3), complement 4 (C4), antistreptolysin O titres (ASO titres) and viral screen (hepatitis B, hepatitis C), cryoglobulin assay and lactate dehydrogenase and even peripheral smear to look for schistocytes (in cases of hemolytic uremic syndrome) will be required **(Tables 4.9 to 4.11)**.

In renal biopsy specimens, immunohistochemistry studies may be needed to assess for IgA nephropathy. In renal transplant recipients biopsy specimens are examined for BK virus or other viral inclusion bodies and to identify rejection C4d and histopathology is utilized. In these cases identification of Decoy cells in urine to identify BK virus infection, urinary or circulating proteins and cytokines, circulating soluble interleukin-2 (IL-2) receptor, the urinary concentration of soluble adhesion molecules, or cellular activation with urinary flow cytometry may be helpful in diagnosing acute allograft rejection. Also latest polymerase chain reaction (PCR) analysis and DNA microarrays are utilised along with renal biopsy to help in early diagnosis of acute rejection **(Table 4.9)**.

SUMMARY

Despite proper history, clinical examination and strong clinical suspicion of renal disease, tailor made biochemical analysis is an absolute necessity to unravel the nature and severity of renal disease for planning the appropriate management.

Multiple Choice Questions

1. **Which biochemical test is known as the noninvasive renal biopsy:**
   a. Urine analysis b. Serum creatinine
   c. Serum electrolytes d. Renal imaging

2. **Urine proteinuria can be:**
   a. Glomerular b. Tubular
   c. Overflow d. All of the above

3. **The ideal substance for glomerular filtration rate should have the following qualities:**
   a. No tubular reabsorption b. Constant production
   c. No tubular secretion d. All of the above

4. **The ideal substance to estimate glomerular filtration rate is:**
   a. Inulin b. Creatinine
   c. Urea d. Cystatin

5. **The gold standard for GFR estimation now is:**
   a. Inulin b. Isotope GFR estimation
   c. Creatinine d. Urea

6. **Proximal tubular function is estimated by:**
   a. Phosphate loss b. Aminoaciduria
   c. Glycosuria d. All of the above

7. **Water deprivation test is used for:**
   a. Diabetes mellitus b. Dehydration
   c. Diabetes insipidus d. Diarrhea

8. Endocrine functions of kidney occur through these hormones:
a. Renin-angiotensin system
b. Vitamin D3
c. Erythropoietin
d. All of the above
e. None of the above

9. Renal failure is associated with:
a. Hyperkalemia
b. Metabolic acidosis
c. a and b
d. Metabolic alkalosis

10. Negative urinary anion gap or low urinary osmolal gap is seen in:
a. Distal renal tubular acidosis
b. Type IV renal tubular acidosis
c. Proximal renal tubular acidosis
d. None of the above

Answers

1. a	2. d	3. d	4. a	5. b	6. d	7. c	8. d
9. c	10. c						

SUGGESTED READING

1. Cooper ME, Harris RC, Skorecki KL, Berl T, DuBose T, Mount DB, et al. Integrated control of body fluid volume and composition. In: Brenner BM (Ed). Brenner and Rector's The Kidney, 8th edn. Philadelphia, PA: Saunders. 2007: Chapter 11-17.
2. Davenport A. Clinical investigation of renal disease. In: Warrell DA, Cox TM, Firth JD (Eds). Oxford Textbook of Medicine, 5th edn. New York: Oxford University Press, 2015:Chapter 21.4.
3. Inker LA, Perrone RD. Assessment of kidney function. In: Post TW (Ed), Up ToDate, Waltham, MA, 2015.
4. Stevens LA, Shastri S, Levey AS, et al. Investigation of renal function. In: Floege J, Johnson RJ, Feehally J (Eds). Comprehensive Clinical Nephrology, 4th edn. Philadelphia, PA: Elsevier/Saunders, 2010.
5. Ypersele CV. The patient with fluid, electrolyte and divalent ion disorders. In: Davison AM, Cameron JS, Grunfeld JP, Ponticelli C, Ritz E, Winearls CG, Ypersele CV (Ed). Oxford Textbook of Clinical Nephrology, 3rd edn. New York: Oxford University Press, 2015:213-346.

URINALYSIS

Sishir Gang

INTRODUCTION

Urine analysis is one of the most frequent and rewarding investigations in clinical medicine. Careful examination is helpful to detected renal parenchymal disease and also ascertains their progression and regression. Urine examination should be considered as an extension of physical examination in all patients.

METHOD OF COLLECTION OF URINE SAMPLE

The first voided morning specimen is the most concentrated and most suitable for routine urinalysis. Urine should be tested promptly to avoid changes in pH and multiplication of contaminating bacteria. The formed elements degenerate over period of time. **Table 4.13** provides the guidelines for collecting urine sample.

Routine urine analysis consists of two major components.

1. *Physiochemical analysis:* Appearance, specific gravity, reagent strip (glycosuria, proteinuria, blood, leukocyturia, infection).
2. *Bright field or phase contrast microscopy:* Hematuria, pyuria, cast and crystalluria.

URINE APPEARANCE

Normal urine is clear and yellow in color due to urochromes. Its color deepens as it becomes more concentrated. Altered urine color is seen in various pathological conditions and in presence of drugs. It is important to observe the color of supernatant and sediment before and after centrifugation. Suspended particles may render the urine turbid and it would settle on centrifugation. **Table 4.14** lists conditions associated with change in color of urine.

Table 4.13 Guidelines for collecting midstream urine sample
• Explain the procedure to the patient • Ensure privacy • Wash hands
Women • Hold labia well separated during collection of the specimen • Gently cleanse the periurethral area from anterior to posterior with wet gauze pieces
Men • Hold the retracted fore skin back throughout the collection • Clean the urethral meatus with moist gauze
Ask patient to pass first part of urine stream into the toilet/bedpan/bottle. At least 100 mL should be passed before a midstream urine specimen is collected without interruption of the flow of urine. Catch midstream specimen in sterile specimen container or sterile kidney dish. Take care not to contaminate the specimen. Allow patient to void remainder of urine.

Table 4.14 Urine color and diagnostic significance

Urine color	*Condition*
Red sediment	Hematuria
Red supernatant Heme negative	Beeturia, phenazopyridine, Porphyria
Red supernatant Heme positive	Myoglobinuria—clear plasma Hemoglobinuria—red plasma
Black upon standing	Alkaptonuria—homogentistic aciduria, imipenem cilastatin, methyl dopa, metronidazole, porphyria (porphobilinogen), melanoma (melanogen)
Black	Hemoglobinuria
Yellow-brown	Hyperbilirubinemia, chloroquine, nitrofurantion
Orange	Rifampicin, Senna
Green-blue	Methylene blue, propofol, amitriptyline, triamterene
Milky White	Pyuria, chyluria

URINE ODOUR (TABLE 4.15)

Table 4.15 Urine odour

Odour	*Condition*
Offensive	Urinary tract infection urea splitting bacteria and ammonia production
Musty or mousy	Phenylketonuria
Sweet, fruity	Ketones
Sweaty feet	Isovaleric acidemia
Maple syrup	Maple syrup urine disease
Fishy or rancid	Hypermethioninemia, tyrosinemia

SPECIFIC GRAVITY

Specific gravity depends upon the number and weight of the particles dissolved in urine. Urine osmolality is a colligative property of matter and depends only on the number of particles dissolved in urine. In practice urine specific gravity is often used as a surrogate for urine osmolality. However, for evaluation of dysnatremia patients it is desirable use osmolality rather than specific gravity.

Specific gravity of 1.010 connotes isosthenuria, i.e. it has the same specific gravity as plasma. Under physiologic condition specific gravity varies from 1.001 to 1.030, which correlated with osmolality of 50 to 1000 mOsmol/L.

Methods used to measure specific gravity are hydrometer, refractometer and dipstick.

Isothenuria is seen in patients with chronic kidney disease or acute tubular necrosis where the ability to concentrate the urine is impaired. Low specific gravity is associated with dilute urine and diabetes insipidus. Whereas high specific gravity indicates dehydration, glycosuria or radio contrast administration.

CHEMICAL COMPOSITION OF URINE

Routine Dipstick Testing

Dipsticks are plastic strips embedded with multiple small pads containing a reagent. When dipped in urine color change in the reagent pad allows recognition and semi-quantification of the analyte present by visually comparing it with standard charts. It is sensitive and rapid test, which can easily be performed in clinician office **(Table 4.16)**.

Table 4.16 Dipstick testing of urine

Test	*Reagent*	*Reaction*	*Remarks*
pH	Methyl red and bromothymol blue	Dyes change color with change in pH	Range is 4.5–8. Useful in patient with metabolic acidosis to determine if renal acidification mechanism is intact. Urine *Proteus* infection can increase the urine pH above 7
Protein	Tetrabromo-phenol blue	Color change of pH indicator is different in presence of protein	Dipstick is more sensitive to albumin and less to globulin and other proteins. Hence negative dipstick does not rule out proteinuria. Heat and acid test detects all proteins. False positive test may occur in alkaline urine and in presence of quaternary ammonium compounds
Glucose	Glucose oxidase/ peroxidase	Gluose oxidase generates hydrogen peroxide	False positive test may be seen with peroxidase strip but not with oxidase strip. Large doses of vitamin C will cause false positive results
Ketones	Sodium nitroprusside	Acetoacetic acid reacts with sodium nitroprusside to produce maroon color	Reagent strips detect acetoacetic acid and acetone but do not detect B-hydrxoybutyric acid
Occult blood	Organic peroxide	Hemoglobin and peroxide oxidizes the chromogen. Orange to green to dark blue	Detects hematuria, hemoglobinuria and myoglobinuria. It is a very sensitive test. Detection needs confirmation by microscopic examination
Bilirubin	Diazonium salt	Azobilirubin. Tan colored	Test should be done on fresh urine sample. On standing bilirubin is converted to biliverdin and the test would be negative.

Contd...

Contd...

Urobilinogen	p-Dimethyl-aminobenzal-dehyde	Red colored azo dye	
Nitrite	p-arsanilic and quinolone	Diazonium compound, pink color	Common organism (*E. coli, Klebsiella, Proteus, Enterobacter*) that cause UTI reduce urinary nitrate to nitrite. Should be checked on fresh sample so as prevent bacteria from multiplying. Negative test does not rule out infection
Leukocyte esterase	Indoxyl or pyrole	Neutrophil esterases reacts with indoxyl or pyrrole and produces lavender to purple color	Test detects the presence of neutrophils in urine. False positive results are seen with detergents, formalin or contamination with vaginal discharge

URINE MICROSCOPY

"When the patient dies the kidneys may go to the pathologist, but while he lives the urine is ours. It can provide us day-by-day, month by month, and year-by-year with a serial story of the major events within the kidney. The examination of the urine is the most essential part of the physical examination of any patient..." wrote Thomas Addis (1881–1949) who championed the role of urine microscopy in care of patients with renal disease.

Urine microscopy is cheap, noninvasive and quick test that provides critical information if performed properly in a patient with kidney disease.

Sample Collection for Urine Microscopy

Collect midstream urine in a sterile container. It should be processed immediately to avoid lysis of cellular elements **(Figs 4.2A to F)**. Collect an aliquot of 10 mL and centrifuge at 1500 rpm. Discard 9.5 mL of supernatant and resuspend the sediment in 0.5 mL of urine. Transfer the suspended sediment on the glass slide and cover it with a cover slip.

Bright field microscopy provides limited information on unstained preparation. Staining helps to delineate the cellular elements better. Phase contrast microscopy is ideal and obviates the need of staining.

The constituents of the urinary sediment either originate from the blood circulation or from the urinary tract. **Table 4.17** shows the classification of various constituent of urinary sediment.

Cells

Red Blood Cells

Red blood cells (RBCs) are round cells without a nucleus. They appear swollen in dilute urine and uniformly crenated in concentrated urine. Normally, they

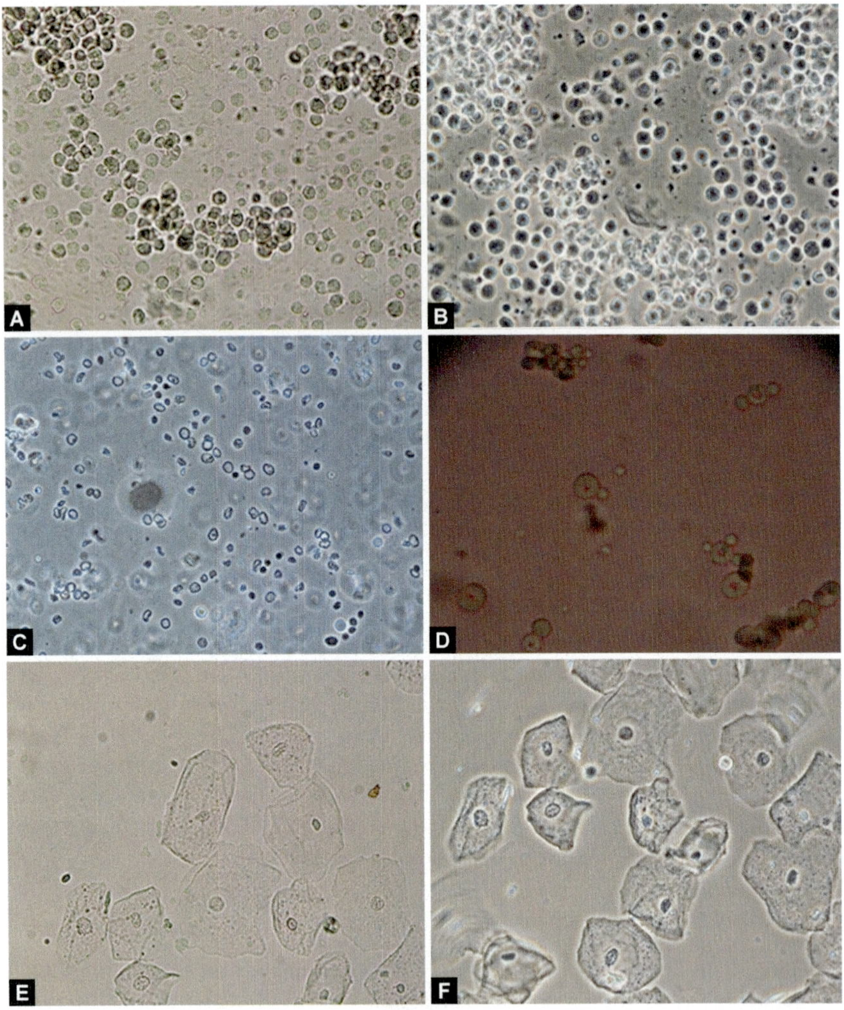

Figures 4.2A to F Cellular elements in urine: (A) Pus cells, light microscopy (LM); (B) Pus cells phase contrast; (C) RBC, phase contrast; (D) Dismorphic RBCs, LM, 400x (E) Epithelial cells, LM; (F) Epithelial cells phase contrast (All images, 400x)
(*Courtesy:* Dr Shailesh Soni and Dr Amit Jojera)

are less than 2/hpf. RBCs can originate from anywhere in the urinary tract. Cells originating from the glomerulus are often dysmorphic, i.e. they are irregular in shape due to their passage through the glomerulus and tubules.

White Blood Cells (Leukocytes)

Normally there are not more than 5 leukocytes per high power field. Pyuria refers to presence of leukocytes in the urine. Neutrophils are the predominant leukocytes and are recognized by their multilobed nucleus and granular cytoplasm. They indicate upper or lower urinary tract infection. Sterile pyuria

Table 4.17 Urine sediment

Cells	*Casts*	*Crystals*			*Organism/ artifacts*
		Nonpathological		**Pathological**	
		Acid urine	**Alkaline urine**	**Acid urine**	
White blood cells	Hyaline	Uric acid	Calcium phosphate	Cystine	Yeast
Red blood cells	Red blood cells	Amorphous urates	Triple phosphate	Leucine	Parasite
Tubular epithelial cells	Granular	Calcium oxalate	Amorphous phosphates	Tyrosine	Sperm
Epithelial cells Squamous and transitional	Tubular cell	Hippuric acid	Calcium carbonate	Cholesterol	Bacteria
	White blood cell		Ammonium biurate		Fibers
	Waxy				Starch

Table 4.18 Urinary casts

Type of cast	*Composition and features*	*Remarks*
Hyaline	Tamm-Horsfall protein—a glycoprotein secreted by the cells of thick ascending limb of the loop of Henle	Homogenous, translucent and smooth. They are nonspecific and do not indicate any disease
Granular	*Fine granular*: Altered serum protein *Coarse granular*: Degeneration of embedded cells	Are nonspecific and are seen in variety of renal disease
Waxy or broad	Higher refractive index then hyaline. Their edges are hard and indented. Broad cast form in dilated and atrophic tubules	Their presence denote advanced renal disease
Erythrocyte	Red blood cells	Suggests glomerular bleeding. Frequently seen in proliferative glomerulonephritis and occasionally in tubulointerstitial nephritis. Frequently associated with granular cast, dysmorphic RBCs and proteinuria
Leukocyte	White blood cells	Pyelonephritis, glomerulonephritis, interstitial nephritis, renal inflammatory processes
Epithelial	Renal tubule cells	Acute tubular necrosis, interstitial nephritis
Fatty	Lipid-laden renal tubule cells	Nephrotic syndrome, renal disease, hypothyroidism

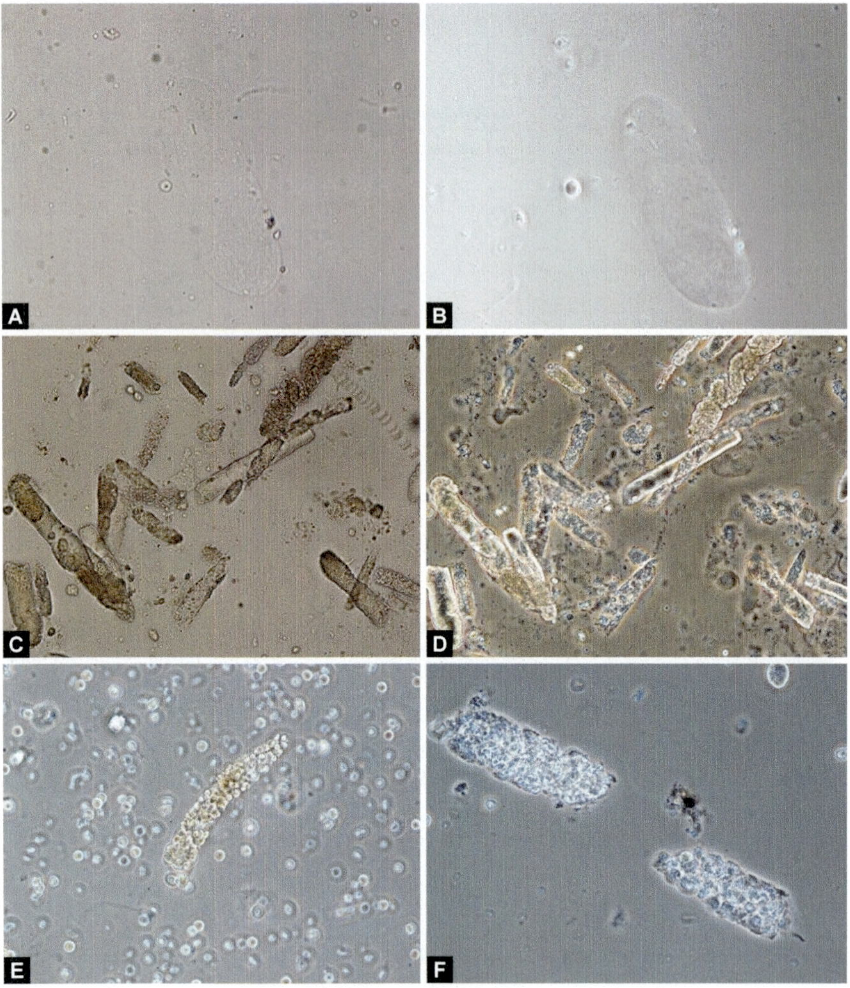

Figures 4.3A to F Urinary casts: (A) Hyaline cast, LM; (B) Hyaline cast phase contrast; (C) Granular and waxy cast, LM; (D) Granular and waxy cast phase contrast; (E) RBC cast phase contrast; (F) WBC cast, phase contrast (All images 400x)
(*Courtesy:* Dr Shailesh Soni and Dr Amit Jojera)

refers presence of pyuria with routine cultures being negative. It may indicate tuberculous infection. They may also be seen in noninfective inflammatory conditions such as glomerulonephritis and interstitial nephritis.

Epithelial Cells

- *Renal tubular epithelial cells* are usually larger than leukocytes. They have a large nucleus placed eccentrically. Their numbers may increase in acute tubular necrosis, interstitial nephritis and nephrotic syndrome. In nephrotic syndrome they are laden with numerous refractile fat droplets.

- *Uroepithelial cells* (transitional epithelial cells) originate anywhere from renal calyses to proximal urethra. They are large rounded cells and often appear in clumps.
- *Squamous epithelial cells* originate from distal urethra or as contamination from external genitalia. They are large flat cells with small nuclei.

Casts

Urinary casts are cylindrical elements, consisting of a matrix of Tamm-Horsfall glycoprotein. They are formed in the lumen of distal renal tubules and collecting ducts. Different elements get embedded in them giving it various morphological features and names. They are best seen in acidic urine and should be examined promptly **(Table 4.18** and **Figs 4.3A to F)**.

Crystals

As detailed in **Table 4.17** and **Figures 4.4A to C** several types of crystals can be identified based on their morphology in polarized light. Their formation is pH dependent. Most of them are of no clinical consequence except some like cystine which always suggests cystinuria.

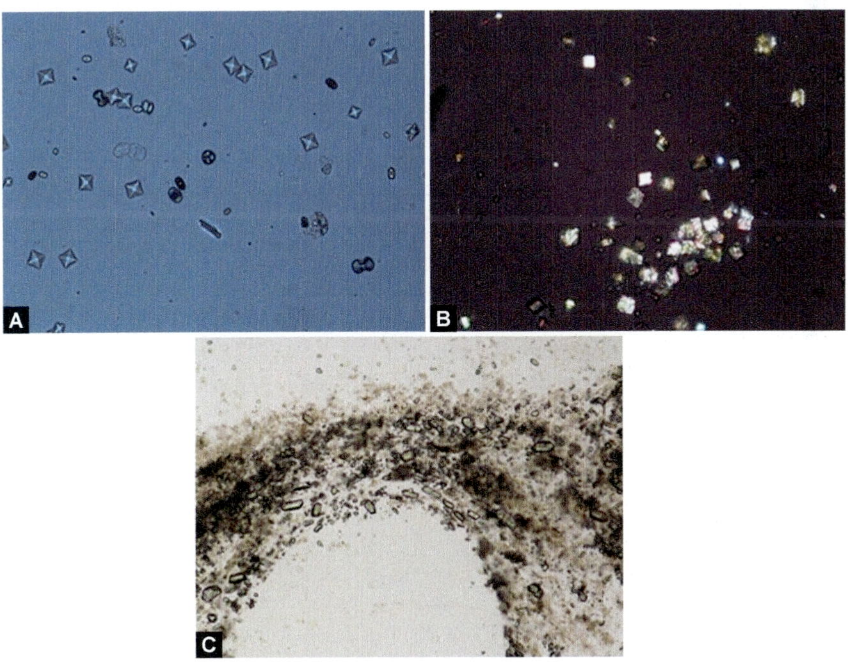

Figures 4.4A to C Urinary crystals: (A) Oxalate crystals polarized; (B) Uric acid crystals, polarized; (C) Triple phosphate LM (All images, 400x
(*Courtesy*: Dr Shailesh Soni and Dr Amit Jojera)

HEMATURIA

Hematuria is defined as more than two RBCs per high power field in a centrifuged specimen. Hematuria by dipstick should always be confirmed by microscopy **(Figs 4.2A to F)**. Microscopic hematuria is one that does not stain the urine red but is detected only by dipstick or microscopic examination. In macroscopic hematuria the urine appears red or smoky brown. **Flow chart 4.1** provides the algorithm for work of hematuria.

PROTEINURIA

Plasma contains about 6–8 g/L of protein. About 1000 liters of plasma passes through the kidney per day. Healthy adult excretes less than 150 mg of protein per day in urine. The glomerular filtration barrier restricts the protein excretion and proximal tubule reabsorbs and degrades most of the protein which escapes the filtration barrier. The composition of normal urine is shown in **Table 4.19. Flow chart 4.2** shows algorithm for evaluation of proteinuria.

Flow chart 4.1 Algorithm for evaluation of hematuria

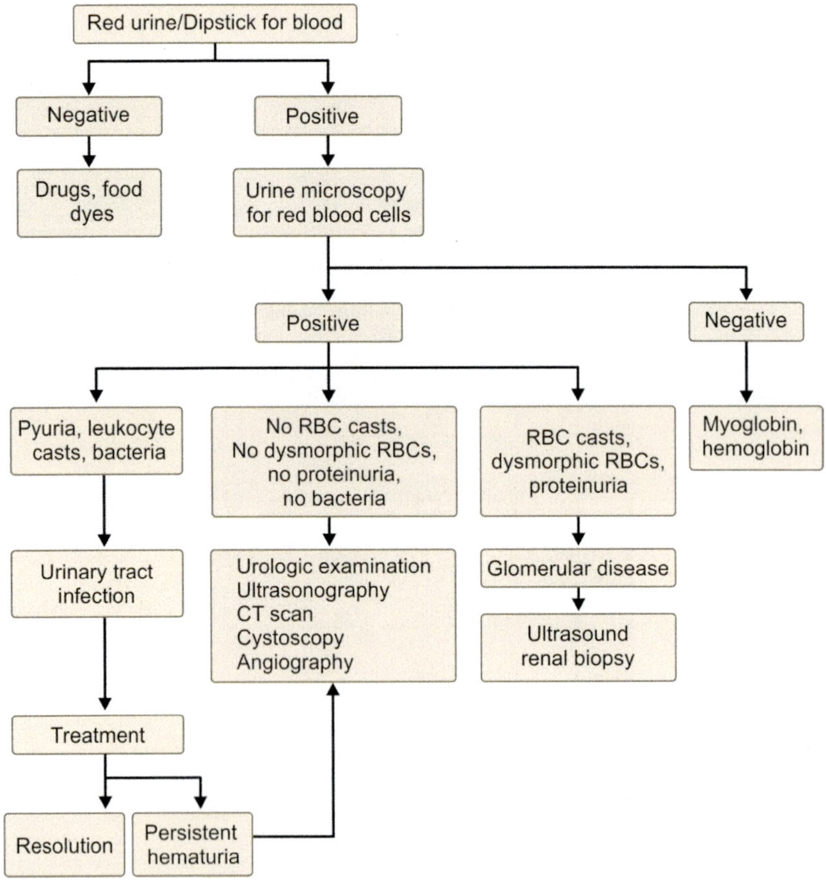

Table 4.19 Protein composition of normal urine

Plasma proteins	*Excretion (mg/day)*
Plasma proteins	
Albumin	12
Immunoglobulin G	3
Immunoglobulin A	1
Immunoglobulin M	0.3
Light chains	
κ	2.3
λ	1.4
β - microglobulins	0.12
Other plasma proteins	20
All plasma proteins	40
Nonplasma proteins	
Tamm-Horsfall protein	40
Other nonrenal-derived proteins	<1
All nonplasma proteins	40
Total proteins	80 ± 24 (SD)

From Glassock R; Proteinuria. In Massry SG, Glassock RJ (eds); Textbook of Nephrology, 3rd edn. Baltimore, Williams and Williams, 1995.

Flow chart 4.2 Algorithm for evaluation of proteinuria

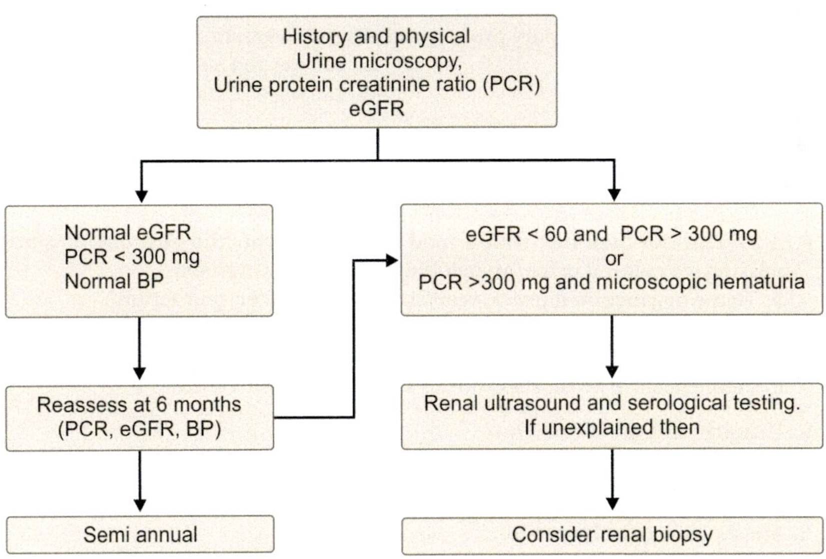

The origin of abnormal protein can be from:

- *Glomerular pathology:* Excess protein crosses the damaged glomerular basement membrane and overwhelms the tubular reabsorptive capacity, e.g. primary or secondary glomerular disease.
- *Tubular pathology:* Damaged tubules failure to reabsorb the normally filtered protein or secretes an excess amount, e.g. interstitial nephritis, hereditary nephritis
- *Overflow of an abnormal plasma protein:* Filtered protein exceeds the resorptive capacity of the tubules, e.g. multiple myeloma. Dipstick which detects albumin may be negative in this case.

SUMMARY

- Urinalysis is one of the most common diagnostic investigations for renal diseases.
- Correct method of urine collection is very important for accurate analysis.
- Urinary sample should be analyzed at the earliest and storage and transportation time must be minimized.
- Macroscopic, chemical and microscopic examination constitute complete urinalysis.
- It helps in differentiating various types of disease affecting the kidneys and guide further investigation and appropriate management.

Multiple Choice Questions

1. **Best urine sample to examine is:**
   a. First void, midstream, clean catch
   b. Second void, midstream, clean catch
   c. Random sample
   d. All of the above

2. **Approximate daily urinary protein and albumin excretion respectively is:**
   a. 100 mg and 50 mg
   b. 200 mg and 50 mg
   c. 150 mg and 30 mg
   d. 250 mg and 100 mg

3. **Urine in isosthenuria has specific gravity of:**
   a. 1.020
   b. 1.010
   c. 1.015
   d. 1.012

4. **A 37-year-old man met with a road traffic accident. The next day he started passing tea colored urine. Myoglobinuria will be proven by:**
   a. Heme negative on dipstick, reddish discoloration of spun serum
   b. Heme negative on dipstick, no discoloration of spun serum
   c. Heme positive on dipstick, reddish discoloration of spun serum
   d. Heme positive on dipstick, no discoloration of spun serum

5. **Urinary casts are formed in:**
   a. Proximal convoluted tubules
   b. Glomerulus
   c. Distal tubules and collecting ducts
   d. Descending limb of Henle's loop

6. **Musty urine odor is seen in:**
   a. Isovaleric acidemia
   b. Maple syrup urine disease
   c. Ketonuria
   d. Phenylketonuria

7. **A 67-year-old patient with history of type 2 diabetes mellitus and BPH presents with history of fever with chills, dysuria, frequency and urgency. His urinalysis will show:**
   a. Positive nitrite test
   b. Pyuria
   c. Positive leukocyte esterase test
   d. All of the above

8. **A 16-year-old boy presents with history of passing cola colored urine ten days after an episode of sore throat. Which one of the following will support glomerular origin of hematuria in this case:**
   a. Red blood cell casts
   b. Dysmorphic RBCs on phase contrast microscope
   c. Both a and b
   d. None of the above

9. **Leukocyte casts are seen in:**
   a. Pyelonephritis
   b. Interstitial nephritis
   c. Glomerulonephritis
   d. All of the above

10. **Most common urinary crystals are:**
    a. Calcium oxalate crystals
    b. Urate crystals
    c. Calcium carbonate crystals
    d. Triple phosphate crystals

Answers

1. a	2. c	3. b	4. d	5. c	6. d	7. d	8. c
9. d	10. a						

SUGGESTED READING

1. Fogazzi GB, Ponticelli C, Ritz E. The Urinary Sediment: An Integrated View, 2nd edn. Oxford: Oxford University Press, 1999.
2. Graff L. A Handbook of Routine Urinalysis. Philadelphia: JB Lippincott Co., 1983.
3. Henry JB (Ed). Clinical Diagnosis and Management by Laboratory Methods, 20th edn. Philadelphia, WB Saunders Co., 2001.

RADIOLOGICAL EXAMINATION OF KIDNEYS

Ashish Nandwani, Pranaw Kumar Jha

INTRODUCTION

Imaging is one of the key investigations to evaluate the patient with kidney and urinary tract disorders. Kidney is usually not accessible on physical examination due to its retroperitoneal position, unless it is markedly enlarged in size due to cystic diseases or mass lesions. In such situations, imaging becomes necessary to know the size, shape, position and other information to reach at diagnosis. Various conditions which are diagnosed on renal imaging include renal stones, urinary tract obstructions leading to hydronephrosis, vesicoureteral reflux, renal cystic diseases or mass, congenital disorders with altered renal anatomy and renal vascular diseases. Besides diagnosis, imaging techniques are commonly used for interventional studies, especially ultrasound for kidney biopsy and percutaneous nephrostomy.

Imaging for kidney diseases has changed significantly over the years. It is important to understand the benefits, limitations, and the diagnostic yields of these imaging modalities. Because of safety, ease of performing and relatively low-cost ultrasound is most preferred renal imaging study at present. The most frequently used imaging modalities are summarized in **Table 4.20.**

RECOMMENDED IMAGING MODALITIES FOR KIDNEY DISEASES

The American College of Radiology (ACR) Appropriateness Criteria® (November 2015) are evidence-based guidelines to assist physicians in making the most appropriate imaging or treatment decision for a specific clinical condition. Employing these guidelines helps physicians enhance quality of care and contribute to the most efficacious use of imaging. The recommended imaging modalities for kidney disease are summarized in **Table 4.21.**

A brief discussion regarding the use of imaging studies in the evaluation of patients with a variety of suspected renal disorders is given.

Table 4.20 Commonly used renal imaging modalities
Ultrasonography, including color Doppler
Computed tomography
Magnetic resonance imaging
Voiding cystourethrography
Retrograde or antegrade pyelography
Intravenous urography
Renal angiography
Nuclear medicine studies

Table 4.21 The American College of Radiology—Appropriateness Criteria[*] for Kidney Diseases

Kidney disease	*Imaging of choice*
Acute onset flank pain—urolithiasis	CT abdomen and pelvis without contrast
Acute pyelonephritis	CT abdomen and pelvis without and with contrast
Proteinuria	USG kidneys
Hematuria	USG kidneys and bladder, CT
Renal mass	CT abdomen with or without contrast, MRI
Acute kidney injury/chronic kidney disease	USG kidneys and bladder
Renal transplant dysfunction	USG transplant kidney
Renovascular hypertension	MR angiography without or with contrast CT angiography with contrast
Renal artery/vein thrombosis	CT with contrast
Lower urinary tract infection	X-ray/CT cystography

PLAIN FILM OF THE ABDOMEN

The plain film of the abdomen, also known as the kidney, ureter and bladder (KUB) radiograph was previously used to be the first investigation for kidney diseases. Plain film of KUB may be useful to determine the renal size, contour, calcifications and radiopaque stones. Nephrocalcinosis may be cortical or medullary and is diffuse or localized. The information provided by plain radiograph is usually inadequate, requiring intravenous iodinated contrast material for the opacification of the kidneys and urinary tract.

INTRAVENOUS UROGRAPHY

The intravenous urography (IVU) had been the standard imaging procedure for evaluating the renal excretory function and anatomy of the urinary tract in the past; however, it has been increasingly replaced by contrast CT urography. An IVU necessitates the injection of iodinated contrast agent and is contraindicated in patients with history of allergic reaction with contrast agent and glomerular filtration rate <60 mL/min in view of risk of nephrotoxicity and poor images due to decreased excretion. IVU provides detailed view of the pelvicaliceal system, assess renal size and shape, detect renal stones, and assess renal function. Calculi that are radiolucent on plain films are usually detected as filling defects on IVU. It is particularly useful in diagnosing certain rare disorders, such as medullary sponge kidney and papillary necrosis **(Fig. 4.5)**.

RETROGRADE OR ANTEGRADE PYELOGRAPHY

These are invasive procedures requiring placement of percutaneous nephrostomy in antegrade pyelography and placement of ureteral catheter under cystoscopic guidance in retrograde pyelography and injecting contrast agent. This is done to evaluate the cases of hydronephrosis and ureteral obstruction. These procedures

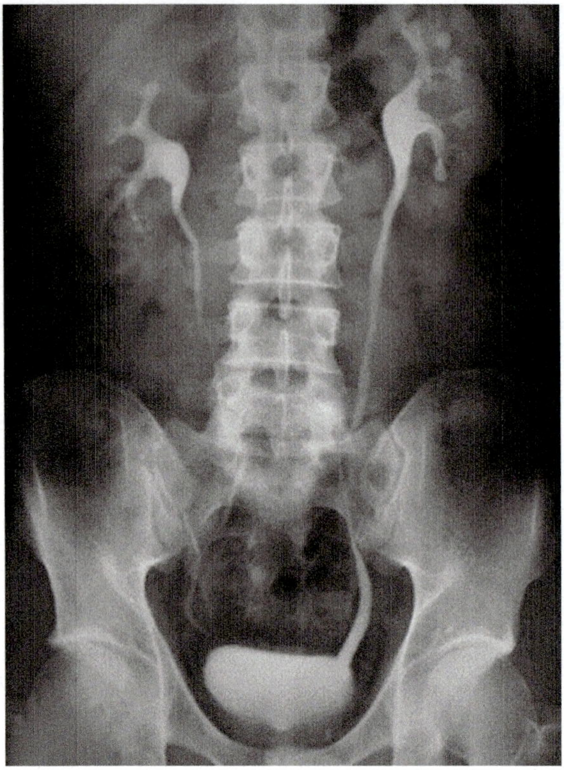

Figure 4.5 Intravenous urogram showing renal outline and pelvicalyceal system

are used in patients with poor renal functions, who cannot be given intravenous iodinated contrast agents.

CYSTOGRAPHY

Radiographic evaluation of bladder can be done by cystography, in which urethral catheter is placed and contrast agent is infused and bladder is filled under fluoroscopic guidance. Voiding cystography is used to assess the bladder function and identify the ureteral reflux. Cystogram can identify bladder stones, diverticula and ureterocele.

ULTRASOUND

Basic Ultrasound Concepts

Ultrasound (USG) is a high-frequency vibration, which travels through tissue at high speed, close to 1540 m/s. In clinical application, ultrasound is generated and detected by piezoelectric crystals, which are contained in small hand-held transducers. Echoes are produced by transmitted ultrasound pulses at tissue interfaces and are the basic sources of information. These are displayed on monitor in diagnostic ultrasound. The Doppler effect is a very sensitive and accurate detector of motion. It is commonly used to study blood flow in vessels, but it can also be employed to measure tissue motion. Doppler images and spectrograms are produced in realtime, making them very useful for the study of physiological function.

Anatomy of Kidney

The length of the normal adult kidney is usually 9–12 cm, but there is a wider range of 7–14 cm in patients with normal renal function. Renal sizes vary with sex, age and build of the individual. The length can even vary in the same individual between scans depending sagittal and transverse planes at the time of measurement. Characteristic of normal kidney is shown in **Table 4.22 and Figure 4.6**.

A number of congenital anomalies of the kidneys can be detected by ultrasound. Agenesis of kidney is associated with an empty renal fossa along with an elongated ipsilateral adrenal gland. Hypertrophy of the contralateral

Table 4.22 Characteristics of normal kidney

Size	9–12 cm (average 11 cm)
Echogenicity	Right: Less than or equal to that of the liver Left: Less than that of the spleen
Parenchyma	Homogeneous (except for hypoechoic pyramids)
Renal sinus	Hypoechoic
Surface and contour	Smooth
Renal pelvis	Anechoic

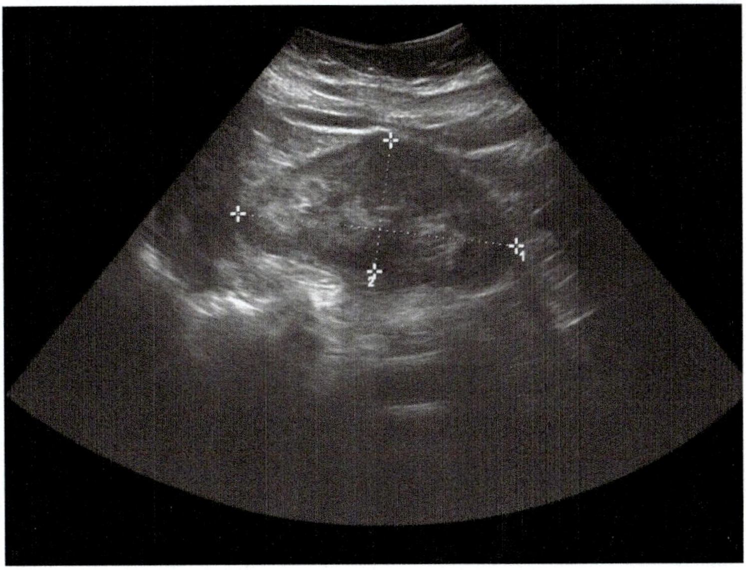

Figure 4.6 Normal sagittal renal ultrasound image

kidney is usually present in such cases. Kidney can also be present at ectopic site, commonly inferior to renal fossa, often in pelvis. Pelvic kidneys are almost always malrotated with the renal hilum directed anteriorly. Fusion anomalies are commonly (1 in 250) detected on ultrasound. The most common fusion anomaly is the horseshoe kidney **(Fig. 4.7)**. It appears as a variably thick band of renal tissue extending from both the lower poles to connect anterior to the aorta below the level of the inferior mesenteric artery. It should be suspected when the axis of the kidney is distorted and the lower poles of the kidneys are directed medially or are hard to image sonographically. Crossed, fused renal ectopia may appear as an unusually large kidney with a duplicated renal sinus or as a mass arising from the lower pole. Duplication anomalies are the most commonly detected on ultrasound. Complete ureteral duplication refers to two ureters that insert into the bladder or other pelvic structures separately.

Large kidneys (>12 cm) are usually associated with polycystic kidney disease, infiltration (myeloma, lymphoma, amyloid), hydronephrosis or renal vein thrombosis. The common causes of small kidneys (<9 cm) are congenital hypoplasia, renal artery stenosis, chronic glomerulonephritis, chronic interstitial nephritis and reflux nephropathy. These abnormalities may be unilateral or bilateral.

Various renal parenchymal diseases can be diagnosed on ultrasound. These include change in size of kidneys. Kidneys may swell in acute disorders, such as acute tubular necrosis and acute pyelonephritis and tend to contract with chronic kidney diseases. The altered echogenicity of cortex is a sensitive marker of the renal parenchymal diseases. Increased parenchymal reflectivity is associated with inflammatory infiltration; decreased reflectivity with edema. Loss of corticomedullary differentiation is seen with medullary inflammation or early calcinosis. Increased echogenicity is a nonspecific finding seen with many

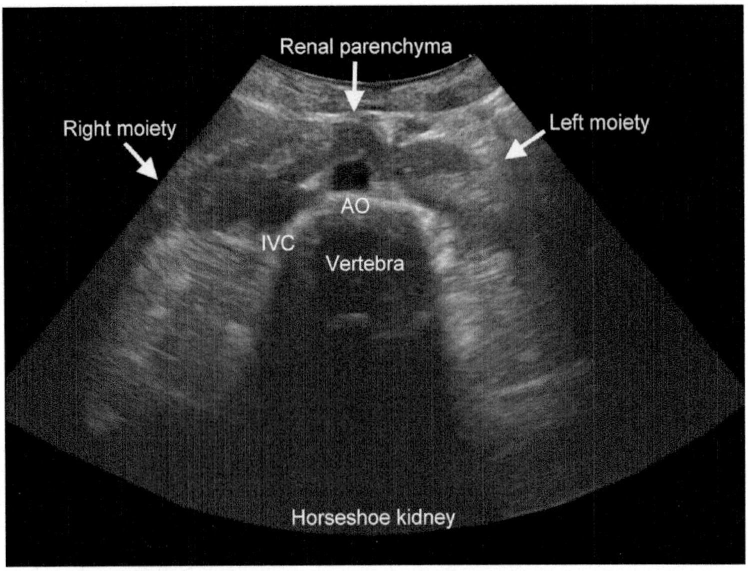

Figure 4.7 Horseshoe kidney ultrasound image

diffuse renal diseases that does not necessarily indicate irreversible disease. In contrast, the combination of increased echogenicity and kidney length <9 cm almost always indicates irreversible disease **(Fig. 4.8)**. The normal renal contour is smooth. Cortex has uniform thickness with slightly more thicker at poles. Scarring occurs in the cortex of a renal lobule due to reflux nephropathy or pyelonephritis. Doppler ultrasound shows an elevated resistive index in the intrarenal arteries in the majority of patients with renal parenchymal diseases. Ultrasound is indicated for renal infections in children, adult males, or females with recurrent infections. Lobar nephronia is focal inflammation in the renal parenchyma. Renal abscess refers to collection of pus and necrotic material within the renal parenchyma whereas pyonephrosis develops in infected and obstructed collecting system.

Ultrasound, in the majority of affected patients, diagnoses hydronephrosis and often establishes its cause. The sonographic diagnosis of obstruction relies on the detection of a dilated collecting system this appears as anechoic spaces that conform to the expected location and shape of the renal calices and infundibula and communicate with a dilated renal pelvis. Marked hydronephrosis (grade 3) refers to severe dilatation that is associated with cortical thinning. Moderate hydronephrosis (grade 2) refers to dilatation of the collecting system that is readily evident but is not associated with cortical thinning. Mild hydronephrosis (grade 1) refers to minimal amounts of urine producing slight distention of the collecting system. The cause of obstruction due to stones or pelviureteric junction abnormalities can also be detected on ultrasound.

Ultrasound is useful tool to detect renal cyst and mass lesions. It can be useful in differentiating a simple, benign renal cyst from a more complex cyst. It is used to screen for and diagnose polycystic kidney disease. Simple renal cysts **(Fig. 4.9)** are the most common renal mass lesions. Their prevalence increases with age; are usually asymptomatic and are diagnosed incidentally on abdominal

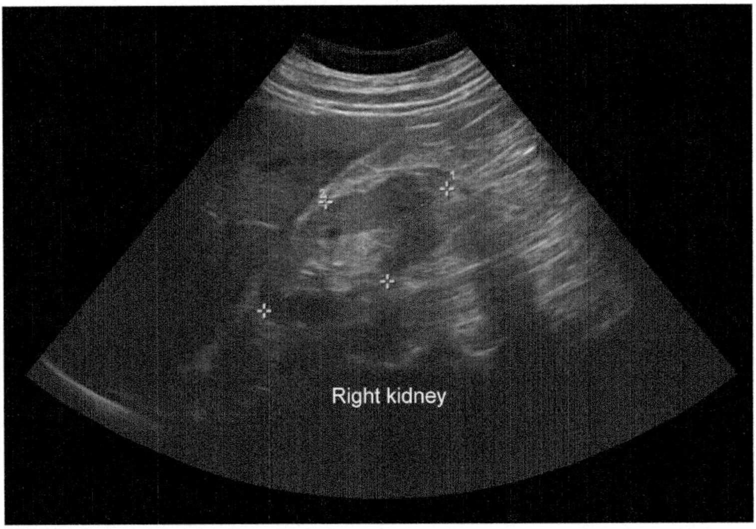

Figure 4.8 Sagittal ultrasound image showing small kidney with increased echogenicity and lost corticomedullary differentiation in a patient with chronic kidney disease

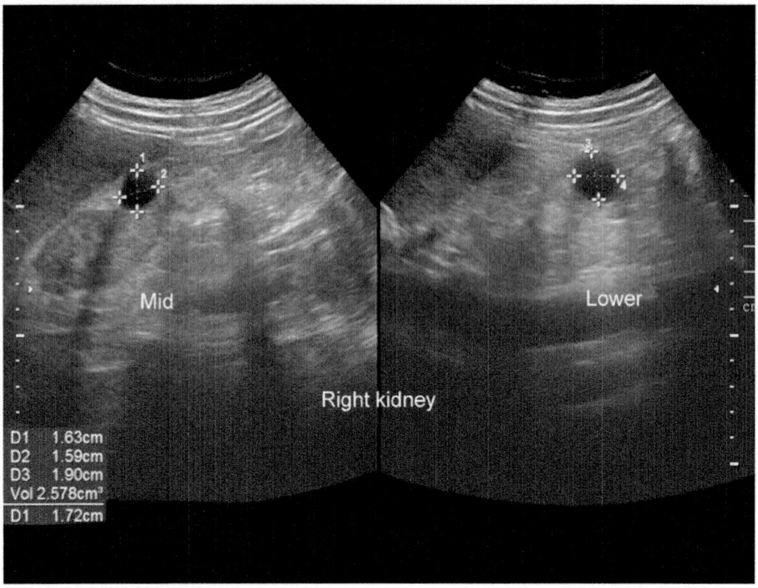

Figure 4.9 Ultrasound showing simple cortical renal cyst

Table 4.23 Ultrasound Criteria for Diagnosis of ADPKD (Revised Unified Diagnostic criteria)

Age (years)	*Number of cyst*
15–29	≥3 cysts, unilateral or bilateral
30–39	≥3 cysts, unilateral or bilateral
40–59	≥2 cysts in each kidney
≥60	≥4 cysts in each kidney

sonography. These are anechoic and have thin or imperceptible wall and no signal on Doppler. Complicated renal cyst refers to any cyst that does not display entirely simple features. These may contain calcifications, septations and nodules. These are likely to have hemorrhage, infection or malignancy. Bosniak renal cyst classification system is used to classify them further for management and require contrast enhanced CT for the same.

Acquired cystic kidney disease is associated with dialysis and prevalence rise with increasing length of dialysis. Cysts are of 0.5–3.0 cm and form in failing kidneys that are not otherwise cystic. These are usually asymptomatic. Autosomal dominant polycystic kidney disease (ADPKD) is a multisystem disorder characterized by multiple bilateral renal cysts with enlarged kidneys with cyst in other organs as well. The diagnostic criteria for ADPKD are in **Table 4.23**. Various causes of renal cyst are given in **Table 4.24**.

Renal cell carcinoma (RCC) appears as a solid tumor mass, distorting the normal renal architecture often with a 'ball' pattern of growth rather than an infiltrative pattern. Reflectivity of cortex may be increased, decreased or similar when compared to the normal renal cortex. The larger tumors are more likely to

Table 4.24 Cystic disease of kidney
Simple renal cyst
Complicated renal cyst
Acquired cystic disease of kidney
Autosomal recessive polycystic kidney disease
Autosomal dominant polycystic kidney disease
Multicystic dysplastic kidney
Von Hippel–Lindau disease
Tuberous sclerosis

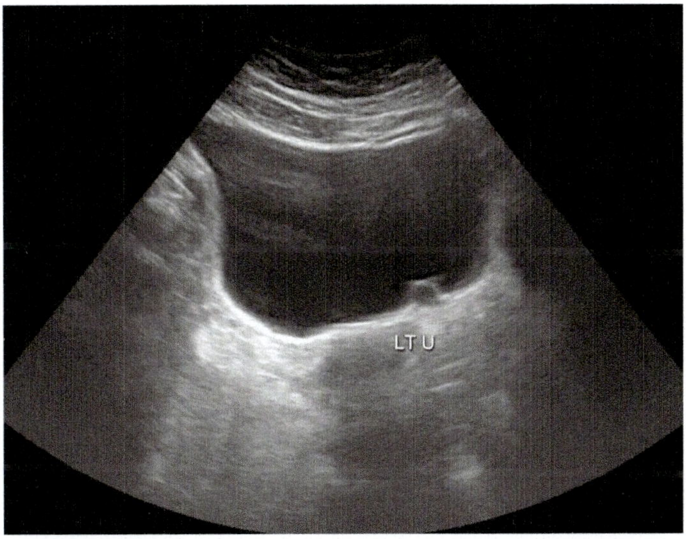

Figure 4.10 Ultrasound urinary bladder showing ureterocele

have central necrosis or hemorrhage Calcification is found in 30% of RCCs but not in angiomyolipoma. This calcification may be rim-like but is more commonly central. Ultrasound may also be used to detect abnormalities, such as ureterocele **(Fig. 4.10)**.

DOPPLER ULTRASONOGRAPHY

Doppler ultrasonography is used for renal vascular anatomy and can be used to evaluate renal artery stenosis, renal vein thrombosis, and renal infarction. The narrowing of renal artery will cause velocity change and waveform change commensurate with the degree of the stenosis. The waveform becomes dampened downstream the stenosis site. This leads to decrease in the resistive index (RI). Doppler ultrasonography is used to obtain the renal resistive index, which is calculated from the following formula:

(Peak systolic velocity–end diastolic velocity) ÷ Peak systolic velocity

The normal renal resistive index is <0.7. A high renal resistive index can be observed in a wide variety of disorders and is dependent primarily on extrarenal hemodynamic rather than intrarenal factors.

Features of significant renal artery stenosis:

- *Elevated peak systolic velocity*: Velocities in the stenotic segment >1.8–2.0 m/s correlate well with stenosis of >60% diameter reduction
- *Renal artery/aorta ratio*: An RAR >3.5 correlates with stenosis >60%
- *Acceleration time*: An AT >0.07 s correlates with a stenosis >60%
- *Loss of the early systolic peak (ESP)*: Proximal stenosis results in changes to the intrarenal waveform with loss of the ESP and a 'tardus parvus' appearance.

Color Doppler examination is useful in confirming the lack of venous flow in the main renal veins and within the kidney parenchyma in severe cases of renal vein thrombosis. In more severe cases the renal artery flow reduces to the baseline in diastole, or may even show reverse diastolic flow. In patients with occlusion of segmental intrarenal veins, venous Doppler signals may still be apparent within the renal parenchyma and the only clue to venous thrombosis may be a decrease in arterial diastolic flow, secondary to the increased intrarenal vascular resistance.

COMPUTED TOMOGRAPHY

Computed tomography (CT) is the computerized reconstruction of X-ray-generated image which depicts a slice through the body area being studied. The X-ray tube produces a highly collimated fan-bean and is mounted opposite the electronic detectors. This system rotates in tandem around the patient. The detector system collects hundreds of thousands of samples representing the X-ray attenuation along the line formed from the X-ray source to the detector as the rotation occurs. These data are transferred to a computer, which reconstructs the image. The image is displayed on a computer monitor or transferred to radiograph film for reviewing. Hounsfield unit (HU) scale is used to detect the relative densities of common substances compared to distilled water at standard pressure and temperature and is defined as 0 HU.

CT of kidneys is now the investigation of choice for the patients with stone diseases **(Fig. 4.11)**, hydronephrosis **(Fig. 4.12)**, pelviureteric junction abnormalities, renal masses, retroperitoneal masses, renal abscess, acute pyelonephritis, hematuria and to locate ectopic kidneys. Noncontrast CT is usually the first investigations for nephrolithiasis and renal cystic disease. CT urography (CTU) involves injection of iodinated contrast agent and assesses the anatomy of kidney along with function and perfusion. It also evaluates the excretory patterns. Early phase scans leads to arterial phase assessment (12–15 seconds). Scanning at 25–30 seconds yields a combined arterial-venous phase with clear corticomedullary differentiation. Nephrogenic phase imaging of the kidneys is obtained at 90–100 seconds. Nonenhanced areas may be caused by scars, pyelonephritis, infarction or mass lesions. Delayed imaging, typically at 3–7 minutes, provides excretory phase images with evaluation of calyces, renal pelvis, ureters, and bladder. Delayed excretion is found in cases of obstruction caused by stones or strictures.

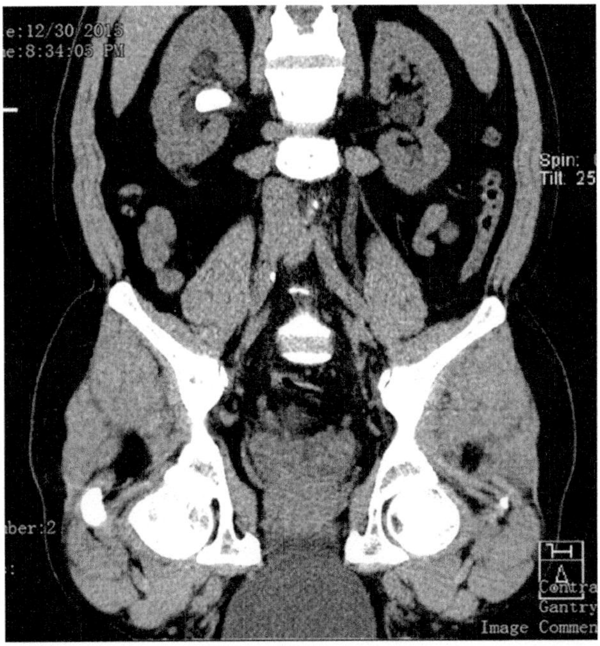

Figure 4.11 CT image of right renal stone in renal pelvis

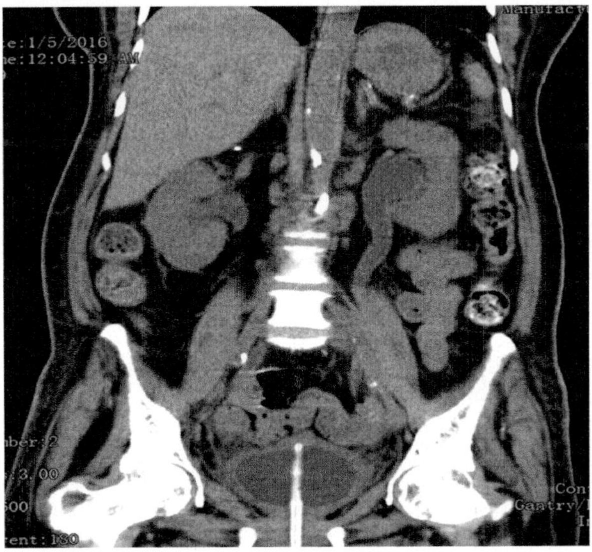

Figure 4.12 CT image showing hydroureteronephrosis

CT angiography (CTA) provides information regarding arterial and venous anatomy. CTA is commonly used for renal donor for evaluating the number, size and location of renal arteries and veins. CTA has sensitivity of 96% and specificity of 99% for detection of hemodynamically significant renal artery stenosis.

CTA can also diagnose fibromuscular dysplasia with sensitivity of 87%. Renal artery and renal vein thrombosis can be diagnosed on CTA **(Fig. 4.13)**. Contrast-enhanced CT and CTA are contraindicated in patients with allergy to iodinated radiographic contrast agents and low glomerular filtration rate. Patients should be adequately hydrated with intravenous saline to decrease the risk of contrast-induced nephrotoxicity.

Contrast-enhanced CT scan is also used to characterize the type of renal cyst and identify the presence of complexity if any, which has important bearing in decision making for cysts **(Table 4.25)**.

■ MAGNETIC RESONANCE IMAGING

MRI is usually not the first modality of imaging in renal disease. Nevertheless, it can be useful in variety of clinical settings and can be an important tool for

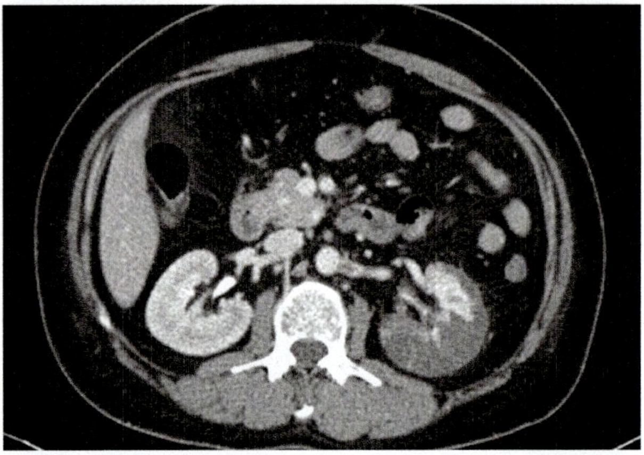

Figure 4.13 CT image of left renal artery thrombosis leading to infarct

Table 4.25 Bosniak renal cyst classification

Category	*CT features*	*Significance*
I	• Thin wall, water density and does not enhance • No septa, calcification or solid component	Benign
II	• Thin septa with "perceived" enhancement • Fine or slightly thick calcification • High attenuation nonenhancing cyst <3 cm	Benign
IIF	• Thick regular septa with "perceived" enhancement • Thick regular wall with "perceived" enhancement • Thick nodular and irregular calcification	Likely benign Follow-up required
III	• Thick smooth or irregular septa • Thick smooth or irregular wall • With measurable enhancement	About 50% malignant
IV	• Criteria of category III • Enhancing mass independent of wall or septa	Malignant cystic carcinomas

evaluation of various renal diseases. Noncontrast-enhanced MRI can be used in patients with renal dysfunction. Also, it can be used in patients where radiation exposure needs to be avoided. It is helpful if patient is allergic to iodinated iv contrast media.

Principle

MRI makes use of a strong magnetic field to align spins of hydrogen nuclei present in human body producing measurable *magnetic moment*. The nuclei will precess in the direction of magnetic field (termed as *Larmor precession*). The magnetic field used is usually between 0.5 and 1.5 Tesla.

A radiofrequency (RF) pulse is applied perpendicular to the strong magnetic field. This leads to tilting of magnetic moment away from the previous magnetic field. Once the radiofrequency pulse is removed, the nuclei realign and magnetic moment returns to equilibrium known as *relaxation*. During relaxation nuclei lose energy and emit their own RF signal. This is measured and processed to obtain MR images. These signals are encoded for each dimension to produce a 3D image.

The presence of contrast in an MR image depends on longitudinal relaxation time T1 and transverse relaxation time T2. T1 is the time required for the magnetic moment to return to equilibrium while T2 is time required for free-induction response signal decay. Fast spin echo (FSE) is a rapid sequence variant of T2. In a T1 weighted (T1W) image fat and protein rich fluid appears bright while air, dense bone and fluid such as urine, CSF appears dark. In a T2W image, cyst, edema, CSF and water appears bright while fat and solid lesion appears dark. Kidneys in a T1W image has higher signal in cortex than medulla.

Most commonly used intravenous contrast in MR imaging is gadolinium. MRI used to detect blood flow and many other anatomical structures do not need contrast due to the varying properties of blood and tissue acts as natural contrast. Gadolinium contrast although safe in patients with mild renal dysfunction, in those with severe renal dysfunction (such as end stage renal disease patients on dialysis), it can lead to nephrogenic systemic fibrosis.

Magnetic Resonance Angiogram

MR angiogram can be used to detect renal artery stenosis. A gadolinium contrast-enhanced MRI has very high sensitivity and specificity (>90%) while a non-contrast image has poor sensitivity and specificity. MRA is a very good alternative in cases with mild renal dysfunction where use of iodinated contrast can lead to contrast-induced nephropathy or if there is allergy to iodinated contrast material. It can help detect arterial or venous thrombosis.

Magnetic Resonance Urogram

There are two types of MR urogram:

1. *Dynamic*: Here repeat T1W images are taken after administration of intravenous contrast. It is also known as excretory MRU. Contrast is filtered and excreted by kidneys thereby giving some idea about renal function.

2. *Static*: As urine contains water, a T2W image will appear bright and stand out against darker soft tissue background. Presence of ascites or fluid elsewhere in pelvis or abdomen can interfere with the images.
   CT urogram should be used if one is suspecting calculus in urinary tract as cause of obstruction while, MR urogram is used if there is a high suspicion of noncalculous obstruction **(Fig. 4.14)**.

Magnetic Resonance Imaging for Evaluation of Renal Masses

A solid or cystic lesion can be detected and further delineated in patients by using MRI. MRI has higher sensitivity and specificity for detection of such lesions when compared to ultrasound. It can differentiate between simple and complex cysts. It is also helpful in assessing the extent of lesion in perirenal tissue **(Fig. 4.15)**.

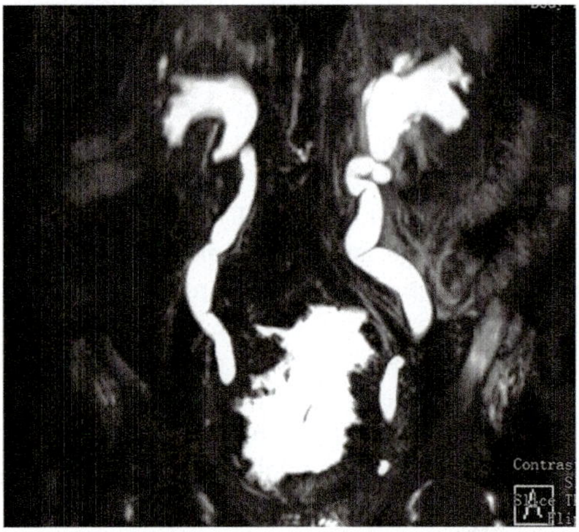

Figure 4.14 MR urogram showing bladder mass with bilateral hydroureteronephrosis

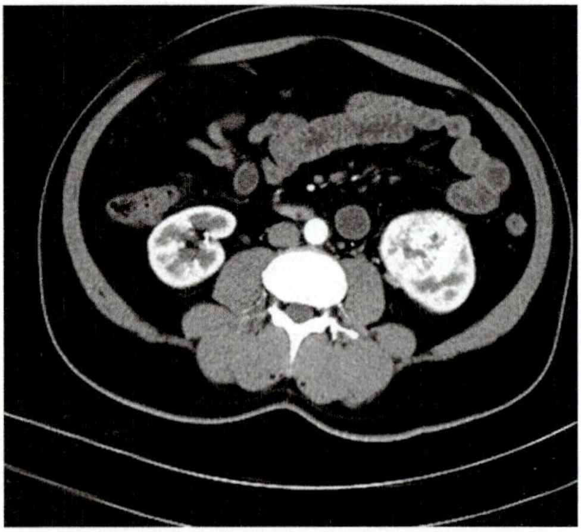

Figure 4.15 MRI showing left renal mass

SUMMARY

- Radiological imaging is an important tool for diagnosis of renal disease
- Judicious and timely use is helpful in patient management
- One should know which imaging modality to prefer in various clinical condition
- Unnecessary use of intravenous contrast should be avoided in patients with renal disease to avoid contrast-induced nephropathy.

ACKNOWLEDGMENTS

We would like to acknowledge Dr Vivek Sharma and Dr Rajiv Yadav for the images provided for this chapter.

Multiple Choice Questions

1. **Which of the following will qualify for diagnosis for ADPKD by Unified diagnostic criteria?**
   a. ≥ 3 cysts unilateral of bilateral in a patient 15–39 years
   b. ≥ 2 cysts in each kidney in a patient 40–59 years
   c. ≥ 4 cysts in each kidney in a patient ≥60 years
   d. All of the above

2. **Normal resistive index on renal artery doppler is:**
   a. <0.7 b. <0.8
   c. <0.9 d. <1

3. **Features of significant RAS on renal Doppler include:**
   a. Velocities in the stenotic segment >1.8–2.0 m/s
   b. Renal artery/aorta ratio > 3.5
   c. Acceleration time >0.07 s
   d. All of the above

4. **A 24-year-old patient Mr RM presents with colicky right lumbar pain radiating towards groin. He has past history of renal stone disease. Best imaging modality for detecting renal stone disease in such a patient is:**
   a. Plain X-ray abdomen b. Ultrasound KUB
   c. Computed tomography scan d. Magnetic resonance imaging

5. **Nephrogenic phase images in a CT urogram is obtained at:**
   a. 12–15 seconds b. 25–30 seconds
   c. 90–100 seconds d. 120–150 seconds

6. **A 67-year-old patient Mr RN, who is a known case of type 2 diabetes mellitus, hypertension and peripheral vascular disease presents with worsening hypertension despite using full dose of four different antihypertensives. Suspecting renal artery stenosis he underwent CT angiogram. Sensitivity and specificity of CT angiogram for detection of hemodynamically significant renal artery stenosis is:**
   a. 90% and 95%, respectively b. 96% and 99%, respectively
   c. 93% and 98%, respectively d. 95% and 90%, respectively

7. MRI is useful if:
  a. Radiation exposure is to be avoided
  b. Patient is allergic to iodinated iv contrast
  c. In case of renal dysfunction to avoid contrast-induced nephropathy
  d. All of the above

8. Which of the following appears bright on T1W MRI?
  a. Air
  b. Fat
  c. Bone
  d. Urine

9. Which of the following appears dark on T1W MRI?
  a. Cyst
  b. Edema
  c. Solid lesions
  d. CSF

10. Large kidneys (>12 cm) on ultrasound is associated with:
  a. Polycystic kidney disease
  b. Infiltrative disease
  c. Renal vein thrombosis
  d. All of the above

Answers

1. d 2. a 3. d 4. c 5. c 6. b 7. d 8. b
9. c 10. d

SUGGESTED READING

1. American College of Radiology. Appropriateness criteria. Available at: http://www.acr.org/ac.
2. Amis ES, Hartman DS: Renal ultrasonography: A practical overview. Radiol Clin North Am. 1984;22(2):315-32.
3. Bosniak MA.The small (less than or equal to 3.0 cm) renal parenchymal tumor: detection, diagnosis, and controversies. Radiology. 1991;179:307.
4. Caoili EM, Cohan RH, Korobkin M, et al. Urinary tract abnormalities:initial experience with CT urography. Radiology. 2002;222:353-60.
5. Hattery RR, Williamson Jr B, Hartman GW, et al. Intravenous urographic technique. Radiology. 1988;167:593-9.
6. Israel GM, Bosniak MA. An update of the Bosniak renal cyst classification system. Urology. 2005;66:484-8.
7. O'Neill WC, Bardelli M, Yevzlin AS. Imaging for renovascular disease. semin Nephrol. 2011;31:272-82.
8. Page JE, Morgan SH, Eastwood JB, et al. Ultrasound findings in renal parenchymal disease: Comparison with histological appearances. Clin Radiol. 1994;49: 867-70.
9. Pei Y, Obaji J, Dupuis A, et al.Unified criteria for ultrasonographic diagnosis of ADPKD.J AM Soc Nephrol. 2009;20:205-12.
10. Tublin ME, Bude RO, Platt JF. Review—The resistive index in renal Doppler sonography: Where do we stand ? Am J Roentgenol. 2003;180:885-92.

NUCLEAR MEDICINE IMAGING IN NEPHROLOGY

Arun Kumar Reddy Gorla, Harbir Singh Kohli, Bhagwant Rai Mittal

INTRODUCTION

Nuclear medicine is a distinct division of medical imaging that involves the utilization of radionuclides in minute concentrations to evaluate disease settings. Its uniqueness lies in the fact that it involves administration of radiolabeled substances that functionally mimic physiological molecules, which is then followed by assessment of dynamics of this substance in the body using external (imaging/counting) instrumentation. Thus, unlike conventional anatomical imaging modalities, nuclear medicine involves appraisal of physiological processes and pattern of alterations in these processes under pathological situations. In the present generation of medical imaging, functional imaging using radiolabeled tracers has increasing importance due to the emergence of hybrid imaging modalities including SPECT/CT and PET/CT.

Renal pathologies were one of the earliest disorders evaluated using radionuclide imaging as early as 1924. Advances in instrumentation and availability of novel radiopharmaceuticals and techniques lead to the increased use of radionuclide imaging in these disorders. Despite poor resolution, scintigraphic techniques are unique in that they can provide differential renal function. Additional advantages of being non-invasive, relatively non-operator dependent nature and involvement of minimal risk facilitated widespread application of these techniques. This chapter is intended to familiarize the physicians with various applications of radionuclide imaging in nephrology. We will discuss the basic principles of radionuclide renal imaging, various radiopharmaceuticals, types of scintigraphic techniques available, utility of these techniques in various clinical indications (including renal failure, renovascular hypertension, transplant kidney evaluation, infective conditions of kidney and vesicoureteric reflux) and concludes by briefly summarizing the role of PET imaging in nephrology.

Principles of Radionuclide Renal Imaging

Excretory function is the most important domain among the several different functions of the kidney. In renal nuclear medicine, specific radiolabeled molecules (most common radionuclide being ^{99m}Technetium) are administered that proceed through various physiological pathways of renal excretion (including glomerular filtration, tubular secretion and tubular reabsorption) and the distribution and dynamics of these tracers is recorded using external instrumentation (usually a gamma camera/well counter). Specific tracers are combined with appropriate imaging/counting techniques to monitor the status and changes in a given physiological process.

Radiopharmaceuticals

Radiopharmaceuticals available for assessment of renal function can be categorized into three basic types: (a) Tracers excreted by glomerular filtration, (b) Tracers that are actively excreted by tubular secretion, and (c) Tracers that are reabsorbed by tubular cells from the lumen. The characteristics of different radiopharmaceuticals are depicted in **Tables 4.26 and 4.27**.

Techniques of Radionuclide Renal Imaging

Dynamic Renal Scintigraphy

It involves the acquisition of sequential images immediately after the administration of rapidly excreted renal radiopharmaceuticals, such as ^{99m}Tc-DTPA, ^{99m}Tc-EC and ^{99m}Tc-MAG3. This technique allows the visualization of the various phases of tracer dynamics from the vascular compartment to the urinary collecting system via the renal parenchyma. This technique can simultaneously provide qualitative evaluation of the overall renal function, the differential renal function (split function), and the patency status of urinary tract. Tracer dynamics follow three phases during the dynamic renal imaging: the perfusion phase, that represents the blood flow to the kidneys (first minute); followed by cortical phase, representing the extraction of tracer by the renal parenchyma (subsequent 2–3 min); and the excretory phase, representing the outflow into the collecting system. The dynamic study is usually followed by static sequences in pre-void, post-void and delayed phases until adequate clearance of the activity is noted.

These renograms provide an overview of the renal function and drainage at a glance. In normal individuals, the perfusion phase is characterized by the visualization of both kidneys simultaneously within 3–5 seconds of the aortic visualization (aorto-renal interval); cortical phase by rapid renal uptake (through glomerular filtration/tubular extraction) of tracer from the vascular pool reaching the maximum by 2–3 min (depending upon the extraction fraction of the tracer) and the subsequent drainage phase by prompt clearance of tracer from the kidneys into the pelvicalyceal-ureteric drainage pathway. **Figure 4.16** depicts a normal dynamic renal study showing the three phases of the renogram curve. In addition to qualitative interpretation, quantification of renal function (in the form of GFR or ERPF depending upon the tracer utilized) is feasible using computational algorithms applied to ROI based counting after correction for background, attenuation and normalization to the injected activity. Although not completely accurate, these values are sufficiently reliable. This form of typical dynamic renal scintigraphy can be enhanced by addition of a pharmacological challenge to the study in the form of a diuretic or an angiotensin converting enzyme (ACE) inhibitor. These pharmacological-challenge enhanced scintigraphic studies (called as diuretic renography and ACE-I renography respectively) are utilized to evaluate specific disease settings and will be discussed in greater detail in subsequent sections.

Static Cortical Scintigraphy

This technique involves the administration of slowly excreted renal radiopharmaceuticals that are characterized by prolonged cortical retention

Table 4.26 Renal radiopharmaceuticals classified on the basis of predominant mode of renal handling

Category	*Radiopharmaceutical*	*Predominant mode of renal handling*	*Extraction fraction*	*Plasma protein binding*	*Renal parameter assessed*
Glomerular tracers	^{99m}TcDTPA	Glomerular filtration	~20%	< 5 %	GFR
	^{51}Cr-EDTA		–	< 5 %	
	^{125}Iothalamate/diatrizoate		–	–	
	^{14}C/^{3}H – Inulin		–	–	
Tubular tracers	^{123}I/^{131}I Hippuran	Tubular secretion	~90%	~95%	ERPF
	^{99m}Tc EC		~55–65%	~50%	
	^{99m}Tc MAG3		~40–50%	~70%	
Cortical tracers	^{99m}Tc DMSA	Tubular cell reuptake	~ 40% @ 3 hrs§		DRF, cortical morphology
	^{99m}Tc Glucoheptonate*		~20% @ 3 hrs§	~90 %	

Abbreviations: GFR: Glomerular filtration rate, ERPF: Effective renal plasma flow, DRF: Differential renal function

*Glucoheptonate can also be used for dynamic renal scintigraphy (See text)

§Renal cortical binding at 3 hrs; extraction fraction is in the range of 0.5–2%

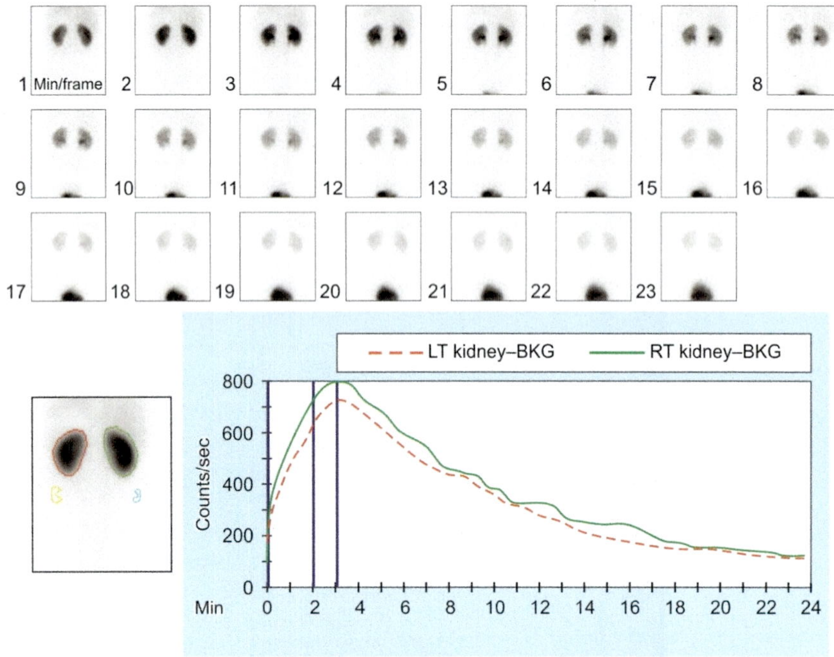

Figure 4.16 Dynamic renal scintigraphy showing normal kidney function; good tracer uptake and clearance

(such as ^{99m}Tc-DMSA) followed by imaging after few hours. Accumulation of tracer is limited to the functioning tubules and thus tracer uptake represents the distribution of the functional renal mass. This enables the assessment of renal morphology and simultaneously facilitates the calculation of differential renal function.

Static imaging is usually performed in anterior and posterior views at least 2–3 hours after intravenous administration of the radiopharmaceutical. The radiopharmaceutical gets trapped in the proximal tubular cells after its slow and progressive uptake from the tubular lumen. A normal cortical scintigraphy is characterized by homogenous tracer uptake in the bilateral renal cortices with uniform cortical margins and negligible background tracer activity. Impairment in renal function is noted as diffuse or patchy areas of reduced tracer uptake (in diseases like pyelonephritis, infarction, scarring, etc.) depending upon the underlying etiology. This may be associated with raised background activity and liver uptake when the renal insufficiency is severe enough. Its ability to visualize the functional renal mass enables the evaluation of various renal anomalies including agenesis, ectopia, horseshoe kidney, dysplasia, etc.

Radionuclide Cystography

Radionuclide cystography (RCG) can be performed using two approaches:

1. *Direct radionuclide cystography (DRCG)*: The technique is similar to voiding cystourethrography (VCUG) requiring bladder catheterization followed by

luminal instillation of a low activity of a radiopharmaceutical (such as ^{99m}Tc-sodium pertechnetate, sulphur colloid or DTPA) and fluids (amount of which is calculated using age related formulas) for maximal distension of the bladder. Images are acquired during filling, voiding and post-void phases and are visual interpreted for reflux of tracer activity. Main limitations of DRCG are the relative invasive nature, and non-physiological emulation of bladder filling. An alternative methodology practiced at some centers involves instillation of the radiopharmaceutical into distended clinically palpable bladder using a thin gauge needle of adequate length through suprapubic route.

2. *Indirect radionuclide cystography (IRCG)*: This technique usually follows a dynamic renal scintigraphy and does not require bladder catheterization. In the presence of normal cortical function, tracer activity is significantly cleared from the kidneys by the end of dynamic study. The accumulated tracer activity in the bladder may be utilized to emulate the fluid filled bladder with instilled radiopharmaceutical of DRCG. Imaging is obtained during voiding and post-void phases to look for retrograde movement of tracer activity along the ureters. Main limitations of IRCG are the need for toilet-trained patients and interference of tracer activity from ongoing renal clearance. Due to the limitation of poor anatomical detail, RCG is only indicated as per current guidelines in evaluation of established VUR after medical management, after antireflux surgery and during serial follow-up.

Radionuclide Techniques for Clearance Estimation

Evaluation of renal function has a pivotal importance in nephrology practice. GFR is one of the most representative objective parameter for the estimation of renal function. Estimation of GFR is useful in assessment of degree of renal impairment and monitoring of renal function over a period of time. Renal function can be assessed by two different techniques:

1. *Serum/plasma markers*: Historically, urea concentration in the blood was used as marker of renal function. Later, creatinine has been shown to be more consistent than urea. Several formulae have been proposed to calculate GFR based on serum creatinine concentration, some of which in routine clinical use (e.g. Cockcroft-Gault formula, MDRD equation).
2. *Clearance based markers*: Renal clearance is the volume of plasma from which all the substance might have been cleared in a given minute. Renal clearance of a substance is given by the formula: Clearance = (UV/P) Where U: urinary concentration V: Volume of urine P: plasma concentration of the substance. The renal clearance of a substance which is freely filtered and neither reabsorbed nor excreted in the tubules gives the GFR. Similarly, renal plasma flow is defined for a substance extracted exclusively by tubular secretion. Two types of methods are described for the estimation of renal clearance:
   - *Non-radionuclide based*: Inulin clearance is considered the gold standard for the estimation of GFR. However, estimation of GFR through inulin clearance has phased out after the introduction of radionuclide methods like ^{51}Cr-EDTA.

- *Radionuclide based techniques*: These techniques involve injection of a radiolabeled tracer in a single bolus dose followed by serial blood sampling at regular intervals. This facilitates the measurement of plasma concentration of the tracer over time and thus can estimate the rate of disappearance of the tracer, which gives the clearance of the tracer.

Alternatively, when radionuclides with favorable imaging properties are used (e.g. ^{99m}Technetium) external imaging instrumentation (gamma camera) can be employed to assess the rate of clearance of tracer. Also, this method facilitates the calculation of split renal function and thus provides objective functioning of individual kidneys. However, an inherent limitation is that the values derived through camera based method are usually at a lower level than assessed by plasma sampling based clearance assessment methods. Depending on the use of either glomerular or tubular agents used, GFR or RPF (renal plasma flow) can be calculated. For estimation of renal plasma flow (more exactly ERPF) tubular tracers like ^{99m}Tc MAG3, ^{99m}Tc EC, ^{123}I/^{131}I Hippuran are utilized.

Clinical Applications

Radionuclide renal imaging holds a unique role in the clinical practice of nephro-urology. This importance stems from the fact that it can provide functional information regarding the perfusion of the kidneys, their functioning (of even individual kidneys) and urinary tract dynamics simultaneously. Fair insight in to the renal pathophysiology and knowledge regarding limitations and potential technical pitfalls is essential in deducing complete information from these studies.

Urinary Tract Dilatation

The need for evaluation urinary tract dilatation is to rule out obstruction as the cause, which if left untreated can lead to renal impairment. However, it is not uncommon to have dilated urinary system with no real obstruction (dilated nonobstructive systems). Hence, to differentiate a dilated non-obstructed urinary system from a true obstruction, a state of forced diuresis is created using pharmacological intervention by furosemide during the dynamic renal scintigraphy, called the diuretic scintigraphy.

Urinary tract dilatation in adults is always considered pathological as obstruction is contemplated in most of the cases and is only rarely due to undetected congenital abnormalities. However, in children, it can be due to various pathological or non-pathological disease entities, including obstruction but either vesicoureteric reflux (VUR) or other para-physiological situations, although the most worrisome condition is an obstructive system. Diuretic scintigraphy plays an impactful role in the evaluation of urinary tract dilatation by discriminating between obstructed and non-obstructed system, as well as assessing the functional and urodynamic results of a corrective surgery.

For diuretic renography, tubular excreted tracers such as ^{99m}Tc-MAG3, ^{99m}Tc-EC and ^{123}I-OIH are generally preferred over glomerular agents like ^{99m}Tc-DTPA because of their higher renal extraction fraction and rapid plasma clearance, especially in patients with impaired renal function. The usual recommendation is that diuretic renography be delayed until the age of 4 weeks as renal tubules are immature and may be unable to respond to the effect of furosemide. Furosemide is often used at a dose of 1 mg/kg, up to a maximum of 20 mg in children and 40 mg in adults (SNMMI and EANM guidelines). Effect of furosemide begins 1–2 min after administration and usually peaks at 10 min of the study.

Response to diuretic is usually evaluated using visual and quantitative interpretation of the dynamic acquisition. Post-voiding images are required to rule out distended bladder delaying the drainage. Bladder catheterization is not routinely indicated but is strongly advised in neurogenic, dysfunctional, or low-capacity bladder. Adequate hydration and renal function are also important determinants of response to furosemide. Background-corrected renogram curves are utilized to assess urinary drainage and to calculate differential renal function. Unobstructed system is characterized by prompt tracer washout whereas a rising curve will be highly suggestive of true obstruction.

Time from peak to half the peak (diuretic T1/2) is a helpful parameter, albeit its drawbacks. Normally, it is usually less than 10 min. A value greater than 20 min strongly suggests obstruction. Values in between 10 and 20 are considered equivocal. Several other quantitative parameters like 20 min/peak ratio, 20 min/3 min ratio, output efficiency, pelvic excretion efficiency, parenchymal transit time, normalized residual activity are proposed to aid in the visual interpretation, although none stands valid comprehensively. An F-15 study, with furosemide administered 15 min prior to tracer administration is recommended to clarify equivocal studies. Differential renal function represents individual contribution of each kidney to the overall renal function and has a normal range of 45–55%. A value below 40% or a decrease of more than 5% on serial diuretic studies is generally considered indicative of deterioration. False-negative results are rare and can occur due to highly compliant renal pelvis or presence of marked diuretic response masking a partially obstructed system.

Chronic obstruction can result in loss of renal parenchymal function due to increased backpressure. Using tubular excreted tracers, this is usually manifested as reduced slope of the curve and reduction in differential renal function. However, fallacious reduction in DRF can occur due to compensatory enlargement of the contralateral non-affected kidney, although the actual function of the affected kidney is actually stable. GFR measured using blood sampling ^{51}Cr-EDTA and differential renal function measured during renography can be combined to obtain a single-kidney GFR which remains the gold standard for surveillance of deterioration in renal function.

Renovascular Hypertension

Renovascular hypertension (RVH) is characterized by elevated blood pressure secondary to a stenotic lesion within the main renal artery or its proximal branches. It is estimated to be the cause in ~1–3% of all hypertensive patients and 15–30% of patients with refractory hypertension. However, not all stenotic lesions are accountable for RVH as essential hypertension coexisting with an innocuous renal artery stenosis is a familiar entity. Hence, the final diagnosis of RVH is always retrospective, confirmed only after improvement/resolution of hypertension following revascularization.

Inhibition of the renin-angiotensin-aldosterone (RAA) pathway using ACE inhibitors (ACEi) and demonstration of resultant reduction in renal perfusion constitutes a simple and effective pharmacological challenge test in the evaluation of a stenotic lesion. An ACEi enhanced renography involves performance of two scintigraphic studies (baseline and challenge tests) either on same or different days (single day/two day protocol). After adequate patient preparation (hydration, medication withdrawal, 4 hours fasting for solids; baseline dynamic renal scintigraphy is performed using ^{99m}Tc-DTPA or ^{99m}Tc-MAG3/EC. ACEi challenge renography is performed 60 min after administration of Captopril (25–50 mg, p.o; 0.5 mg/kg in children) or 15 min after Enalaprilat administration (40 μg/kg, IV; maximum of 2.5 mg). ACEi blocks the compensatory RAA activation, by reducing activation of angiotensin II thereby decreasing the GFR due to withdrawal of constrictive influence on efferent arteriole. Most specific criterion for interpretation is the demonstration of change in renogram following ACEi. Absolute or relative reduction in renal uptake is noted in affected kidney with glomerular filtered tracers while increased cortical retention is the salient feature when tubular tracers are utilized (Refer to SNMMI guidelines for further reading). Findings are reported as low, intermediate and high probability for RVH. An overall sensitivity and specificity of above 90% is reported in detection of RVH when the affected kidney has normal or minimally reduced function. However, in azotemic patients lower values are observed. **Figure 4.17** represents a captopril positive renal scintigraphy in a hypertensive patient, indicating high probability of RVH.

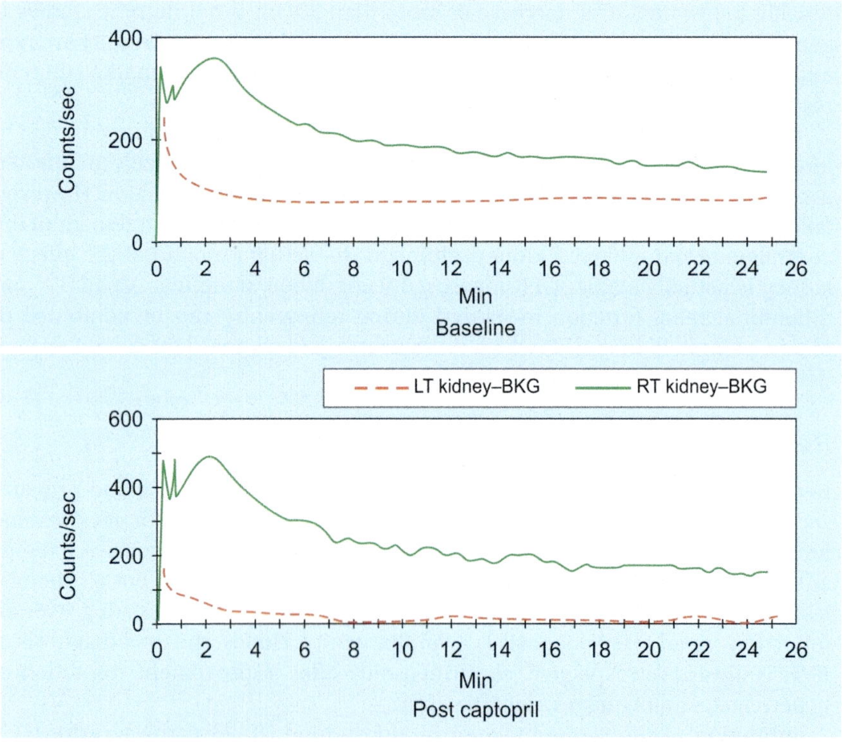

Figure 4.17 Captopril renal scintigraphy, upper baseline and lower post-captopril, showing deterioration in left kidney function

Transplant Kidney Evaluation

With the increasing incidence of ESRD, renal transplantation has become a customary procedure. In the recent decades, remarkable improvement is noted in the short-term graft survival due to advances in immunosuppressive therapy, surgical techniques and monitoring modalities. Advancement in imaging modalities has a notable contribution to this betterment. Early transplant complications such as repeated episodes of acute rejection and delayed graft function are considered to be predecessors of chronic allograft dysfunction, which is the most common cause for long-term graft loss. Rapid diagnosis and management of these early post-transplant complications is of paramount importance for overall graft survival. Although increasing utilization of renal biopsy has subdued the role of transplant renal scintigraphy, it still bears important role in specific clinical settings.

Transplant renography **(Fig. 4.18)** is essentially similar to the typical dynamic renal scintigraphy except that the gamma camera is positioned anteriorly over the pelvic region (to obtain best possible proximity with the transplanted kidney in right iliac fossa). Since perfusion phase is the key, higher activity of bolus tracer administration is required. Quantitative perfusion parameters including K/A ratio (ratio of the slope of the ascending portions of the renal and iliac arterial curves; Normal: 0.64–1.16) and Hilson's perfusion index (ratio of the AUC of the arterial curve to peak and renal curve to peak; N < 1.5) can be calculated to provide objective assessment of perfusion. Additional challenge with diuretics and ACEi may be incorporated into the study to address specific clinical settings of suspected RAS or obstructed drainage.

Several patterns of findings may be noted some of which overlap between various complications and therefore interpretation should be done keeping in mind the age of the transplant, current clinical question, ongoing medications, type of allograft (more incidence of vasomotor nephropathy in cadaveric). Normally, perfusion phase usually depicts intense tracer pooling in the initial seconds with slow progressive uptake in further study. Transplant kidney usually clears slightly slower than a healthy native kidney (living related better than cadaveric). **Table 4.28** lists the various complications and the pattern of scintigraphic findings. Both vasomotor nephropathy and acute rejection present as reduced function and marked cortical retention with a reduced initial slope of the renogram curve and progressive raise indicating accumulation of cortical tracer activity with delayed visualization of collecting system. However, perfusion phase is normal in vasomotor nephropathy while impaired perfusion is noted in acute rejection. Also, on serial imaging, improvement of function is noted in vasomotor nephropathy while deterioration after initially documented normal function is suggestive of evolving acute rejection. Worsening function in vasomotor nephropathy often suggests simultaneous alternate pathology like acute rejection. Availability of initial perfusion study at 24–48 hours following transplant (though not commonly performed), is very helpful in differentiating persistent vasomotor nephropathy and acute rejection with high confidence. Immunosuppressive drug toxicity also presents with rapid tracer uptake and cortical retention in a pattern similar to vasomotor nephropathy. Timing after transplantation is helpful in differentiating the two complications.

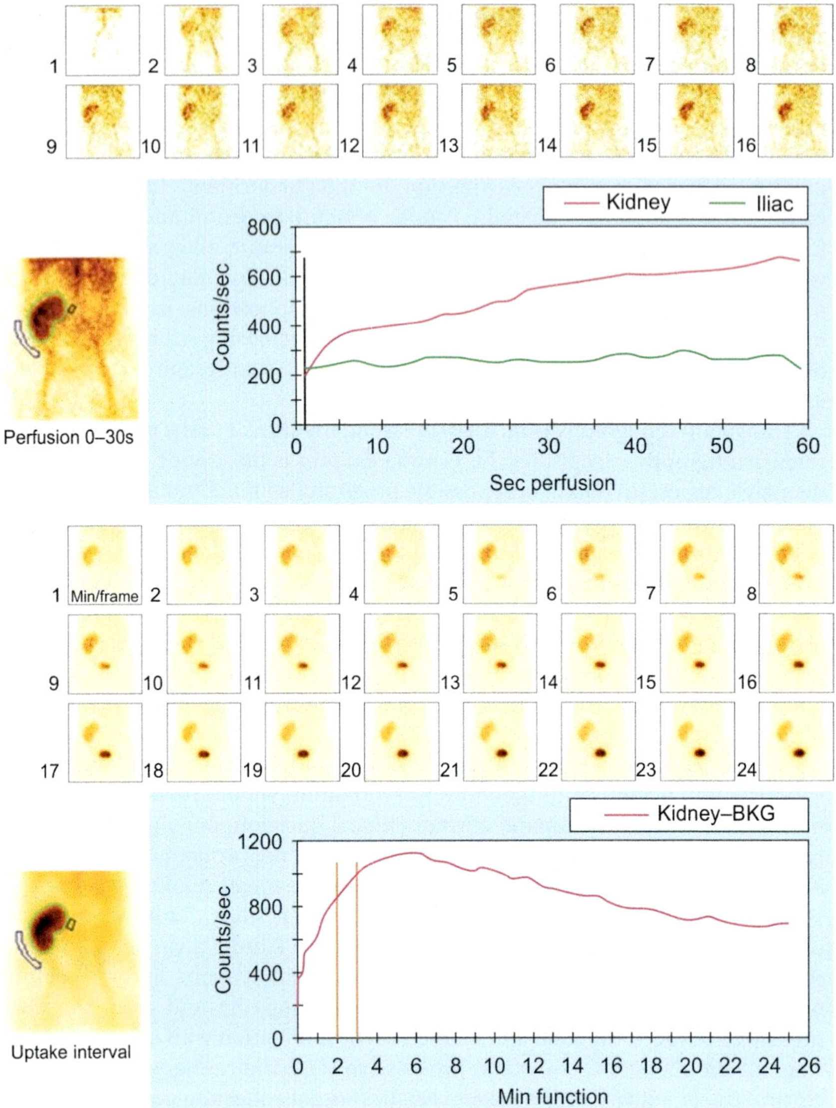

Figure 4.18 Dynamic renal scintigraphy in a post-renal transplant recipient showing normal kidney function

Perfusion and cortical uptake may appear normal in early chronic allograft nephropathy. However, on serial imaging, deterioration in quantitative parameters (like ERPF, GFR) is usually noted along with increasing cortical retention is seen. Renal artery occlusion/venous thrombosis are relatively rare events, but however, needs to be suspected in patients with anuria. Negligible perfusion is noted with a large photopenic area on cortical phase in renal artery occlusion. Renal vein thrombosis is characterized by the classic appearance of an enlarged kidney with intense cortical retention although has variable appearance

Table 4.27 Renal radiopharmaceuticals classified on the basis of predominant mode of renal handling

Radiopharma-ceuticals	*Modes of renal handing / extraction fraction*	*Imaging / sampling*	*Renal parameters derived*	*Protein binding*	*Clinical indications*
^{99m}TcMAG3	Tubular secretion (40–50%)	Imaging	ERPF	~95%	To diagnose upper urinary tract obstruction. To differentiate obstructed from dilated non-obstructed system For decision making to determine which patients will benefit from surgery and which can be safely managed conservatively
^{99m}Tc EC	Tubular secretion (55–65%)	Imaging	ERPF	~50%	
123I / 131I Hippuran	Tubular secretion (80%) + glomerular filtration (20%) (EF = 90%)	Imaging	ERPF	~70%	
^{14}C / ^{3}H – PAH	Tubular secretion + glomerular filteration (90%)	Sampling	ERPF		
^{99m}TcDTPA	Glomerular filteration (20%)	Imaging	GFR + ERPF	<5%	Monitoring of drugs that may cause nephrotoxicity. Calculation of dose in chemotherapy. Detection of renal failure Assessment of potential live donors for transplantation Evaluation and follow-up of renal function in patients with chronic glomerulopathies
^{51}Cr-EDTA	Glomerular filteration	Sampling	GFR	<5%	
^{125}Iothalamate/ Diatrizoate	Glomerular filteration	Sampling	GFR		
^{14}C/^{3}H – Inulin	Glomerular filteration	Sampling	GFR		
^{99m}Tc DMSA	Cortical binding (40% at 1 hrs)	Imaging	Renal morphology and differential function	~95%	For detection of pyelonephritis during a suspected acute attack.
^{99m}Tc Glucoheptonate	Cortical binding + glomerular filteration (20% at 2 hrs)	Imaging	Renal morphology and differential function	~95%	Gold standard for detection of renal scars 9-12 months following an attack of pyelonephritis

depending on severity and stage of resolution. Lack of venous collaterals in a transplanted kidney yields the appearance as that of renal artery occlusion in renal venous thrombosis unlike native kidneys.

Postoperative leaks result in formation of urinoma, which may attain large sizes before becoming symptomatic. Significant (major) leaks are characterized by active tracer extravasation outside the urinary tract causing abnormal pooling tracer. However, minor leaks may present initially as photopenic defect (due to pre-existing non-radiolabeled urine), which progressively fills on subsequent delayed images. Other collections such as lymphoceles may present with variable patterns of scintigraphic findings and often require correlation with other imaging modalities. An obstructed transplant kidney can present with hydronephrosis or reduced urine output. Diuretic enhanced renography as mentioned previously could be useful in a way similar to that in native kidneys.

Glomerular Filtration Rate Estimation

Estimation of actual value of glomerular filtration rate (GFR) is of paramount importance not only in prospective kidney donors but also in staging of chronic kidney disease (CKD) patients. As described earlier, GFR may be calculated by clearance or uptake (Gate's) method. Gates's method does not provide absolute values but can give percentage function of each kidney and hence GFR contribution by each kidney. This is a good method for follow-up of the same patient. Clearance method is the most common method employed in clinical practice. GFR calculation can be done by taking multiple blood samples after intravenous administration of radiotracer. In a prospective kidney donor, only two samples may be sufficient but in patients with deteriorating renal function, multiple samples, usually 5, are required.

Scintigraphy and GFR calculation combined together not only gives the near true GFR of the healthy kidney donor, but also by providing a differential function helps in decision making regarding the choice of nephrectomy.

Urinary Tract Infections

Urinary tract infections (UTI) includes inflammatory process of the urinary tract (cystitis, pyelitis, etc.) and renal parenchyma as well (pyelonephritis). It is noted more frequently in children and affects girls twice as often as boys. Vesicoureteral reflux (VUR), urinary tract obstruction, renal calculi, and incomplete bladder emptying are the most common predisposing factors for UTI.

Acute pyelonephritis is commonly a consequence of reflux of infected urine. Clinical findings of fever, flank pain, and positive urine cultures can suggest a diagnosis of pyelonephritis, however, these are unreliable especially in children. Ultrasonography has reported very low detection rate for pyelonephritic changes (~38%) and scars (~65%). Cortical scintigraphy with ^{99m}Tc-DMSA has greater sensitivity than ultrasonography in detection of scars. A normal ^{99m}Tc-DMSA scintigraphy shows homogeneous tracer distribution in the renal cortex. In pyelonephritis, cortical tubular dysfunction in conjunction with inflammatory edema and ischemia results in reduced tracer uptake/retention resulting in cold defects. For the detection of pyelonephritis, ^{99m}Tc-DMSA is considered the gold standard imaging modality. Additional SPECT imaging significantly increases the

Table 4.28 Renal scintigraphic findings in various post transplantation complications

Category	*Complication*	*Timing after Tx*	*Perfusion*	*Renogram*
Medical	ATN (Vasomotor Nephropathy)	Min to hrs (usually resolved within 2 weeks)	Relatively preserved	DTPA: Descending, without a peak activity EC: Accumulative. Delayed cortical transit. Delayed time to maximal activity
	AR	5 days to years (most commonly within 3 months)	Decreased perfusion (preserved in low grade AR) EC: Slope of 2nd phase of perfusion curve: ascending/flat/ descending	Similar to ATN. Reduced uptake. Little or no tracer accumulation in the collecting system
	CR	Months to years	Deteriorated	Decrease in uptake
	CNI toxicity	Immediately to months	Usually preserved	Delayed renal transit time
Vascular	Renal artery thrombosi	Days to weeks	No perfusion	Photon deficient area
	Renal vein thrombosi	Days to weeks	No perfusion	Photon deficient area
Surgical	Urinoma	Days or weeks	*Major leaks*: tracer leak outside the urinary tract with abnormal pooling. *Minor leaks*: initially photopenic defect, which progressively fills	
	Lymphocele	2 – 4 months	• Initial photopenic area with a surrounding rim of increased tracer activity that is filled up with tracer on delayed image • Initial photopenic area without a surrounding rim of increased tracer activity, that is filled up with tracer on delayed image. • Persistent photopenia	
	Seroma	Immediately	Persisting photopenia	
	Hematoma	Immediately	Persisting photopenia	
	Ureteral obstruction	Days, months, years	• Normal perfusion. • Usually preserved cortical function. • Progressive increase in tracer accumulation in the PCS	
	Urinary leak	2 weeks	Progressive intense tracer accumulation	

Abbreviations: ATN: Acute tubular necrosis; AR: Acute Rejection; CR: Chronic Rejection, CNI: Calcineurin Inhibitor

sensitivity of ^{99m}Tc DMSA cortical scintigraphy over planar imaging, but requires sedation in children. Serial imaging is often performed to look for the recovery of the lesion(s). A time interval of at least 6 months is recommended to allow recovery. Nearly 80–85% of the lesions show complete recovery or significant improvement. Persistent defect on a follow-up scan is accounted as scarring. Good knowledge of anatomical variations in shape (splenic impression, fetal lobulation, etc.) is required to avoid potential misinterpretation.

Due to its ability to accurately demonstrate the functional renal tissue, cortical scintigraphy has also been used in the evaluation of renal pseudotumor (e.g., prominent column of Bertin noted on ultrasound as a renal mass), ectopic kidney and traumatic kidney injury etc. Tracer uptake is noted in the columns of Bertin but not in true renal mass and thus can differentiate between the two.

Vesicoureteric Reflux

Vesicoureteric reflux (VUR) is more commonly noted in pediatric population with an incidence of up to ~2%. It is usually detected early in life through indirect manifestations like prenatally detected hydronephrosis or UTI during childhood. VUR is commonly evaluated using VCUG and RCG. As briefed previously, RCG is more sensitive than VCUG for detecting reflux and imparts lower radiation dose to the patient. This high sensitivity is the result of the rapid and continuous dynamic imaging, which permits detection of reflux volumes of the order of 1 mL. No retrograde movement of radiotracer is noted into the ureters or kidneys in a normal RCG study. Any retrograde movement of tracer activity is considered abnormal and is detected as activity above the bladder. Grading system has been developed for the interpretation of RCG studies similar to the radiographic grading. RCG Grade I corresponds to the radiological grade I. A RCG grade II includes reflux in to the renal pelvis and corresponds to radiological grades II and III. Visualization of diffusely dilated urinary and pelvicalyceal system on scintigraphy is categorized as RCG grade IV which corresponds to radiological grades IV and V. RCG has relatively lesser sensitivity to grade I reflux, but however, this can be disregarded as it of little significance.

Direct radionuclide cystogram is the recommended investigation of choice now for evaluating suspected reflux in female children, adequacy of antireflux surgery/procedures and serial follow-up of patients on conservative management. VCUG is only currently reserved for the initial work-up of male patients (to exclude anatomical anomalies like posterior urethral valves) and screening of siblings of patients with reflux (40% have increased risk of VUR).

SUMMARY

- Renal radionuclide imaging techniques constitute a significant section of nuclear medicine procedures. They are safe, easy to perform and reproducible procedures, imparting lower radiation doses than their radiological counterparts.
- Despite poor anatomical resolution, they provide functional information and facilitate quantification of the renal function (especially the calculation of GFR and split renal function unlike other modalities).

- Additional strength of these procedures includes the scope for pharmacological challenging tests like diuretic and ACEi scintigraphy in the evaluation of specific disease entities.
- These advantages render radionuclide imaging techniques a special relevance in the clinical practice of nephrourology, especially in conditions, which require a functional comparison before and after a therapeutic intervention and those that require serial imaging during follow-up.

Multiple Choice Questions

1. **Which of the following is not used for dynamic renal scintigraphy:**
   a. ^{99m}Tc-DTPA
   b. ^{99m}Tc-EC
   c. ^{99m}Tc-MAG3
   d. DMSA

2. **Which of the following is used to assess renal morphology:**
   a. ^{99m}Tc-DTPA
   b. ^{99m}Tc-EC
   c. DMSA
   d. ^{99m}Tc-MAG3

3. **For direct radionuclide cystography which of the following can be used:**
   a. ^{99m}Tc-sodium pertechnetate
   b. Sulphur colloid
   c. DTPA
   d. All of the above

4. **For estimation of renal plasma flow which of the following is used:**
   a. ^{99m}Tc MAG3
   b. ^{99m}Tc EC
   c. ^{123}I/^{131}I Hippuran
   d. All of the above

5. **For diuretic renography least preferred agent will be:**
   a. ^{99m}Tc-MAG3
   b. ^{99m}Tc-EC
   c. ^{99m}Tc-DTPA
   d. ^{123}I-OIH

6. **A 56-year-old patient with history of longstanding type 2 diabetes mellitus, coronary artery disease and peripheral vascular disease and also a chronic smoker has presented with history of worsening hypertension despite being on 4 different antihypertensives. He also has history of deteriorating renal functions lately. Physical examination shows renal bruit. Overall sensitivity of ACEi enhanced renogram for detection of clinically significant renal artery stenosis in such a case is:**
   a. 60%
   b. 70%
   c. 80%
   d. 90%

7. **A 11-year-old boy presented with history of fever and painful micturition since 4 days. He also has abdominal tenderness. Urine microscopy shows numerous pus cells. For detection of pyelonephritis, best imaging modality in this case will be:**
   a. ^{99m}Tc-MAG3
   b. ^{99m}Tc-EC
   c. ^{99m}Tc DMSA cortical scintigraphy over planar imaging
   d. ^{99m}Tc-DTPA

8. **Which of the following is used to evaluate VUR:**
   a. VCUG
   b. RCG
   c. ^{99m}Tc DMSA
   d. Both VCUG and RCG

9. Which of the following can be used for the evaluation of a renal pseudotumor:

a. ^{99m}Tc-MAG3
b. ^{99m}Tc DMSA
c. ^{99m}Tc-EC
d. ^{99m}Tc-DTPA

10. Gold standard method for estimation of GFR is:

a. GFR measured using blood sampling of ^{51}Cr-EDTA
b. By serum creatinine using Cockcroft-Gault formula
c. 24 hours urinary creatinine clearance
d. ^{99m}Tc-DTPA

Answers

1. d 2. c 3. d 4. d 5. c 6. d 7. c 8. d
9. b 10. a

SUGGESTED READING

1. Aktaş A. Transplanted Kidney Function Evaluation. Seminars in Nuclear Medicine. 2014;44(2):129-145.
2. Biassoni L, Chippington S. Imaging in Urinary Tract Infections: Current Strategies and New Trends. Seminars in Nuclear Medicine. 2008;38(1):56-66.
3. Blaufox MD, Aurell M, Bubeck B, Fommei E, Piepsz A, Russell C, et al. Report of the Radionuclides in Nephrourology Committee on renal clearance. J Nucl Med. 1996;37(11):1883-90.
4. Boubaker A, Prior JO, Meuwly JY, Bischof-Delaloye A. Radionuclide investigations of the urinary tract in the era of multimodality imaging. J Nucl Med. 2006;47(11):1819-36.
5. Eanm. org. European Association of Nuclear Medicine—Guidelines [Internet]. 2016 [cited 12 January 2016]. Available from: *http://www.eanm.org/publications/guidelines/index.php?navId=37*
6. O'Reilly P, Shields R, Testa H. Nuclear medicine in urology and nephrology. London: Butterworths; 1979.
7. Prigent A, Piepsz A. Functional imaging in nephro-urology. London: Taylor and Francis; 2006.
8. Quaia E. Radiological imaging of the kidney. Berlin: Springer; 2010.
9. Snmmi.org. Procedure Standards—SNMMI [Internet]. 2016 [cited 12 January 2016]. Available from: *http://www.snmmi.org/ClinicalPractice/content.aspx?ItemNumber=6414*
10. Taylor A, Schuster D, Alazraki N. A clinician's guide to nuclear medicine. Reston, VA: Society of Nuclear Medicine; 2006.
11. Taylor A. Radionuclides in Nephrourology, Part 1: Radiopharmaceuticals, Quality Control, and Quantitative Indices. Journal of Nuclear Medicine. 2014;55 (4):608-615.

CHAPTER

5 Acute Kidney Injury

Vivekanand Jha

INTRODUCTION

Acute kidney injury (AKI) is defined as the abrupt loss of kidney function, resulting in the retention of nitrogenous waste products (azotemia). This decline is characteristically over a period of hours to days, differentiating it from "rapidly progressive renal failure" or "subacute renal failure", where this change occurs over days to weeks. The clinical presentation is largely with features of dysregulated extracellular volume, electrolyte, and acid-base balance. In some cases, especially in underdeveloped countries, presentation is delayed until more extreme features such as altered mentation or complications such as infections become apparent. AKI has replaced the older term, acute renal failure (ARF), because of the perception that the latter did not appropriately reflect the importance of acute but small decrements in kidney function on morbidity and mortality.

In this chapter, we discuss the currently accepted definition and classification system, the clinical presentation, evaluation and management. Not discussed are pathophysiology of AKI, details of diseases that may cause or be associated with AKI and their identification and management, which must be done as appropriate depending on the clinical circumstances.

DEFINITION AND CLASSIFICATION

Typically, the diagnosis of AKI is made by observing an increase in serum creatinine and/or a decline in urine output. Until the turn of the century, there was no agreed definition of ARF—there were scores of different definition, making them impossible to compare.

In 2002, the Acute Dialysis Quality Initiative (ADQI) Group, composed largely of nephrologists and intensivists, published the first draft of a new classification system. Risk, injury, failure, loss, end stage kidney failure (RIFLE), it proposed a graded classification of ARF. ADQI was later merged into acute kidney injury network (AKIN), which for the first time proposed replacing the term ARF with AKI, and proposed a 3-stage classification system. Eventually, the Kidney Disease—Improving Global Outcomes (KDIGO) harmonized and reconciled the differences between the two systems, and proposed a modified 3-stage system, which is now widely accepted.

All the systems use changes in serum creatinine and urine output to define and classify AKI—with variations in the degree of elevation in creatinine and

Table 5.1 RIFLE, AKIN and KDIGO classification systems for acute kidney injury

	Serum creatinine criteria			*Urine output criteria*
	RIFLE	*AKIN*	*KDIGO*	
Definition	↑ in serum creatinine >50% over <7 days	↑ in serum creatinine 0.3 mg/dL or >50% over <48 hours	↑ in serum creatinine 0.3 mg/dL over 48 hours or >50% over 7 days	<0.5 mL/kg/hour for >6 hours
Staging				
RIFLE-risk AKIN/KDIGO *stage 1*	↑ in serum creatinine of >50%	↑ in serum creatinine of 0.3 mg/dL or >50%	↑ in serum creatinine of 0.3 mg/dL or >50%	<0.5 mL/kg/hour for >6 hours
RIFLE-injury AKIN/KDIGO *stage 2*	↑ in serum creatinine of >100%	↑ in serum creatinine of >100%	↑ in serum creatinine of >100%	<0.5 mL/kg/hour for >12 hours
RIFLE-failure AKIN/KDIGO *stage 3*	↑ in serum creatinine of >100%	↑ in serum creatinine of >200%	↑ in serum creatinine of >200%	<0.5 mL/kg/hour for >6 hours or anuria for >24 hours
RIFLE-*Loss*	RRT needed for >4 weeks			
RIFLE-*End-stage*	RRT needed for >3 months			

Abbreviation: RRT, renal replacement therapy.

duration as well as volume of decline in urine output **(Table 5.1)**. The clinical utility of all 3 sets of criteria has been tested in a number of clinical studies, with variable results. These studies have validated the criteria by showing a graded increase in mortality as the severity of renal failure increases. Although useful for epidemiological studies and increasing the across-study comparability, there is no agreement on any action plan for management of these condition-based on the classification system. The criteria should be applied only after optimizing volume status and excluding urinary obstruction. Between the urine output and serum creatinine criteria, the one that classifies patients into the higher category should be used.

There is a separate definition and classification system for diagnosing AKI in children.

There have been several concerns with the use of serum creatinine as a marker for identifying AKI and the proposed classification systems **(Table 5.2)**. Despite all the limitations, there is a global consensus in using the KDIGO classification system until some new biomarker or a set of biomarkers of tubular injury are identified and validated.

CLINICAL PRESENTATION

Acute kidney injury is predominantly encountered in two clinical settings—either in community, or amongst already hospitalized patients **(Table 5.3)**.

Table 5.2 Concerns with use of serum creatinine and the current AKI definition and classification systems

•	Serum creatinine does not accurately reflect glomerular filtration rate (GFR) in early stages of AKI and in unstable conditions.
•	Elevation of serum creatinine significantly delays diagnosis, leading to loss of identification at which interventions might have been more helpful.
•	Creatinine is removed by dialysis, further reducing its value.
•	There is lack of agreement of establishing baseline kidney function in whom the baseline serum creatinine is not available.
•	Whether the current or ideal body-weight should be used to apply urine output criteria.
•	The current diagnostic and classification criteria cannot be used to make clinical judgments for patient management.

Abbreviation: AKI, acute kidney injury.

Table 5.3 Community and hospital acquired acute kidney injury

	Community acquired	*Hospital acquired*
Geography	Developing world, especially tropical countries	Developed world and tertiary care hospitals in developing world
Age	Usually younger	Usually elderly
Clinical setting	Tropical infection, volume loss secondary to diarrhea, obstetric accidents, Snake bite or insect stings, Toxic AKI secondary to consumption of nephrotoxic plants or animal products	Already hospitalized with pre-existing illnesses like complex surgeries, sepsis, organ failure
First encounter	Usually in clinics	Usually in ICUs
Pre-existing CKD	Usually absent	Usually present
Organ involved	Kidney often only involved organ, other specific organs involved depending on basis disease	Multiple organs requiring support
Identification	Presentation with advanced kidney failure, in late stages, with complications and imminent need for RRT	Identified on investigations, earlier stages more common
Course of AKI	Usually well-defined, depends on basic illness	Protracted
Long-term outcome	Data poor, recovery likely complete if basic disease recovers	Recovery likely partial, high likelihood of progressive CKD despite improvement of precipitating causes

Abbreviations: AKI, acute kidney injury; CKD, chronic kidney disease.

Acute kidney injury usually does not manifest with unique or tell-tale clinical symptoms. As discussed above, AKI in those already hospitalized is identified by noticing changes in serum creatinine and/or urine output since they are under routine monitoring. In other instances, AKI may be suspected by noticing symptoms and signs resulting from diminished kidney function, such as dyselectrolytemia (hyperkalemia, hyponatremia), acid-base imbalance (high anion gap metabolic acidosis), edema, hypertension or abnormal urinalysis.

Once AKI has been identified, the focus of clinical evaluation and subsequent investigations shifts to identifying the potential cause in particular to ensure removal of any offending factor. AKI can be reversed, if the underlying cause is quickly identified and addressed.

MAJOR CAUSES AND CLASSIFICATION OF AKI

Acute kidney injury can be classified in several ways, but for conceptual understanding as well as developing an implementable management approach, the classification scheme is based on the portion of the renal anatomy that is most affected: prerenal (decreased renal perfusion), intrinsic renal (disease of some element of renal parenchyma—tubules, glomeruli, vasculature or interstitium), or postrenal (obstruction, intratubular or extratubular). Such well-defined divisions are valid only in initial stages. For example, prolonged prerenal azotemia can lead to intrinsic acute tubular necrosis (ATN), and untreated urinary tract obstruction eventually causes interstitial inflammation and fibrosis **(Table 5.4)**.

EVALUATION

A carefully history is important, in particular to establish the timing of onset of AKI and identify the potential precipitating cause. It is important to carefully review the volume status of the patient while interpreting small changes in serum creatinine or recent decline in urine volume. While application of the diagnostic criteria in volume depleted patients may lead to overdiagnosis of AKI, volume expanded patients may show a blunting of the rise in serum creatinine due to dilution effect. A careful assessment of the urinary bladder must be done to rule out acute urinary retention in appropriate clinical settings. Persistent anuria (urine volume <50–100 mL/day) suggests the possibility of severe prolonged shock, rapidly progressive glomerulonephritis, bilateral urinary tract obstruction, bilateral diffuse cortical necrosis, or bilateral renal artery obstruction. Fluctuating urine volume suggests urinary tract obstruction.

A careful review of history and medication use is imperative, to establish etiology. In appropriate clinical settings, especially in AKI that has developed in community, the history must include an assessment of potential causes.

In community acquired AKI in the developing countries, this requires knowledge of local causes, such as plant and chemical toxins, animal bites, obstetric practices or cultural factors. Use of nephrotoxic medications requires a careful chart review in hospitalized subjects and history of over-the-counter medication use.

A physical examination is essential, with particular emphasis on the following:

- *Assessment of volume status*: Signs of volume contraction suggest a prerenal.

Table 5.4 Etiological classification of acute kidney injury

Prerenal	
•	*Volume loss*: Acute hemorrhage, diarrhea, or unreplenished insensible losses.
•	*Low effective arterial volume*: Heart failure, decompensated liver disease (hepatorenal syndrome).
•	*Alerted renal vascular autoregulation*: Caused by nonsteroidal anti-inflammatory drugs, or drugs blocking angiotensin pathway.
Intrinsic renal	
•	*Disease of small vessels*: Vasculitides, TTP/HUS, scleroderma, atheroembolic disease, and malignant hypertension.
•	*Disease of large vessels*: Aortic dissection, systemic thromboembolism, acute renal artery or vein thrombosis.
Glomerular	
•	Acute proliferative glomerulonephritides.
•	Nephrotic syndrome with superimposed hemodynamic insult.
Acute tubular necrosis	
•	After prolonged hypovolemia or renal ischemia.
•	*Toxic*: Drugs, radiocontrast agent, envenomations, hemolysis or rhabdomyolysis, toxic plants.
•	*Tropical infections*: Malaria, scrub typhus, dengue, etc.
•	Tumor lysis syndrome
•	Anticoagulant related nephropathy
•	Acute phosphate nephropathy
Acute interstitial nephritis	
•	Drugs
•	*Infections*: Leptospitosis, hemorrhagic fever with renal syndrome.
Postrenal	
•	*Bladder outlet obstruction*: Prostatic hyperplasia or cancer, metastatic cancer
•	Urothelial malignancy
•	Retroperitoneal fibrosis
•	Urolithiasis
•	*Intratubular obstruction*: Uric acid nephropathy, crystal nephropathy.

- *Cutaneous examination*: Skin rash may suggest AIN, cholesterol emboli or vasculitis.
- Volume overload and signs of heart failure suggest cardiorenal syndrome.
- Jaundice and findings of portal hypertension suggest hepatorenal syndrome.
- Lymphadenopathy and/or hepatosplenomegaly may suggest lympho-proliferative or other disseminated malignancies.
- Assessment may reveal features of pre-existing chronic kidney disease such as hypertension, unexplained anemia, bone disease.

Table 5.5 Urinalysis in differential diagnosis of causes of AKI

Finding	*Likely etiology*
Hematuria, RBC casts, proteinuria	Acute glomerulonephritis, anticoagulant associated nephropathy
Heavy proteinuria with bland sediment	Nonproliferative glomerulopathy with volume depletion or hemodynamic AKI
Granular and dirty brown casts, epithelial cells, minimal proteinuria	Acute tubular necrosis
Pyuria with or without erythrocyturia	Urinary tract infection, renal mucormycosis, interstitial nephritis
Eosinophiluria	Acute interstitial nephritis
Crystals	Intratubular obstruction by oxalate or drug crystals
Normal urinalysis	Urinary tract obstruction, prerenal azotemia or drug induced hemodynamic AKI, hypercalcemia, myeloma cast nephropathy, phosphate nephropathy, cardiorenal or hepatorenal syndromes

Initial testing must include urinalysis unless the patient is anuric. Of particular importance are microscopic examination of appropriately processed urine sample, and quantification of urine protein or albumin. Manual urine microscopy for the assessment of urine sediment is best performed by an experienced operator, and findings provide important diagnostic clues **(Table 5.5)**.

Special tests should be ordered only in appropriate clinical setting. In view of the fact, that there might be little clinical suspicion, it is appropriate to order serum or urine protein electrophoresis at the time of the initial evaluation in those over the age of 40 with unexplained AKI. Evaluation for glomerulonephritis and/or vasculitis should be based on initial clues.

Imaging

Imaging is an integral part of evaluation of AKI, unless the cause is apparent. The main reasons for performing imaging is to quickly establish or exclude urinary tract obstruction and to assess kidney size. In a large number of patients presenting for the first time with azotemia, imaging reveals small kidneys raising the possibility of unrecognized CKD.

The imaging technique of choice in patients with AKI is renal ultrasound since it is safe, easy to perform, and sensitive for obstruction. Special attention should be given to and volume of post-void residual urine.

Non-contrast computed tomography (CT) may be done among patients with possible urolithiasis. Contrast enhanced CT scan is indicated in appropriate situations, such as when infection of renal parenchyma, e.g. fulminant pyelonephritis, emphysematous pyelonephritis or renal mucormycosis are being considered. Magnetic resonance imaging (MRI) with gadolinium should be avoided among patients with AKI, as it can lead to nephrogenic systemic fibrosis.

The results of the urinalysis and ultrasound generally direct the remainder of the diagnostic evaluation **(Flow charts 5.1 and 5.2)**. For patients, who have

Flow chart 5.1 Evaluation of acute kidney injury among hospitalized patients

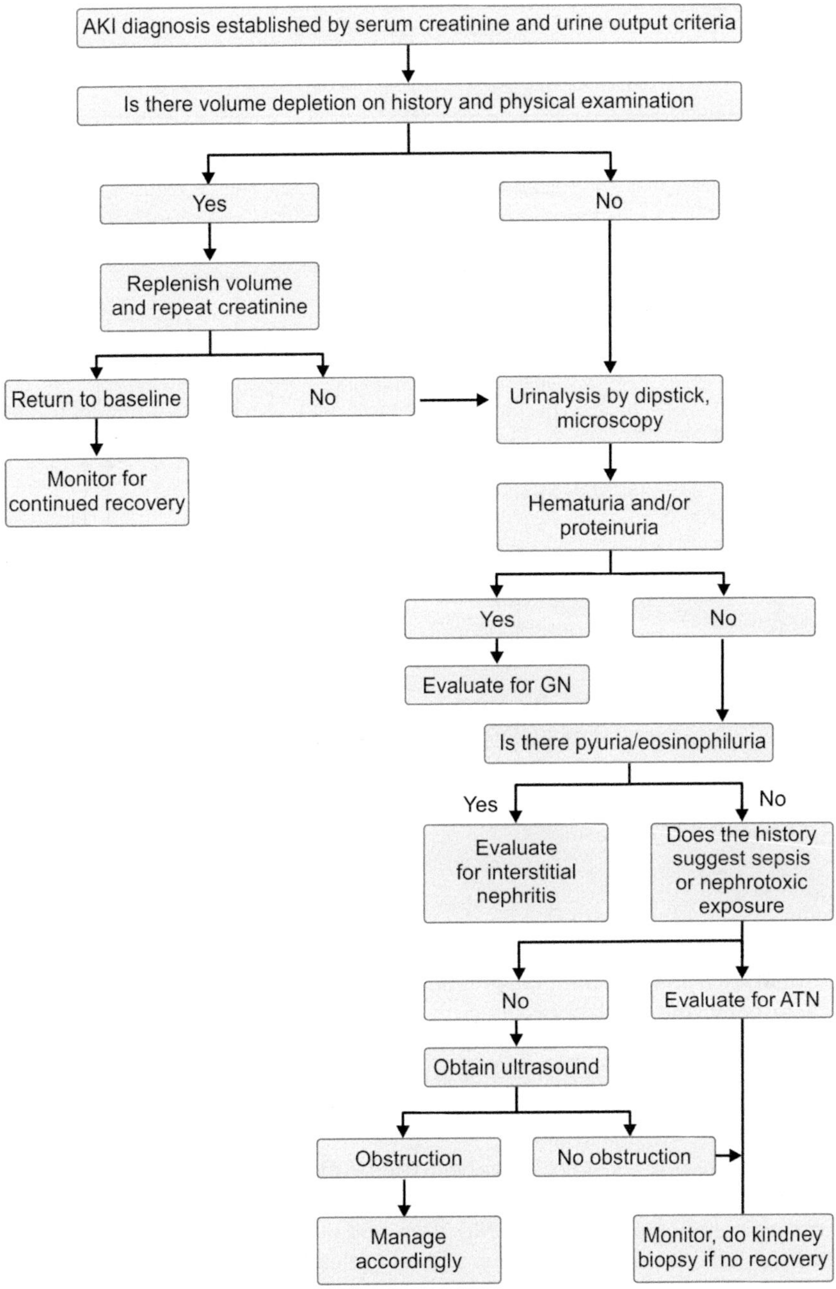

Flow chart 5.2 Evaluation and triaging of community-acquired acute kidney injury

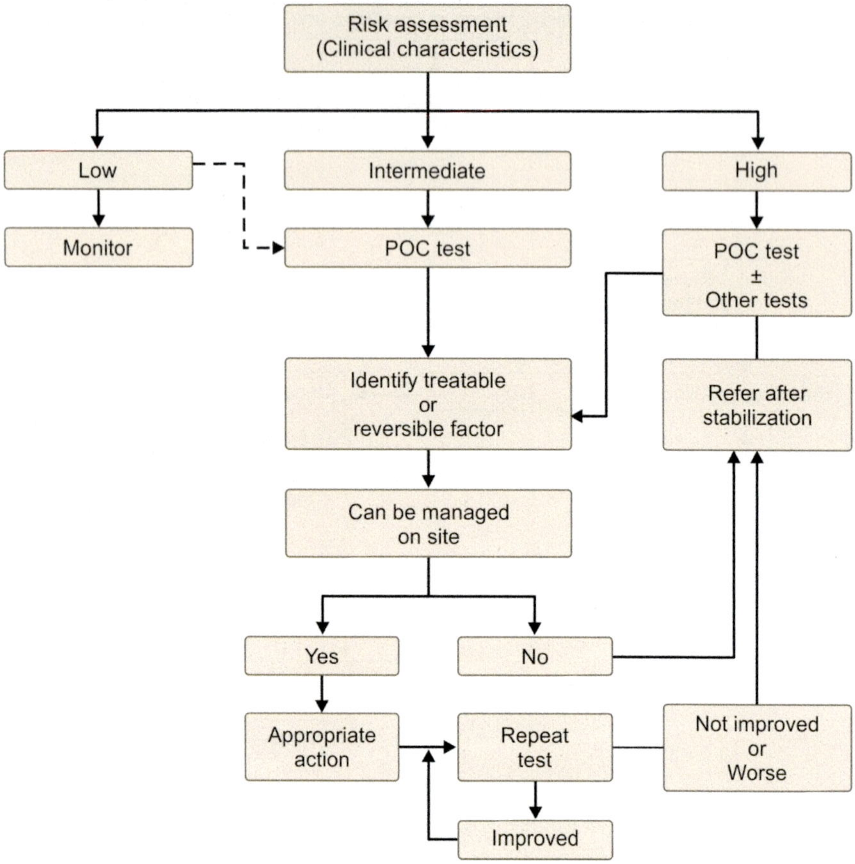

normal renal imaging, minimal proteinuria, benign urine sediment on urinalysis/microscopy, and no clear explanation for AKI, further evaluation is determined by the severity of disease and disease course.

Urinary Indices

Traditionally, urinary indices have been used to distinguish between acute tubular necrosis and prerenal azotemia **(Table 5.6)**. These indices include fractional urinary excretion of sodium (FENa), urea, and other molecules in AKI. Of all the indices, FENa is the preferred one, as it more clearly differentiates between these two conditions than other laboratory tests. It can be calculated as follows:

$$\text{FENa}(\%) = \frac{\text{UNa} \times \text{SCr}}{\text{SNa} \times \text{UCr}} \times 100$$

Table 5.6 Urinary indices for differentiating AKI from prerenal azotemia

Index	*Prerenal azotemia*	*Acute kidney injury*
Urine osmolality (mOsm/kg)	>500	<400
Urine sodium level (mEq/L)	<20	>40
Urine/plasma creatinine ratio	>40	<20
Urine/plasma urea ratio	>8	<3
Fractional excretion of sodium (%)	<1	>2
Fractional excretion of urea (%)	<35	>35

A few caveats need to be mentioned. The cut-off values apply only in patients with advanced AKI. All indices leave grey areas in which the differentiation is uncertain. Some conditions in which the FENa is <1% in the presence of AKI are early ischemic or toxic ATN, ATN superimposed upon a chronic prerenal disease, such as cirrhosis or heart failure, nonoliguric ATN, and radiocontrast media or pigment induced AKI. FEUrea may be helpful in patients who are being treated with diuretics, which can transiently raise the FENa above the diagnostic threshold.

Diuretic challenge: Administration of diuretics has not been shown to improve renal recovery in AKI. However, the increase of urine output often reflects less severe injury, and a single administration of high dose diuretic at appropriate rate can be justified. It also helps establish the diagnosis of prerenal azotemia.

Kidney biopsy: A kidney biopsy is needed when noninvasive evaluation has been unable to establish the correct diagnosis. Biopsy may be deferred if other findings and serologic testing strongly support diagnostic and therapeutic decision making or if the risk of biopsy outweighs the expected benefit. In patients, in whom there are no reasons to suspect glomerular, vascular or interstitial disease, kidney biopsy is usually deferred for 2–3 weeks.

If the creatinine is markedly elevated, worsens after an initial stable mildly increased value, is seen in the context of unexplained systemic disease and does not resolve quickly after withdrawal of potentially offending factors, a kidney biopsy should be considered.

In some cases, clues to the nature of kidney disease can be obtained from tissue diagnosis from other sites, such as a bone marrow biopsy showing multiple myeloma, lymph node biopsy showing lymphoma or malignancy or a fat pad biopsy showing amyloidosis.

MANAGEMENT

Acute kidney injury is the most common nephrological emergency. Patients may present with the following life-threatening complications requiring urgent management:

- Fluid overload
- Hyperkalemia

- Features of advanced uremia, such as pericarditis, unexplained decline in mental status
- Severe metabolic acidosis
- Dyselectrolytemias, e.g. hyponatremia, hypocalcemia

The initial management starts with an assessment of volume status, since both volume depletion and overload need immediate attention.

Volume Depletion

Assessment is done by history (e.g. vomiting, diarrhea, extreme exertion in hot and humid environment), physical examination (dry skin and mucosae, postural hypotension and tachycardia), and urinary indices. In ICUs, new monitoring techniques like ultrasound may be utilized to assess volume status. These patients should be immediately volume resuscitated using crystalloid solutions such as isotonic saline. Potassium-containing solutions, such as Ringer's lactate should be avoided until kidney function is established.

Fluid administration is continued until the initial physiological abnormalities are corrected, e.g. restored blood pressure or urine output. The infusion rate varies depending on the clinical status and comorbidities of the patient, with careful and repeated clinical assessment to assess the response to therapy.

Determination of volume status may be difficult, and invasive monitoring may be required to adequately assess the patient's fluid status to accurately guide the therapy. In the absence of these facilities, it is reasonable to start fluid replacement with intravenous saline at the rate of 75–100 mL per hour while ensuring there is no fluid overload, and the rate of administration is sufficient to keep up with ongoing fluid losses.

Volume Overload

Volume overload is suggested by the history of breathlessness, orthopnea, edema, engorged neck veins or pulmonary rales. Positive fluid balance is associated with mortality in patients with AKI. Short-term use of loop diuretics to relieve hypervolemia is appropriate, but prolonged therapy should be avoided. If there is no increase in urine output, dialysis should be started.

Amongst diuretics, agents that act on the loop of Henle are the preferred agents as they provide a greater natriuretic effect. In patients, who are refractory to high doses of loop diuretics, concomitant administration of a thiazide diuretic may achieve effective diuresis.

Hyperkalemia

Hyperkalemia is a common and potentially life-threatening complication of AKI. Immediate therapy **(Table 5.7)** is warranted for severe hyperkalemia, especially if electrocardiographic changes or neuromuscular abnormalities are present. Treatment is directed at combating the membrane effects of potassium, moving extracellular potassium into the cells, or removing excess potassium from the body. These therapies are temporizing methods in those with established oliguric AKI, and usually requires definitive treatment, e.g. dialysis.

Table 5.7 Management of hyperkalemia

Reversal of membrane actions of potassium	
•	*Intravenous calcium gluconate or chloride*: 500–1000 mg infused over two to three minutes, with constant cardiac monitoring.
Movement of extracellular potassium into the cells	
•	*Insulin and glucose*: 10 units of regular insulin in 500 mL of 10% dextrose, given over 60 minutes.
•	*Sodium bicarbonate (if metabolic acidosis)*: Isotonic solution (150 mEq in one liter of 5% dextrose in water over 2–4 hours)
•	*β2-adrenergic agonists*: Salbutamol, 10–20 mg in 4 mL of saline by nebulization over 10 minutes.
Removal of potassium from the body	
•	Loop or thiazide diuretics, combined with fluid therapy.
•	*Cation exchange resin*: Sodium polystyrene sulfonate (with or without sorbitol) 15–30 g, repeated every four to six hours as necessary.
•	Patiromer (not available in India).
•	Zirconium cyclosilicate (not available in India).
•	Dialysis

Metabolic Acidosis

This develops due to a combination of compromised renal acid excretion, acid overproduction due to sepsis, trauma, and multi-organ failure and loss of bicarbonate from diarrhea or renal tubular acidosis. Treatment includes dialysis and bicarbonate administration.

Dialysis is the preferred choice among volume overloaded patients with pH <7.1. Bicarbonate may be administered to patients who are not volume overloaded and have no other indication for dialysis, especially for non-anion gap acidosis related to diarrhea or in patients with rhabdomyolysis (e.g. Crush syndrome) in order to prevent further renal injury. Bicarbonate administration can precipitate or worsen hypocalcemia or hypernatremia.

It must be pointed out that dialysis alone may not be sufficient to correct the acidosis in those with excessive acid production due to shock, sepsis or exogenous acid administration unless the basic cause is corrected.

Other complications that may need attention include hypocalcemia (especially in those with rhabdomyolysis and acute pancreatitis), hyperphosphatemia (especially in those with evidence of cellular breakdown like tumor lysis syndrome or rhabdomyolysis), and bleeding disorders due to qualitative platelet dysfunction.

Nutrition

All patients with AKI must receive adequate amounts of energy, protein, and other nutrients. The details of therapy depend on the severity of the

Table 5.8 Indications for dialysis in AKI

•	Fluid overload refractory to diuretics.
•	Hyperkalemia (serum potassium concentration >6.5 mEq/L) or rapidly rising potassium levels, refractory to medical therapy.
•	Metabolic acidosis (pH <7.1) in patients in whom the administration of bicarbonate is not indicated.
•	Signs of uremia such as pericarditis, unexplained decline in mental status or bleeding diathesis.
•	Certain alcohol or drug intoxications.

underlying disease, pre-existing nutritional status, and comorbidities. The average caloric requirements are approximately 25–30 kcal/kg per day. Protein requirement depend upon the catabolic state: those with mild to moderate illness require 0.8–1.2 g/kg per day whereas the need goes up to 1.2–1.5 g/kg per day or more in critically ill patients or those on dialysis. Enteral nutrition is preferred because of its lower cost, less frequent and severe complications, less mucosal permeability, greater wound healing, and lower rates of infection.

Metabolic parameters should be monitored in all patients with AKI in ICUs. A suggested frequency is to check serum potassium, sodium, and bicarbonate twice daily. Body weight, serum calcium, phosphate, and albumin should be measured daily in stable patients.

Dialysis Therapy

Accepted indications for dialysis in patients with AKI are shown in **Table 5.8**. All patients with prolonged AKI and advanced azotemia should also receive dialysis. The optimal timing for starting dialysis is not known, and depends on overall clinical picture. In general, dialysis should be started prior to the development of symptoms and signs of renal failure due to AKI. This is based on evidence from observational and comparative studies that initiating dialysis at BUN 90–100 mg/dL, as compared with waiting until the BUN exceeded 150–200 mg/dL might be associated with better outcomes. The studies however suffer from several design limitations, limiting the strength of recommendation.

Dialysis modality: A large number of dialysis modalities are available for patients with AKI, including intermittent hemodialysis (IHD), peritoneal dialysis, continuous renal replacement therapy (CRRT), and hybrid therapies such as sustained low-efficiency hemodialysis (SLED).

Continuous renal replacement therapy (CRRT) include a suite of therapies such as continuous hemofiltration, hemodialysis, and hemodiafiltration, which are primarily driven by convection. Pump-driven venovenous therapies are preferred since they provides higher solute clearances and eliminates the complications associated with arterial cannulation.

There has been a lot of discussion on the choice of dialysis. Compared with HD, CRRT may offer a few advantages **(Table 5.9)**. A number of studies, albeit

Table 5.9 Potential advantages of CRRT over intermittent HD

•	Enhanced hemodynamic stability.
•	Increased net salt and water removal.
•	Enhanced clearance of inflammatory mediators, which may provide benefit in septic patients.
•	Better preservation of cerebral perfusion in those with or at risk of cerebral edema, such as acute brain injury or fulminant hepatic failure.

of variable quality, have looked at this question but failed to demonstrated the superiority of any form of therapy in terms of mortality, hospital stay, or recovery of renal function. Therefore, modality selection should be based upon local expertise and availability of staff and equipment.

Dialysis dose: A number of studies have examined the question of optimal dialysis dose for AKI, both for intermittent and continuous therapies. In general, comparative studies have been unable to show a benefit of more intensive dialysis therapies compared to the current standard of care. The Kidney Diseases: Improving Global Outcomes (KDIGO) Guidelines recommend a Kt/V of 3.9 per week for patients undergoing IHD. Another suggested approach is to give HD three times per week, with a targeted dose of ≥1.2 per treatment. The dialysis frequency may need to be increased if the targeted dose cannot be achieved or if there are other indications (e.g. hyperkalemia).

CRRT should be delivered with an effluent flow rate of ≥25 mL/kg per hour, to ensure a delivered effluent flow rate (sum of hemofiltration rate and dialysate flow rate) of ≥20 mL/kg per hour. This is based on observational studies that have suggested that the actual delivered effluent volume during CRRT is substantially less than the prescribed dose.

As with the two extracorporeal therapies, dose of dialysis has not been shown to effect outcomes in those receiving PD. A suggested minimum dose is a Kt/V of 0.5 per session.

Discontinuation of renal replacement therapy: Renal replacement therapy (RRT) is usually continued until recovery can be documented, as shown by increase in urine output in the initially oliguric cases, a progressive decline in serum creatinine concentration after initial attainment of stable values (before dialysis amongst those on IHD). For more objective assessment, creatinine clearance can be measured via 6-hour urine collections and midpoint sample for serum creatinine. A clearance of <12 mL/min is adequate to allow discontinuation of therapy.

PROGNOSIS

Most patients recover kidney function, as shown by increased urine output and a gradual decrease of the blood urea nitrogen and serum creatinine concentration. However, many patients, in particular those with pre-existing CKD do not return to baseline renal function **(Fig. 5.1)**.

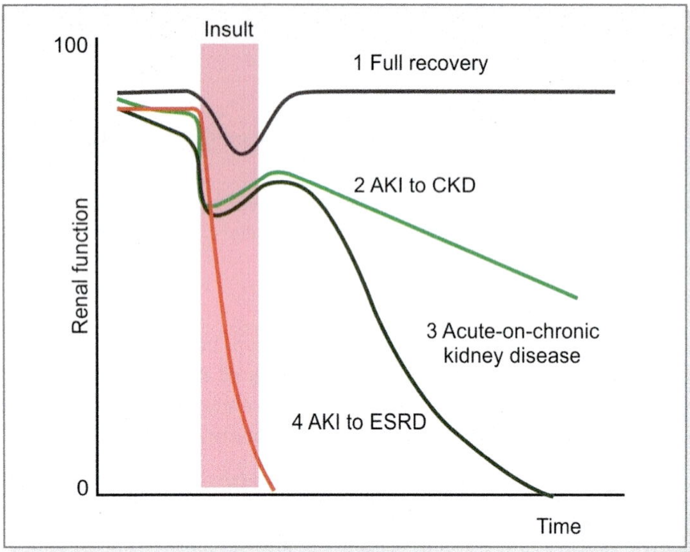

Figure 5.1 Clinical course of patients with acute kidney injury (From Cerda J, CJASN 2008;3:881-6)

BIOMARKERS IN ACUTE KIDNEY INJURY

One of the major limitations in institution of timely preventive measures to reduce complications and mortality due to AKI is the lack of an appropriate biomarker to identify early tubular injury. The absence of a renal "troponin" has been long lamented. Over the last decade, however, a number of molecules have been identified, and are being tested. These include neutrophil gelatinase-associated lipocalin (NGAL), kidney injury molecule 1 (KIM-1), cystatin C, interleukin-18, liver-type fatty acid-binding protein (L-FABP), tissue inhibitor of metalloproteinase-2 (TIMP-2) and IGF-binding protein 7 (IGFBP7). Unfortunately, the clinical utility of such a biomarker remains unclear, because large, prospective, multicenter trials, have failed to show troponin-like diagnostic performance.

In recent studies, the product of TIMP-2 and IGFBP7 predicted the onset of KDIGO stage 2 or 3 AKI within 12 hours with significantly greater accuracy than NGAL, KIM-1, IL-18, L-FABP, or cystatin C. The TIMP-2 × IGFBP7 product had areas under the receiver-operator characteristic curve of 0.8. Though promising, additional studies are needed to define its clinical role.

Despite simplistic comparisons with troponin, it has been pointed out that there are fundamental differences in the pathobiology of AKI and an acute myocardial infarction. Consequently, biomarkers of AKI are likely to be qualitatively different from troponins. It has been suggested that different biomarkers will reflect the different phases of pathophysiology of AKI, and some will be important in determining repair and recovery as well as defining progression to CKD **(Fig. 5.2)**.

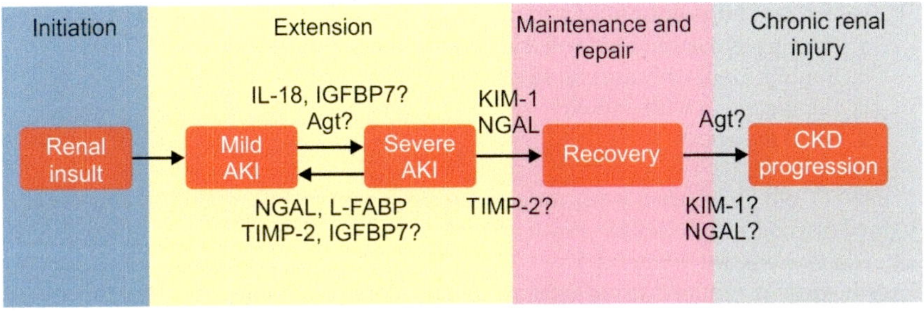

Figure 5.2 Biomarker integrated model of AKI (From CJASN 2015;10:147-55)

Multiple Choice Questions

1. **Diagnostic criteria of acute kidney injury depends on:**
   a. Urine output and serum creatinine
   b. Serum creatinine and blood urea
   c. Urine output and blood urea
   d. All of the above

2. **Concern with use of serum creatinine for defining AKI include:**
   a. It does not accurately reflect GFR in early AKI
   b. Elevation is significantly delayed thereby leading to delay in diagnosis and loss of precious time
   c. It is removed by dialysis, thereby reducing its value
   d. All of the above

3. **Most promising for prediction of AKI onset amongst the following in a patient is:**
   a. Serum cystatin C
   b. NGAL
   c. Product of TIMP-2 and IGFBP7
   d. KIM-1

4. **Target weekly Kt/V for patients undergoing hemodialysis is:**
   a. 2.7
   b. 3.9
   c. 4.9
   d. 5.9

A 30-year-old MR. RM presented with history of recurrent vomiting and loose stools of 2 days duration. He had not passed urine since last 12 hours. On presentation in emergency department his blood pressure was 90/60 mm Hg. He was tachycardic and had dry skin and mucosa. Investigation revealed blood urea 100 mg/dL and serum creatinine of 2 mg/dL, serum sodium 135 mmol/L, serum potassium 4.9 mmol/L.

5. **What is the most likely etiology of renal dysfunction in this case?**
   a. Prerenal AKI
   b. Postrenal obstruction
   c. Intrinsic renal
   d. Chronic kidney disease

6. **Urinary indices in this patient will show all except:**
   a. Urine osmolality 600 mOsm/kg
   b. Urine sodium 5 mEq/L
   c. Fractional excretion of sodium <1
   d. Urine/plasma creatinine ratio <20

7. **How should this patient be treated:**
   a. Prompt replacement of volume deficit with IV Ringer's lactate
   b. Replacement with normal saline
   c. Replacement with colloid
   d. All of the above

A 65-year-old gentleman with long standing hypertension, diabetes and chronic kidney disease with baseline serum creatinine of 1.7 mg/dL had been taking NSAID since one week for bilateral knee joint pain due to osteoarthritis. He presented with history of reduced urine output, nausea, loss of appetite and breathlessness. On examination, he had bilateral pedal edema, BP 170/90 mm Hg, raised JVP and bibasal crepitation on examination. Evaluation showed serum creatinine of 4.3 mg/dL, blood urea 110 mg/dL, serum sodium 127 mmol/L, serum potassium 6 mmol/L. Venous blood gas analysis showed metabolic acidosis with pH 7.14. USG ruled out any obstructive etiology.

8. **What will be the most appropriate next line of treatment?**
   a. IV sodium bicarbonate
   b. IV diuretics
   c. Potassium binding resins
   d. Hemodialysis

9. **Indication for dialysis is this case will be all except:**
   a. Hyperkalemia
   b. Serum creatinine 4.3 mg/dL
   c. Severe metabolic acidosis
   d. Fluid overload

10. **Daily protein requirement in above patient on dialysis will be:**
   a. 0.6–0.8 g/kg
   b. 0.8–1.2 g/kg
   c. 1.2–1.5 g/kg
   d. 1.8–2 g/kg

Answers

1. a	2. d	3. c	4. b	5. a	6. d	7. b	8. d
9. c	10. c						

SUGGESTED READING

1. Fliser D, Laville M, et al. Ad-hoc working group of ERBP. A European Renal Best Practice (ERBP) position statement on the kidney disease improving global outcomes (KDIGOs) clinical practice guidelines on acute kidney injury: part 1: definitions, conservative management and contrast-induced nephropathy. Nephrol Dial Transplant. 2012;27:4263.
2. Bellomo R, Ronco C, Kellum JA, et al. Acute renal failure—definition, outcome measures, animal models, fluid therapy and information technology needs: the Second International Consensus Conference of the Acute Dialysis Quality Initiative (ADQI) Group. Crit Care. 2004;8:R204.
3. Cho KC, Himmelfarb J, Paganini E, et al. Survival by dialysis modality in critically ill patients with acute kidney injury. J Am Soc Nephrol. 2006;17:3132.
4. Cruz DN, Bolgan I, Perazella MA, et al. North East Italian Prospective Hospital Renal Outcome Survey on Acute Kidney Injury (NEiPHROS-AKI): targeting the problem with the RIFLE Criteria. Clin J Am Soc Nephrol. 2007;2:418.
5. Espinel CH, Gregory AW. Differential diagnosis of acute renal failure. Clin Nephrol. 1980;13:73.

6. Esson ML, Schrier RW. Diagnosis and treatment of acute tubular necrosis. Ann Intern Med. 2002;137:744.
7. Kidney Disease: Improving Global Outcomes (KDIGO) Acute Kidney Injury Work Group. KDIGO Clinical Practice Guideline for Acute Kidney Injury. Kidney Int Suppl. 2012;2:1.
8. Koyner JL, Vaidya VS, Bennett MR, et al. Urinary biomarkers in the clinical prognosis and early detection of acute kidney injury. Clin J Am Soc Nephrol. 2010;5:2154.
9. Levin A, Warnock DG, Mehta RL, et al. Improving outcomes from acute kidney injury: report of an initiative. Am J Kidney Dis. 2007;50:1.
10. Liaño F, Pascual J. Epidemiology of acute renal failure: a prospective, multicenter, community-based study. Madrid Acute Renal Failure Study Group. Kidney Int. 1996;50:811.
11. Mehta RL, Chertow GM. Acute renal failure definitions and classification: time for change? J Am Soc Nephrol. 2003;14:2178.
12. Mehta RL, Kellum JA, Shah SV, et al. Acute Kidney Injury Network: report of an initiative to improve outcomes in acute kidney injury. Crit Care. 2007;11:R31.
13. Mehta RL, McDonald B, Gabbai FB, et al. A randomized clinical trial of continuous versus intermittent dialysis for acute renal failure. Kidney Int. 2001;60:1154.
14. Palevsky PM, Liu KD, Brophy PD, et al. KDOQI US commentary on the 2012 KDIGO clinical practice guideline for acute kidney injury. Am J Kidney Dis. 2013;61:649.
15. Bellomo R, Cass A, et al. RENAL Replacement Therapy Study Investigators. Intensity of continuous renal-replacement therapy in critically ill patients. N Engl J Med. 2009;361:1627.
16. Schneider AG, Bellomo R, Bagshaw SM, et al. Choice of renal replacement therapy modality and dialysis dependence after acute kidney injury: a systematic review and meta-analysis. Intensive Care Med. 2013;39:987.
17. Palevsky PM, Zhang JH, et al. VA/NIH Acute Renal Failure Trial Network. Intensity of renal support in critically ill patients with acute kidney injury. N Engl J Med. 2008;359:7.
18. Palevsky PM, Zhang JH, et al. VA/NIH Acute Renal Failure Trial Network. Intensity of renal support in critically ill patients with acute kidney injury. N Engl J Med 2008;359:7.
19. Zarich S, Fang LS, Diamond JR. Fractional excretion of sodium. Exceptions to its diagnostic value. Arch Intern Med. 1985;145:108.

CHAPTER

6 Chronic Kidney Disease

H Sudarshan Ballal, Rohan Augustine, Vishwanath S

INTRODUCTION

Chronic kidney disease (CKD) describes any degree of kidney injury or impaired kidney function that persists for ≥3 months. CKD replaces multiple definitions and terms used earlier because it is easily understood by the clinicians patients and their families. CKD is a nonspecific term that does not include cause of disease or the impaired kidney functions.

DEFINITION OF CHRONIC KIDNEY DISEASE

Chronic kidney disease is defined as the persistent presence (≥3 months) of either:

- Kidney damage and/or structural abnormalities or
- An estimated glomerular filtration rate (GFR) ≤ 60 mL/min/1.73 m^2, even in the absence of evidence of kidney damage and/or structural abnormalities.

Kidney damage refers to microalbuminuria or overt proteinuria, any abnormal urinary sediment or abnormal imaging results.

STAGING/ESTIMATION OF GLOMERULAR FILTRATION RATE IN CHRONIC KIDNEY DISEASE

Estimation of GFR is an essential step in assessing the kidney function which can be done with simple creatinine based equations or by the clearance tests like creatinine clearance. GFR is used to classify patients to one of the five broad classes or stages of CKD **(Table 6.1)**.

The glomerular filtration rate (GFR) measures the volume of plasma filtered at the glomerulus per unit of time. GFR cannot be measured directly and is estimated by the clearance of nonmetabolized markers that are completely filtered at the glomerulus and are neither secreted nor reabsorbed by the tubule. Iothalamate clearance is considered to be the gold standard for estimating GFR but they are impractical in standard clinical use and surrogate measures are used in day to day practice. The standard GFR marker in clinical practice is serum creatinine (SCr) which can be used in several ways to estimate the level of kidney function.

It has been long recognized that serum creatinine is a poor marker for estimating the GFR. The wide range of GFR values indicate that patient characteristics also influence the relationship between serum creatinine and GFR.

Table 6.1 Stages of chronic kidney disease

Stage	*Description*	*GFR (mL/min/1.73 m^2)*
1	Kidney damage with normal or ↑GFR	≥90
2	Kidney damage with mild ↓GFR	60–89
3a	Moderate ↓GFR	45–59
3b	Moderate ↓GFR	30–44
4	Severe ↓GFR	15–29
5	Kidney failure	<15 (or dialysis)
	CKD is defined as either kidney damage or GFR <60 mL/min/1.73 m^2 for ≥3 months. Kidney damage is defined as pathologic abnormalities or markers of damage like abnormalities in blood or urine tests or imaging studies.	

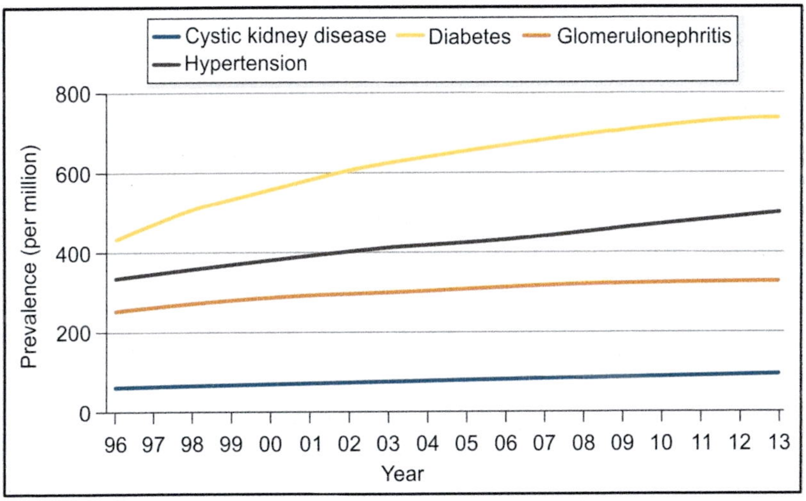

Figure 6.1 Trends in adjusted* prevalence (per million) of ESRD, by primary cause of ESRD, in the US population, 1996–2013

Source: Special analyses, USRDS, ESRD Database.

*Point prevalence on December 31 of each year.

Abbreviation: ESRD, end-stage renal disease

United States Renal Data System. 2015 USRDS annual data report: Epidemiology of kidney disease in the United States. National Institutes of Health, National Institute of Diabetes and Digestive and Kidney Diseases, Bethesda, MD, 2015

These factors are age, sex, body surface area (built of an individual) and race. The various methods of estimating GFR are discussed elsewhere.

ETIOLOGY OF CHRONIC KIDNEY DISEASE

Two causes of CKD end stage renal disease (ESRD) account for over 68% of all incident ESRD cases according to USRDS data **(Fig. 6.1)**. Diabetes accounts for

Table 6.2 Etiologies of end stage renal disease

Condition	*Fraction of patients (%)**	*Fraction of patients (%)***	*Fraction of patients (%)#*
Diabetes mellitus	42	27	30
Hypertension and large vessel disease	25	10	14
Glomerulonephritis—primary and secondary	13	18	19
Hereditary cystic and congenital renal disease	4	3	8
Interstitial nephritis and pyelonephritis	4	35	13
Neoplasm/tumors	2		
Miscellaneous and missing	6	7	16

*USRDS data; **MK Mani et al; #SC Dash and SK Agarwal et al

Table 6.3 Factors contributing to the progression of chronic kidney disease

Degree of systemic and intraglomerular hypertension
Severity of proteinuria
Glomerular hypertrophy with increase of vessel wall stress
Hyperlipidemia (increased LDL cholesterol)
Impaired prostaglandin generation with the use of NSAIDs
High protein diet
Persistent metabolic acidosis and increased ammonia production
Extent of tubulointerstitial disease

over 45% of all new cases of end stage renal failure and hypertension contributes to 24% of cases of end stage renal failure. The individual diseases contributing to ESRD are as in the **Table 6.2**.

PROGRESSION OF CHRONIC KIDNEY DISEASE

Progressive CKD is a maladaptive response that maintains the whole kidney glomerular filtration rate (GFR) in the presence of decreased number of nephrons. **Table 6.3** describes the factors contributing to the progression of CKD.

Individual nephrons surviving the initial injury try to compensate for the decreased number of functioning nephrons by increasing the filtration, secretion and reabsorption of the solutes. This adaptive process that is partially mediated by the activation of RAAS which increases pressure in the glomerulus. The resulting hyper filtration increases the load on individual tubules and contributes to proteinuria. This further increases the workload and hastens further nephron injury and loss.

Reciprocal of Serum Creatinine

Reciprocal of serum creatinine is used to follow the renal progression and also to predict the timeline for development of ESRD. As the GFR is inversely proportional to serum creatinine, the graph of 1/SCr plotted against time is expected to be linear in a person who has constant decline in renal function. If there is a steep decline, then we can look for reversible causes to make any changes in the treatment or to see the effectiveness of interventions to prevent the progression as well **(Fig. 6.2)**.

In short, the process of progressive CKD involves **(Flow chart 6.1)**:

- *Predisposing factors*: Characters that predispose a person to kidney injury for example, genetic factors, age, low birth weight, environmental and social factors like exposure to nephrotoxic drugs.
- *Initiating factors*: Characteristics that cause kidney injury like hypertension, diabetes mellitus, immunological injury and or genetic factors.
- *Progression factors*: Characteristics that cause progressive loss of kidney function such as, high BP, poor glycemic control, activation of RAAS, high dietary protein consumption, proteinuria, smoking, hyperlipidemia, anemia.

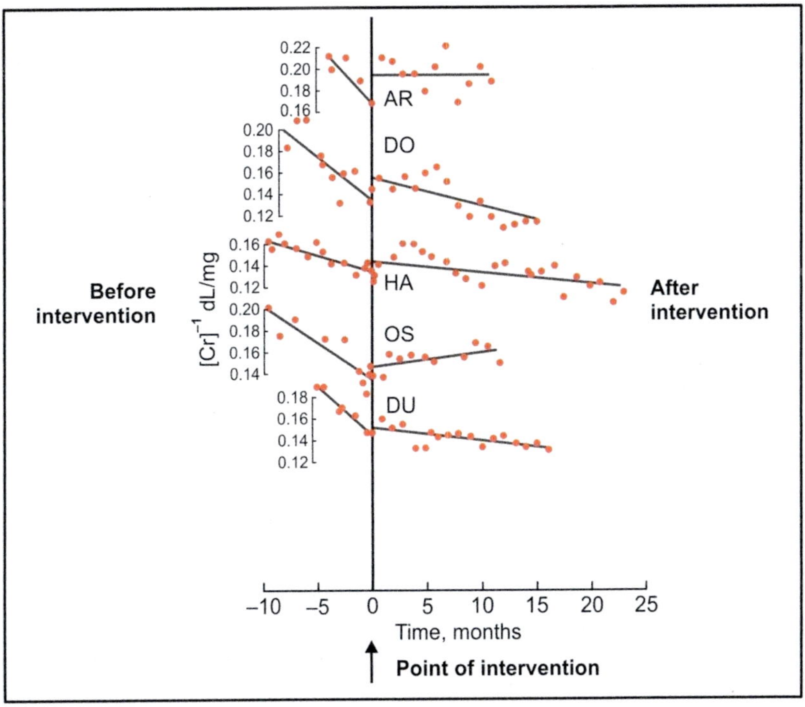

Figure 6.2 How the effect of therapeutic intervention on the progression of CKD was assessed. To the left of vertical line is the slope of 1/cr versus time before intervention and to the right is the slope after intervention. If the slope became less steep, it means beneficial effect of the intervention. If the slope becomes more steep, it means detrimental effect of intervention

Flow chart 6.1 Progression of chronic kidney disease

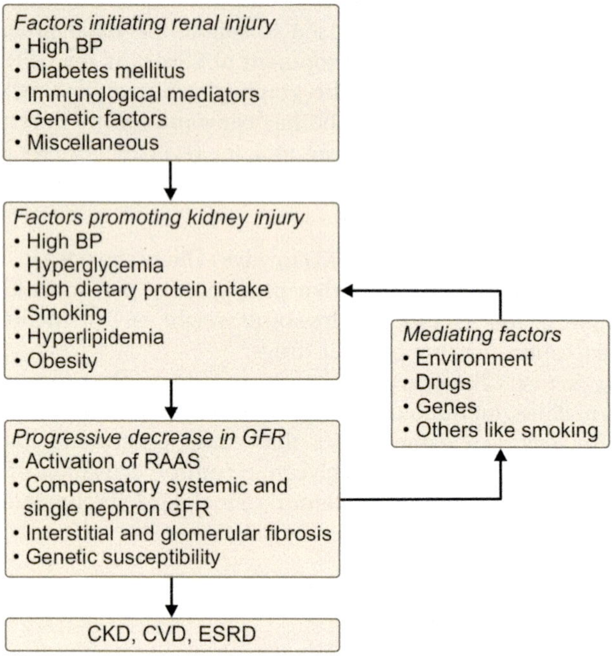

Abbreviations: BP, blood pressure; GFR, glomerular filtration rate; RAAS, renin-angiotensin-aldosterone system

Variable Rates of Progression of CKD

One specific characteristic of progressive kidney damage is that once kidney injury has been initiated the rate of progression is highly variable among individual patients and not everyone losses kidney function continuously. This variable loss of GFR was described in the modification of diet in renal disease (MDRD) study. These data show that progressive CKD is inevitable.

MANIFESTATIONS OF CHRONIC KIDNEY DISEASE

Fluid and Electrolyte Imbalance

Due to reduced GFR and defective tubular functions, there will be an impaired ability to excrete leading to mild or overt expansion in plasma and extracellular fluid volume, salt sensitive hypertension and also edema. Hypertension may also worsen unless intake of salt is restricted to 100 mEq/day. Hyponatremia also may be problem due to dilutional state and fluid restriction to less than 1 L/day would be essential.

Potassium excretion in CKD is maintained in the initial state due to increased excretion by the surviving nephrons and to a small extent by the colonic K^+ secretion. Once the GFR decreases, K^+ elimination is curtailed and hyperkalemia is frequent in CKD.

Acid Base Abnormalities

Metabolic acidosis in CKD is due to defective ammonia genesis and reduced distal H^+ trapping as NH_4^+, which reduces renal bicarbonate regeneration. There could also be proximal HCO_3 loses or reduced distal H^+ secretion. Chronic metabolic acidosis if not corrected will lead to skeletal demineralization. As GFR drops to less than 10 mL/min, there will be retention of organic acids leading to high anion gap with acidosis.

Carbohydrate Intolerance

Insulin is degraded by the liver and kidney. Decrease in insulin clearance is offset by the peripheral insulin resistance. There is a reduced requirement for insulin and oral hypoglycemic agents in diabetics as their renal failure worsen.

Calcium and Phosphate Abnormalities and Metabolic Bone Disease

Phosphate retention and metabolic acidosis ensues once the GFR drops to less than 25 mL/min. Acidosis increases the bone resorption and serum phosphate levels as well. High phosphate levels increases PTH secretion and reduces ionized calcium. This inhibits renal hydroxylation of 25(OH) D_3 to its active metabolite, 1, $25(OH)_2$ D_3 (calcitriol) there by decreasing intestinal calcium absorption. The resulting hypocalcemia further increases PTH. Renal osteodystrophy is classified in **Table 6.4**.

Hematologic Abnormalities

Anemia and uremic bleeding diathesis: Hematocrit falls as the serum creatinine increases >2–3 mg/dL. This is mainly due to progressive loss of nephron function leading to loss of erythropoietin production by the peritubular fibroblasts and anemia sets in.

In uremia, there is a defect in the platelet function which impairs platelet activation and adhesion to endothelium. Anemia exacerbates uremic bleeding. This causes frequent bruising, ecchymosis, and bleeding from mucous membranes as well.

Table 6.4 Different forms of renal osteodystrophy

Type of bone disease	*Prevalence (%)*
High turnover bone disease	
Osteitis fibrosa cystica	50–70
Mixed uremic osteodystrophy	10
Low turnover bone disease	
Adynamic bone disease	30–40
Osteomalacia	<5

Gastrointestinal Abnormalities

Gastrointestinal problems include anorexia, early morning nausea, vomiting. As the renal failure worsens, they develop uremic fetor, esophagitis, gastritis, duodenitis and peptic ulcer disease. Gastroparesis and gastrointestinal bleeding are increased by vascular ectasia and peptic ulcer disease.

Dermatological Abnormalities

Uremic pruritus is related to calcium and phosphorus deposition, hypercalcemia, peripheral neuropathy, dry skin and anemia.

Neuromuscular Abnormalities

Central nervous system (CNS) dysfunction is characterized by decreased attention span, agitation, confusion, insomnia, and reduced memory. They may also develop depression, hallucinations, delusions, hiccups, cramps, asterixis, myoclonus, fasciculation and seizures. Worsening peripheral neuropathy, restless legs syndrome and burning feet are early phases of uremic peripheral neuropathy.

Chronic Kidney Disease and Cardiovascular Disease/Hypertension

Patients with CKD are at greater risk of coronary artery disease, cerebrovascular diseases, peripheral vascular disease, congestive heart failure, poor control of hypertension. All patients with CKD should be considered to be at the highest risk group for cardiovascular disease. Cardiovascular diseases account for 40–50% of all deaths in stage 5 CKD patients and cardiovascular mortality rates in CKD patients is 15 times higher than in general population. 85% of patients at initiation of dialysis have left ventricular hypertrophy by echocardiography.

MANAGEMENT OF CHRONIC KIDNEY DISEASE

The prevalence of chronic kidney disease (CKD) in India is estimated at 7572 per million and end stage kidney disease at 757 per million population. To reduce this burden and to improve patient outcome, CKD should be detected and treated early before the onset of ESRD.

PRINCIPLES OF MANAGEMENT OF CHRONIC KIDNEY DISEASE

Treatment of Reversible Causes of Renal Failure

Patients with CKD and a recent decrease in renal function may have an underlying reversible process, e.g. hypovolemia (vomiting, diarrhea, diuretic use, bleeding); hypotension (due to myocardial dysfunction or pericardial disease); infection (such as sepsis); and drugs (such as nonsteroidal anti-inflammatory drugs [NSAIDs] and angiotensin-converting enzyme [ACE] inhibitors). Among the nephrotoxic drugs aminoglycoside antibiotics and radiographic contrast material are a frequent offenders. Alternative forms of medication are also a major contributor to acute worsening. Certain drugs like cimetidine, trimethoprim, cefoxitin, and flucytosine can interfere with either creatinine secretion or the assay used. Urinary tract obstruction should always be ruled out in patients with unexplained renal dysfunction. Renal ultrasonography is often performed to exclude urinary tract obstruction.

Preventing or Slowing the Progression of Renal Disease

Progression in CKD may be due to secondary factors unrelated to the initial disease. The major factors contributing are intraglomerular hypertension and glomerular hypertrophy, leading to glomerular scarring (glomerulosclerosis). Additional causes may include systemic hypertension, hyperlipidemia, metabolic acidosis, and tubulointerstitial disease.

Early Interventions

- Life style measures
- Blood Pressure lowering, in particular ACEi/ARB
- Salt reduction
- Prevent high protein intake
- Optimal glycaemic control in diabetics
- Lipid lowering
- Uric acid lowering
- Minimizing the risk of contrast induced renal injury
- Avoidance of nephrotoxic drugs.

Lifestyle measures to prevent progression: Patients with CKD should be encouraged to:

- Undertake physical activity (aiming for at least 30 minutes 5 times per week)
- Achieve a healthy weight (BMI 20–25)
- Stop smoking.

Blood pressure management in CKD: Tight blood pressure control is an important for retarding progression of CKD. KDIGO recommends keeping the blood pressure, < 140/90 in nonproteinuric patients and <130/80 in proteinuric CKD with emphasis on ACEi/ARB for their antiproteinuric properties.

	Diabetes			*Nondiabetes*		
ACR	*<30*	*30–300*	*>300*	*<30*	*30–300*	*>300*
BP goal	<140/90	<130/80	<130/80	<140/90	<130/80	<130/80
ACEi/ARB	–	Yes	Yes	–	Yes	Yes

KDIGO BP management in CKD; Kidney Int 2012.
Abbreviation: ACR, Albumin creatinine ratio.

Salt reduction: Low salt improves the effect of ACEi/ARB on survival in non-diabetic and diabetic subjects.

KDIGO recommends lowering salt intake to <90 mmol (<2 g) per day of sodium (corresponding to 5 g of sodium chloride) in adults.

Prevent high protein intake: KDIGO recommends avoiding high protein intake (>1.3 g/kg/day) in adults with CKD with high risk of progression.

KDIGO suggest lowering protein intake to 0.8 g/kg/day in adults with or without diabetes and GFR <30 mL/min/1.73 m^2.

Optimal glycemic control prevents progression of CKD: Various studies like the ADVANCE, ACCORD and the VADT trials have shown that tight glycemic control targeting $HbA_{1c} < 7$ reduces the risk of new onset microalbuminuria by 9–32% and progression to over proteinuria by 30–37%.

KDIGO recommends a target HbA_{1c} ~7% to prevent or delay progression of diabetic kidney disease.

Study	*HbA_{1c} goals*	*New ACR (30–300 mg/g)*	*ACR progression (>300 mg/g)*
Advance	6.5% vs 7.3%	9% less	30% less
ACCORD	6.3% vs 7.6%	21% less	32% less
VADT	6.9% vs 8.4%	32% less	37% less

Patel A, et al. NEJM. 2008;358:2560-72.
Ismail-Beigi F, et al. Lancet. 2010;376:419-30.
Duckworth W, et al. NEJM. 2009;360:129-39.

Lipid management in CKD:

	>50 years		*<50 years*	
GFR	*>60*	*<60*	*>60*	*<60*
LDL goal	?	?	?	?
Statin or Statin/ezitimibe	Yes 1B	Yes 1A	Yes* 2A	Yes* 2A

*In case of DM/CVD history.
KDIGO lipid in CKD, Kidney Int. 2013, Suppl 3.

Lowering of uric acid to prevent progression of CKD: Evidence at present is too limited to support or refute the use of uric acid lowering drugs to prevent progression.

Minimizing risk of contrast injury: In CKD patients undergoing imaging studies KDIGO recommends balancing the risk of acute kidney injury versus the diagnostic and therapeutic implications of the investigation.

Radiocontrast: All CKD patients with GFR <60 mL/min/1.73 m^2 and receiving iodinated radiocontrast media should be managed according to the KDIGO Clinical Practice Guideline for AKI:

- Avoid of hyper osmolar agents
- Use the lowest possible dose of the radiocontrast agent
- Withdrawal all nephrotoxic agents pre- and post-proceedure
- Maintain adequate hydration with saline before, during, and after the procedure
- Measurement of GFR 48–96 hours post-procedure.

Gadolinium-based contrast media

- Gadolinium-containing contrast media are not recommended with GFR <15 mL/min/1.73 m^2.
- Patients who require gadolinium based contrast media and have GFR <30 mL/min/1.73 m^2 are preferentially offered a macrocyclic chelate preparation.

Bowel preparation: Oral phosphate-containing bowel preparations are not recommended with a GFR <60 mL/min/1.73 m^2.

Treatment of the Complications of Renal Failure

The progression of CKD results in disorders of fluid and electrolyte balance, volume overload, hyperkalemia, metabolic acidosis, and hyperphosphatemia. The resulting hormonal or systemic dysfunction leads to symptoms like anorexia, nausea, vomiting, fatigue, hypertension, anemia, malnutrition, hyperlipidemia, and bone disease.

Later Interventions

- Low protein intake
- Management of volume status
- Management of metabolic acidosis
- Prevent hyperkalemia
- Management of CKD-MBD
- Management of malnutrition
- Management of renal anemia
- CKD and CVD management
- CKD and vaccination.

The impact of low protein diet on progression: KDIGO recommends lowering protein intake to 0.8 g/kg/day in adults with or without diabetes and GFR <30 mL/min/1.73 m^2.

Management of volume status: Sodium and intravascular volume balance are usually maintained until the eGFR falls <10–15 mL/min per 1.73 m^2. Patients with CKD and volume overload generally respond to the combination of dietary sodium restriction and diuretic therapy.

CKD and metabolic acidosis: Patients with CKD have an increasing tendency to retain hydrogen ions leading to metabolic acidosis, with the serum bicarbonate concentration stabilizing between 12 mEq/L and 20 mEq/L. Metabolic acidosis may be treated with bicarbonate supplementation. Bicarbonate supplementation requires careful monitoring of volume status because bicarbonate is co-administered with sodium. KDIGO recommends supplementing oral bicarbonate to normalize the plasma levels in CKD patients with bicarbonate <22 mmol/L.

Hyperkalemia: The ability to maintain potassium excretion at near normal levels is generally maintained in patients with renal disease until late in the disease (GFR <10 mL/min). Hyperkalemia generally develops in patients who are oliguric, has a high-potassium diet, increased tissue breakdown, or hypoaldosteronism (administration of an ACE inhibitor or ARB). Measures to prevent hyperkalemia include ingestion of a low-potassium diet (e.g. <40–70 mEq/day [1500–2700 mg/day]), potassium binders and avoiding, if possible, the use of drugs that raise the serum potassium concentration.

Chronic kidney disease and metabolic bone disease: To maintain calcium and phosphate balance, the hypersecretion of parathyroid hormone (PTH) is initially appropriate to correct both hyperphosphatemia and hypocalcemia (trade off hypothesis). As a result, normal serum phosphate concentration is generally maintained up to an eGFR of 30 mL/min per 1.73 m^2.The price paid is secondary hyperparathyroidism and the development of renal osteodystrophy.

Monitoring chronic kidney disease-mineral and bone disorders

- KDIGO recommends monitoring serum levels of calcium, phosphorus, PTH, and alkaline phosphatase activity in CKD stage 3.
- Reasonable monitoring intervals would be:

Frequency of monitoring biomarkers of CKD-MBD					
CKD stage GFR (mL/min/1.73 m^2)	*Calcium*	*Phosphorus*	*PTH*	*Alkaline phosphatase*	*25 (OH)D (Calcidiol)*
Stage 3 30–59	Every 6–12 months	Every 6–12 months	Based on baseline level and CKD progression	NA	Measure with repeated testing determined by baseline values
Stage 4 15–29	Every 3–6 months	Every 3–6 months	Every 6–12 months	Every 12 months, or more frequently in the presence of elevated PTH	Measure with repeated testing determined by baseline values
Stage 5 or 5D <15	Every 1–3 months	Every 1–3 months	Every 3–6 months	Every 12 months, or more frequently in the presence of elevated PTH	Measure with repeated testing determined by baseline values

KDIGO clinical practice guideline for the diagnosis, evaluation, prevention and treatment of chronic disease-mineral and bone disorder (CKD-MBD). Kidney Int. 2009;756:S1-S130.

- Vitamin D (calcidiol) levels should be measured in patients with CKD 3-5D and should be corrected using treatment strategies mentioned below:

Estimate of vitamin D status	
Vitamin D status	*25(OH) D (ng/mL)*
Replete	>30
Insufficiency	16–30
Mild deficiency	5–15
Severe deficiency	<5

- Bone mineral densitometry (BMD) testing is not recommended in patients with CKD stages 3-5D, because BMD does not predict fracture risk and the type of renal osteodystrophy.
- Measurements of serum PTH or bone-specific alkaline phosphatase can be used in patients with CKD stages 3-5D, to evaluate mineral bone disease. Markedly high or low values predict underlying high and low bone turnover respectively.
- A lateral abdominal radiograph can be used to detect the presence or absence of aortic calcification, and an echocardiogram can be used to detect the presence or absence of valvular calcification, in patients with CKD stages 3-5D.

Treatment of CKD-MBD targeted at lowering high serum phosphorus and maintaining serum calcium:

Treatment target ranges			
CKD stage GFR mL/min/1.73 m^2	*Target phosphorus*	*Target calcium*	*Target PTH*
Stage 3 30–59 Stage 4 15–29 Stage 5 ND <15	Maintain within normal range*	Maintain within normal range*	If serum PTH is rising and remains above the upper limit of normal despite addressing modifiable factors, treat with calcitriol or vitamin D analogs
Stage 5D	Treat toward the normal range*	Maintain within normal range*	Two to nine times the upper limit of the normal range*

*Normal ranges may differ by laboratory.
KDIGO clinical practice guideline for the diagnosis, evaluation, prevention and treatment of chronic disease-mineral and bone disorder (CKD-MBD). Kidney Int. 2009;756:S1-S130.

- Dietary phosphate intake must be limited in patients with hyperphosphatemia in combination with other treatments.
- Phosphate-binding agents are recommended in the treatment of hyperphosphatemia refractory to diet control.
- The dose of calcium based phosphate binders needs restriction in:
  - Presence of persistent or recurrent hypercalcemia
  - In the presence of arterial calcification
  - Adynamic bone disease
  - Serum PTH levels are persistently low.

Treatment of abnormal PTH levels in CKD-MBD:

- The optimal PTH level is not known in patients with CKD stages 3-5 (ND). Patients with intact PTH (iPTH) levels above the upper normal limit are first evaluated for hyperphosphatemia, hypocalcemia, and vitamin D deficiency.
- Patients with progressively rising PTH despite correction of modifiable factors, merit treatment with calcitriol or vitamin D analogs.
- The iPTH levels in CKD stage 5D is to be maintained in the range two to nine times the upper normal limit for the assay.

- In CKD stage 5D patients with rising PTH; calcitriol, or vitamin D analogs, or calcimimetics, or their combination can be used to lower PTH.
- Parathyroidectomy can be offered to patients with severe hyperparathyroidism (HPT) who fail to respond to medical/pharmacological therapy.

Treatment of bone with bisphosphonates, other osteoporosis medications, and growth hormone:

- Patients with CKD stages 1–3 with normal PTH with osteoporosis and/or high risk of fracture are managed as for the general population.
- In patients with CKD stage 3-5D with biochemical abnormalities of CKD-MBD/low BMD, treatment must include reversal of the biochemical abnormalities with a low threshold for bone biopsy especially prior to therapy with antiresorptive agents.
- In children and adolescents with CKD stages 2–5D and growth retardation, malnutrition and biochemical abnormalities of CKD–MBD needs to be treated prior to considering recombinant human growth hormone.

Malnutrition: Malnutrition is common in patients with advanced CKD because of poor food intake, decreased absorption and metabolic acidosis. A low plasma concentration of albumin may be indicative of malnutrition. To best assess nutritional status, the serum albumin concentration, anthropometric measurements and body weight should be measured serially every 1–3 months for those with eGFRs <20 mL/min per 1.73 m^2 and more frequently for those with eGFRs ≤15 mL/min per 1.73 m^2.

CKD and anemia: The anemia of CKD is normocytic and normochromic, and is primarily due to reduced production of erythropoietin by the kidney (a reflection of the reduction in functioning renal mass) and to shortened red cell survival. Anemia becomes increasingly common as the eGFRs decline <60 mL/min per 1.73 m^2 and is more common among diabetics.

- For CKD patients with anemia not being treated with an ESA, KDIGO recommends
  - measuring Hb concentration when clinically indicated
  - at least every 3 months in patients with CKD 3–5ND and CKD 5PD
  - at least monthly in patients with CKD 5HD
- Diagnosis of anemia is made when the Hb concentration is <13.0 g/dL in males and <12.0 g/dL in females.
- The following tests are recommended in initial evaluation of the anemia
  - Complete blood count (CBC), which should include Hb concentration, red cell indices, white blood cell count and differential, and platelet count
  - Absolute reticulocyte count
  - Serum ferritin level
  - Serum transferrin saturation (TSAT)
  - Serum vitamin B_{12} and folate levels

Iron supplementation:

- A trial of IV iron (or trial of oral iron for 1–3 months in CKD ND patients) is recommended for anemic CKD patients not on iron or ESA therapy, if:
  - an increase in Hb concentration without ESA is desired and
  - TSAT is <30% and ferritin is <500 ng/mL

- For patients on ESA therapy a trial of IV iron is recommended if:
  - an increase in Hb concentration or a decrease in ESA dose is desired and
  - TSAT is <30% and ferritin is <500 ng/mL (<500 mg/L)
- Iron status (TSAT and ferritin) is to be evaluated every 3 months during ESA therapy
- Administering IV iron is to be avoided in patients with active systemic infections.

ESA initiation:
- The potential benefits of reducing blood transfusions and anemic symptoms must be weighed against the risks (e.g. stroke, vascular access loss, hypertension) while initiating ESA treatment.
- Exercise caution in patients with active malignancy, a history of stroke, or a history of malignancy.
  - ESA therapy need not be initiated for adult CKD (ND) patients with Hb concentration >10.0 g/dL.
  - For CKD (ND) patients with Hb concentration <10.0 g/dL, the decision to initiate ESA therapy is individualized based on the
    - rate of fall of Hb,
    - response to iron therapy,
    - the need for transfusion, and
    - presence of symptoms attributable to anemia.
  - The Hb concentration falling below 9.0 g/dL must be avoided by starting ESA therapy when the hemoglobin is between 9.0 g/dL and 10.0 g/dL in adult CKD 5D patients.

ESA maintenance therapy:
- ESAs should not be used to maintain Hb concentration above 11.5 g/dL in adult patients with CKD.
- ESAs should not be used to intentionally increase the Hb concentration above 13 g/dL.

Use of red cell transfusion in chronic anemia:
- Avoid red cell transfusions to minimize the general risks related to their use.
- Red cell transfusions must be avoided in patients eligible for organ transplantation, to minimize the risk of allosensitization.

CKD and CVD management: Cardiorenal syndrome is defined as the coexistence of cardiac and renal dysfunction, in which an acute or chronic deterioration of one of the two organs leads to an acute or chronic worsening of the other **(Fig. 6.3)**.

All patients with CKD should be considered to be at an increased risk for cardiovascular disease. Adults with CKD are at risk for atherosclerotic events and should be offered treatment with antiplatelet agents unless contraindicated.

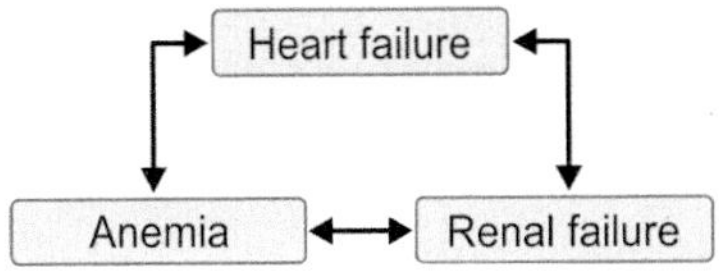

Figure 6.3 Cardiorenal anemia syndrome

In patients with CKD and heart failure, any escalation in therapy should be accompanied with monitoring of eGFR and serum potassium.

Measures for prevention and treatment

General measures
Early and correct optimization of heart failure medication Close monitoring of hemodynamics and renal function (clinical/biomarkers) Correct usage of diuretics • Diuretic combinations of different categories for sequential nephron blockade • Avoidance of diuretic combinations of the same category • Avoidance of thiazides when GFR <15–20 mL/min • Avoidance of extremely high doses Avoidance of hypovolemia Avoidance of excess salt and fluid intake Avoidance of nephrotoxic agents
Specific measures in acute conditions
Inotropes (dopamine, dobutamine, levosimendan) Renal replacement therapy (ultrafiltration) Mechanical circulatory support
Novel/investigational agents
Nesiritide Vasopressin antagonists Adenosine antagonists

Caveats when interpreting tests for CVD in people with CKD:

- *BNP/N-terminal-proBNP (NT-proBNP)*: Serum concentrations of BNP/NT-proBNP should be interpreted with caution with GFR <60 mL/min/1.73 m^2 in the diagnosis of heart failure and assessment of volume status.
- *Troponins*: Serum concentrations of troponin should also be interpreted with caution with GFR <60 mL/min/1.73 m^2 to diagnose acute coronary syndrome.

CKD and vaccination:

- All adults with CKD should be offered annual vaccination with influenza vaccine.
- Adults with eGFR < 30mL/min/1.73 m^2 and at risk of pneumococcal infection (e.g. nephrotic syndrome, diabetes, on immunosuppression) should receive vaccination with polyvalent pneumococcal vaccine. Those who have received pneumococcal vaccination should be offered revaccination within 5 years.
- All patients with GFR <30 mL/min/1.73 m^2 and those at high-risk of progression should be immunized against hepatitis B and the response confirmed by checking the antibody titer.

PRE END-STAGE INTERVENTIONS

- Referral for specialist care
- Preparation for renal replacement therapy
  - Transplantation
  - Dialysis
  - Conservative treatment
- Conservative management.

Referral to Specialist Care

KDIGO recommends referral of patients with CKD to specialist care, according to this diagram **(Fig. 6.4)**.

Patients with CKD also need to be referred for specialist care in case of acute kidney injury or abrupt sustained fall in GFR.

- Progressive CKD
- Urinary red cell casts
- CKD and hypertension refractory to ≥4 antihypertensives
- Persistent hyperkalemia
- Hereditary kidney disease.

Preparation for and Initiation of Renal Replacement Therapy

Choice of renal replacement therapy: Once the need for renal replacement therapy is confirmed, the patient should be counseled about various RRT options, their advantages and disadvantages; namely of hemodialysis, peritoneal dialysis (continuous or intermittent modalities), and renal transplantation (living or deceased donor). The 2006 (K/DOQI) guidelines recommend that patients with an (eGFR) <30 mL/min per 1.73 m^2 should be educated about these issues.

			Persistent albuminuria categories description and range		
			A1	A2	A3
			Normal to mildly increased	Moderately increased	Severely increased
GFR categories (mL/min 1.73 m^2) description and range			<30 mg/g <3 mg/mmol	30–300 mg/g 3–30 mg/mmol	>300 mg/g >30 mg/mmol
G1	Normal or high	≥90		Monitor	Refer
G2	Mildly decreased	60–89		Monitor	Refer
G3a	Mildly to moderately decreased	45–59	Monitor	Monitor	Refer
G3b	Moderately to severely decreased	30–44	Monitor	Monitor	Refer
G4	Severely decreased	15–29	Refer	Refer	Refer
G5	Kidney failure	<15	Refer	Refer	Refer

Figure 6.4 Recommendation for referral of CKD patients based on GFR and albuminuria Levey AS, et al. Kidney Int. 2011;80:17-28.

Preparation for transplantation: Kidney transplantation is the treatment of choice for ESRD. A successful kidney transplant improves the quality of life and reduces the mortality risk. Patients deemed fit and anticipated to need RRT within the next year should be referred to a renal transplant program.

In patients who are not transplant candidates, factors such as availability, convenience, cost, co-morbidities, ability to tolerate ultrafilteration should be taken into consideration while deciding between hemodialysis or peritoneal dialysis.

Preparation for hemodialysis: In patients planned for hemodialysis, a vascular access needs to be created to gain access to the blood stream. The access is preferably placed in the non-dominant upper extremity. There is an increased risk of infection and arterial steal syndrome with lower extremity grafts.

There are three major types of vascular access: Primary arteriovenous (AV) fistulas; synthetic arteriovenous grafts; and cuffed tunneled catheters. Patients should be referred to a vascular access surgeon when the eGFR is <20–25 mL/min/1.73 m^2.

Preparation for peritoneal dialysis: For Peritoneal dialysis, the PD catheters are placed surgically into the abdominal cavity. It is preferable to wait for at least 2 weeks after placement before beginning dialysis. If prior dialysis is needed, small volume exchanges in the recumbent position is recommended to minimize the risk of leak.

Conservative Management of ESRD

Patients may choose to withhold dialysis. The 2012 (KDIGO) guidelines recommend that conservative management of end-stage renal disease (ESRD) should be an option for all patients who decide not to pursue renal replacement therapy. Conservative care includes the management of symptoms, advance-care planning, and provision of appropriate palliative care.

Timing the Initiation of Renal Replacement Therapy

The indications for initiation of dialysis include symptoms or signs caused by kidney failure (like pericarditis, acid-base or electrolyte abnormalities, pruritus); inability to control volume status; a progressive deterioration in nutritional status, or cognitive impairment. This often occurs when the GFR ranges between 5 and 10 mL/min/1.73 m^2.

Preemptive renal transplantation should be considered when the GFR is <20 mL/min/1.73 m^2, and there is progressive worsening renal function over the preceding 6–12 months.

Multidisciplinary CKD Clinic

Patients with CKD need to be managed in a multidisciplinary setting. The multidisciplinary team should emphasise on dietary care, education and counseling on RRT modalities, transplant options, vascular access surgery, and ethical, psychological and social care.

Levels of Evidence

Grade	*Quality of evidence*	*Meaning*
A	High	We are confident that the true effect lies close to that of the estimate of the effect.
B	Moderate	The true effect is likely to be close to the estimate of the effect, but there is a possibility that it is substantially different.
C	Low	The true effect may be substantially different from the estimate of the effect.
D	Very low	The estimate of effect is very uncertain, and often will be far from the truth.

Multiple Choice Questions

1. **Which of the following statements regarding chronic kidney disease (CKD) is true?**
   a. Measurement of 24-hour creatinine clearance is more accurate than estimating GFR from the modification of diet in renal disease (MDRD) equation
   b. Interventions to slow progression of kidney disease, and measures to reduce cardiovascular disease should begin in CKD stage 3
   c. CKD is defined as a glomerular filtration rate (GFR) of <30 mL/min/1.73 m^2 for 3 months
   d. Persistently increased proteinuria with normal or increased GFR is classified as stage 1 CKD

2. **Which of the following statements regarding the management of CKD is false?**
   a. Patients with CKD initially have high anion gap metabolic acidosis, and over time develop a normal anion gap metabolic acidosis
   b. The parathyroid hormone level in CKD rises, resulting in fairly normal serum calcium and phosphate levels
   c. Potassium balance is generally maintained until the GFR falls to <10 mL/min
   d. The patient has achieved the goal for salt intake when a patient is normotensive and maintains a constant weight with only trace edema.

3. **Which of the following statements is true regarding assessment of renal function?**
   a. A serum creatinine within the normal range indicates that the patient's GFR has declined by less than 25%
   b. Averaging the urea and creatinine clearance values will provide a more accurate estimation of GFR than use of the creatinine clearance value alone
   c. Use of creatinine clearance, by 24-hour urine collection, can lead to an underestimation of the GFR in CKD
   d. The Cockcroft-Gault formula estimates GFR while taking into account the increase in creatinine production with age.

4. **Which of the following statements is true regarding the etiology and management of chronic renal insufficiency?**
   a. Alkali therapy can help treat the acidosis but is unlikely to improve the hyperkalemia
   b. The target hemoglobin value to initiate erythropoietin therapy in CKD ND is Hb 10.0-11 gm/dL
   c. The target hemoglobin value to initiate erythropoietin therapy in CKD 5D is Hb <9 gm/dL
   d. For adult CKD patients on ESA therapy who are not receiving iron supplementation, a trial of IV iron is recommended if the Tsat >30% and ferritin <500 ng/mL.

5. **Which of the following statements is true regarding the appropriate measures to slow progression of renal disease?**
   a. The targeted blood pressure in proteinuric CKD should be below 140/90 mm Hg
   b. Microalbuminuria is predictive of progression of renal disease only in diabetic CKD
   c. Aggressive control of hyperglycemia is more likely to slow progression of renal disease in patients with type 1 diabetes mellitus than in patients with type 2 diabetes mellitus
   d. Smoking is a risk factor for microalbuminuria because of its association with hypertension.

6. **Which of the following statements regarding chronic kidney disease is false?**
   a. The incidence of new cardiovascular disease in CKD patients is the same as the normal population for any given age
   b. Anemia is usually evident once the serum creatinine level >3 mg/dL
   c. The decline in hematocrit is largely the result of a reduction in the production of erythropoietin by the kidney
   d. The newer cyclooxygenase-2 (COX-2) non steroidal anti-inflammatory drugs (NSAIDs) can adversely affect renal function.

7. **Which of the following is the most effective intervention to prevent progression of CKD and CVD?**
   a. Use of uric acid lowering agent
   b. Use of ACE-inhibitor or ARB
   c. Use of statin or statin
   d. Vitamin D supplementation.

8. **Which of the following statements regarding management of early CKD is not correct?**
   a. To start an ACE-inhibitor or ARB for ACR of 30–300 mg/g, independent of the presence of diabetes
   b. Independent of the level of albuminuria, it is recommended to lower the blood pressure if it is >130/80
   c. To start an ACE-inhibitor or ARB for ACR of >300 mg/g, independent of the presence of diabetes
   d. A low sodium diet (<90 mmol/day or <5 gr NaCl/day) is recommended.

9. **Preemptive renal transplant should be considered when the GFR is:**
   a. < 5 mL/min/1.73 m^2
   b. <10 mL/min/1.73 m^2
   c. <15 mL/min/1.73 m^2
   d. <20 mL/min/1.73 m^2.

10. Decision to start ESA in a CKD patient not on dialysis should be based on:
   a. Rate of fall of Hb
   b. Response to iron therapy
   c. The need for blood transfusion and symptoms attributable to anemia
   d. All of the above.

Answers

1. d	2. a	3. b	4. c	5. c	6. a	7. b	8. b
9. d	10. d						

SUGGESTED READING

1. Agarwal SK, Dash SC, Irshad M, et al. Prevalence of chronic renal failure in adults in Delhi, India. Nephrol Dial Transplant. 2005;20:1638-42.
2. K/DOQI Clinical practice guidelines for chronic kidney disease: Evaluation, Classification and stratification. *www.kidney.org/professionals/kdoqi/guidelines_ckd/*.
3. KDIGO 2012 Clinical Practice Guideline for the Evaluation and Management of Chronic Kidney Disease; 2013;3(1).
4. KDIGO Clinical Practice Guideline for Anemia in Chronic Kidney Disease. 2012;2(4).
5. KDIGO Clinical Practice Guideline for the Diagnosis, Evaluation, Prevention and Treatment of Chronic Kidney Disease-Mineral and Bone Disorder (CKD-MBD); 2009;76(Supp 113).
6. Mani MK. Chronic renal failure in India. Nephrol Dial Transplant. 1993;8:684-9.
7. Mitch WE, Buffington GA, Lemann J, et al. A simple method of estimating progression of chronic renal failure. Lancet. 1976;2:1326-8.
8. United States Renal Data System. 2015 USRDS annual data report: Epidemiology of kidney disease in the United States. National Institutes of Health, National Institute of Diabetes and Digestive and Kidney Diseases, Bethesda, MD, 2015.

CHAPTER

7 Electrolyte Disorders

HYPONATREMIA AND HYPERNATREMIA

Gokulnath, Ram R, Vinod Kumar K

INTRODUCTION

Water is the predominant constituent of the human body. In healthy individuals, it makes up 60% of a man's body weight and 50% of a woman's body weight. Body water is distributed in two compartments, the intracellular fluid (ICF) compartment, containing 55–65%, and the extracellular fluid (ECF) compartment, containing the remaining 35–45%. The ECF is further subdivided into the interstitial space and the intravascular space. The interstitial space comprises approximately three-fourths of ECF, whereas the intravascular space contains one-fourth. Disorders of water balance and sodium balance are commonly seen in our clinical practice. The following terms are commonly used when discussing disorder of water and sodium balance.

Extracellular fluid (ECF) volume: The ECF volume is regulated by alterations in urinary sodium excretion that are primarily mediated by variation in the activity of renin-angiotensin-aldosterone and sympathetic nervous systems, which promote sodium retention, and the secretion of natriuretic peptides, which promote sodium excretion.

Effective arterial blood volume: The hormonal changes that regulate ECF volume are mediated by sensors in the renal afferent glomerular arterioles (for renin), carotid sinus (for sympathetic activity) and atria and ventricles (for natriuretic peptides) that respond to change in pressure.

Intracellular fluid volume: Changes in the intracellular fluid volume primarily occur when there are changes in plasma tonicity, resulting in water movement into or out of the cells. The intracellular and brain volumes usually increase with hyponatremia and decreases with hypernatremia.

Plasma osmolality (pOsm): Is determined by the ratio of plasma solute and water. 90% of the plasma osmolality is contributed by sodium salts which is the major ECF cation with lesser contributions from other ions (e.g. potassium, calcium), glucose and urea.

The normal pOsm is 275-290 mOsmol/kg

The plasma osmolality can be estimated from the following equation:

$$pOsm = 2 \times [Na^+] + [Glucose]/18 + [Blood\ Urea\ Nitrogen]/2.8.$$

REGULATION OF SODIUM AND WATER BALANCE

The kidney plays an important role in the regulation of water and sodium balance. Plasma tonicity (also called effective plasma osmolality) is of primary importance in osmoregulation. Changes in plasma tonicity is sensed by osmoreceptors in the hypothalamus. These receptors affect both water intake and water excretion by influencing thirst and the release of antidiuretic hormone (ADH) respectively. ADH is the primary physiologic determinant of the rate of free water excretion. Its major renal effect is to augment the water permeability of the luminal membranes of principal cells in the cortical and medullary collecting tubules thereby promoting water reabsorption.

ADH acts via vasopressin 2 (V2) receptors, initiates a sequence of intracellular events resulting in the expression of preformed cytoplasmic vesicles that contain unique water channels (aquaporin 2) on the luminal membranes thereby allowing water to be reabsorbed.

Thus, regulation of plasma tonicity is achieved by alterations in water balance. Suppression of ADH release is the primary protective mechanism against water retention and the development of hyponatremia, while thirst is the primary protective mechanism against water loss and development of hypernatremia. In humans, the osmotic threshold for ADH release is about 280-290 mOsmol/kg. Below this level, there is little if any circulating ADH and above the threshold, there is a progressive and relatively linear rise in ADH secretion. This system is so efficient that the plasma osmolality usually does not vary by more than 1-2%, despite wide fluctuations in water intake. Normal individuals can attain a maximum urine volume of over 10 L/day depending on the water load. Individuals should not develop hyponatremia unless water intake exceeds this value, which occurs most often in psychotic patients with primary polydipsia.

HYPONATREMIA

Hyponatremia is defined as plasma sodium less than 135 meq/L: Its incidence in the hospitalized setting is 1.5-2.5%. Serum sodium reflects the relative proportion of sodium and water. Hyponatremia usually means water overload and not sodium deficit. In normal individuals, a water load results in dilutional fall in serum osmolality, which suppresses the release of antidiuretic hormone and thereby allowing excretion of the excess water in a dilute urine.

In contrast to the response, in normal individuals, patients who develop hyponatremia typically have impairment in renal water excretion, most after due to an inability to suppress ADH secretion. An uncommon exception occurs in patient with primary polydipsia who can become hyponatremic because they drink such large quantities of fluid that overwhelm the excretory capacity of the kidney even though ADH release is appropriately suppressed.

ETIOLOGY AND CLASSIFICATION

Translocational Hyponatremia

This is seen in patients with diabetic ketoacidosis. Glucose cannot move freely across cell membranes in the absence of insulin, and with an increase in glucose, water moves from the cells to the ECF, leading to cellular dehydration and lowering serum sodium. For every 100 mg/dL increase in the glucose, the expected decrease in the sodium is by 1.6 mmol/L.

Pseudohyponatremia

Occurs when the solid phase of plasma is increased by large increments in either lipid or proteins (e.g. in hypertriglyceridemia and paraproteinemia). Serum osmolality is normal in pseudohyponatremia.

True Hyponatremia

True hyponatremia is classified based on the volume status of the patient as *hypovolemic, euvolemic, or hypervolemic.*

Hypovolemic Hyponatremia

- *Gastrointestinal and third space sequestered losses*: Diarrhea, vomiting. *Sequestration of fluid in the third spaces*: In the peritoneal cavity with peritonitis or pancreatitis, in the bowel lumen with ileus.
- *Diuretics*: One of the most common causes of hypovolemic hyponatremia. Thiazide diuretics cause more profound hyponatremia than loop diuretics.
- *Salt losing nephropathy*: Seen in patients with chronic renal impairment due to interstitial disease.
- *Mineralocorticoid deficiency*: Associated with hypovolemia, hyponatremia and hyperkalemia.
- *Osmotic diuresis*: Seen with mannitol or patients with diabetic ketoacidosis, starvation, and alcoholic ketoacidosis.
- *Cerebral salt wasting*: It is a syndrome primarily seen in patients with subarachnoid hemorrhage. The primary defect is salt wasting from the kidneys with subsequent volume contraction, which stimulate vasopressin release. The exact mechanism is not understood, but it is postulated that brain natriuretic peptide increases urine volume and Na^+ excretion.

Hypervolemic Hyponatremia

Here the total body water is increased more than the total body Na^+. Seen in,

- Congestive heart failure
- Hepatic failure
- Nephrotic syndrome
- Advanced chronic renal impairment.

Euvolemic Hyponatremia

It is the most common dysnatremia in hospitalized patients:

- *Glucocorticoid deficiency*: It causes impaired water excretion in patient with primary or secondary adrenal insufficiency. This can be corrected by physiologic doses of corticosteroids.
- *Hypothyroidism*: It occurs in patients with severe hypothyroidism, who usually meet the clinical criteria for myxedema coma. It is readily reversed by treatment with levothyroxine sodium.
- *Postoperative hyponatremia*: Mainly is a result of excessive infusion of electrolyte-free water (hypotonic saline or 5% dextrose in water) and the presence of vasopressin, which prevents water excretion.
- *Drug-induced hyponatremia*: It is becoming the most common cause of hyponatermia. Thiazide diuretics are the most common cause, probably followed by selective serotonin reuptake inhibitors (SSRIs). It is mediated by enhancing the vasopressin release of by potentiating the action of vasopressin.
- *Syndrome of inappropriate antidiuretic hormone (SIADH) secretion:* Despite the most common cause of hyponatremia in hospitalized patients, the syndrome of inappropriate ADH secretion is a diagnosis of exclusion. A defect in osmoregulation causes vasopressin to be inappropriately stimulated, leading to urine concentration. Causes of SIADH are mentioned in **Table 7.1**. The diagnostic criteria for SIADH are summarized in **Table 7.2**.

Cerebral salt wasting (CSW) and SIADH share many features **(Table 7.3)**. Both conditions present with low serum osmolality, high urine osmolality, and a high urine sodium level. The principle difference between the two processes is the extracellular fluid volume status.

CLINICAL MANIFESTATIONS OF HYPONATREMIA

Most patients with a serum [Na^+] above 125 mmol/L are asymptomatic. Hyponatremia induces generalized cellular swelling, a consequence of water movement down the osmotic gradient from the hypotonic ECF to the ICF. The symptoms of hyponatremia are primarily neurologic, due to the development of cerebral edema. Early symptoms can include headache, yawning, lethargy, nausea, reversible ataxia, psychosis and can progress to seizures and coma. Rarely increased intracerebral pressure leads to tentorial herniation, respiratory depression, and death. Acute hyponatremia is a medical emergency and in patient with untreated severe hyponatremia, mortality is as high as 50%.

DIAGNOSTIC APPROACH IN HYPONATREMIA (FLOW CHART 7.1)

Major steps in initial evaluation of hyponatremia:

- Plasma osmolality
  Low: True hyponatremia
  Normal or elevated: Pseudohyponatremia or renal failure.
- *Urine osmolality:* Less than 100 mOsm/kg or specific gravity <1.003-dilute urine suggest primary polydipsia with normal water excretion.

Table 7.1 Causes of syndrome of inappropriate antidiuretic hormone (SIADH) secretion

Central nervous system diseases	*Neoplasias*	*Pulmonary disorders*	*Drugs that stimulate AVP release*	*Drugs that potentiate the effects of AVP action (primarily facilitates peripheral action of ADH)*	*Drugs with an uncertain mechanism*	*Drugs with antidiuretic action*	*Other causes*
• Acute psychosis	Pulmonary—Lung carcinoma and mesothelioma	Acute bronchitis/ bronchiolitis	Acetylcholine	Clofibrate	Antineoplastic agents—Cisplatin, melphalan, methotrexate, imatinib	Cyclophosphamide	Exercise-induced hyponatremia
• Acute intermittent porphyria	Gastrointestinal—Carcinomas of the duodenum, pancreas, and colon	Acute respiratory failure	Antineoplastic agents—Adenine arabinoside, cyclophosphamide, ifosfamide, vincristine, vinblastine	Griseofulvin	Ciprofloxacin		Giant cell arteritis
• Brain abscess	Genitourinary—Adrenocortical carcinoma; carcinomas of cervix, ureter/ bladder, and prostate; and ovarian tumors	Aspergillosis (cavitary lesions)	Barbiturates	Hypoglycemic agents—Metformin, phenformin, tolbutamide	Clomipramine		HIV infection-Idiopathic

Contd...

Contd...

Central nervous system diseases	*Neoplasias*	*Pulmonary disorders*	*Drugs that stimulate AVP release*	*Drugs that potentiate the effects of AVP action (primarily facilitates peripheral action of ADH)*	*Drugs with an uncertain mechanism*	*Drugs with antidiuretic action*	*Other causes*
• Cavernous sinus thrombosis	Other-Brain tumors, carcinoid tumors, Ewing sarcoma, leukemia, lymphoma, nasopharyngeal carcinoma, neuroblastoma (olfactory), and thymoma	Asthma	Bromocriptine	Oxytocin (large doses)	Ecstasy		
• Cerebellar and cerebral atrophy		Atelectasis	Carbachol	Prostaglandin synthetase inhibitors (inhibit renal PGE_2 synthesis)—Indomethacin, aspirin, nonsteroidal anti-inflammatory drugs	Phenoxy-benzamine		
• Cerebrovascular accident		Bacterial pneumonia	Chlorpropamide	Theophylline	Sodium valproate		

Contd...

Contd...

Central nervous system diseases	*Neoplasias*	*Pulmonary disorders*	*Drugs that stimulate AVP release*	*Drugs that potentiate the effects of AVP action (primarily facilitates peripheral action of ADH)*	*Drugs with an uncertain mechanism*	*Drugs with antidiuretic action*	*Other causes*
• CNS lupus		Chronic obstructive lung disease	Clofibrate	Triiodothyronine	SSRIs (e.g. sertraline, fluoxetine, paroxetine)		
• Delirium tremens		Cystic fibrosis	Cyclopropane	Vasopressin analogs (e.g. AVP, DDAVP)	Thiothixene		
• Encephalitis (viral or bacterial)		Emphysema	Dibenzazepines (e.g. carbamazepine, oxcarbazepine				
• Epilepsy		Empyema	Halothane				
• Guillain-Barré syndrome		Pneumonia (viral, bacterial [mycoplasmal], fungal)	Haloperidol				
• Head trauma		Pneumothorax	Histamine				
• Herpes zoster (chest wall)		Positive pressure ventilation	Isoproterenol				

Contd...

Contd...

Central nervous system diseases	*Neoplasias*	*Pulmonary disorders*	*Drugs that stimulate AVP release*	*Drugs that potentiate the effects of AVP action (primarily facilitates peripheral action of ADH)*	*Drugs with an uncertain mechanism*	*Drugs with antidiuretic action*	*Other causes*
• Hydrocephalus		Pulmonary abscess	Lorcainide				
• Hypoxic ischemic encephalopathy		Pulmonary fibrosis	Opiates e.g. morphine				
• Meningitis (viral, bacterial, tuberculous, and fungal)		Sarcoidosis	Nicotine (inhaled tobacco)				
• Midfacial hypoplasia		Tuberculosis	Nitrous oxide				
• Multiple sclerosis		Viral pneumonia	Phenothiazines (e.g. thioridazine)				
• Perinatal hypoxia			Thiopental				
• Rocky Mountain spotted fever			Monoamine oxidase inhibitors (e.g. tranylcypromine)				

Contd...

Contd...

Central nervous system diseases	*Neoplasias*	*Pulmonary disorders*	*Drugs that stimulate AVP release*	*Drugs that potentiate the effects of AVP action (primarily facilitates peripheral action of ADH)*	*Drugs with an uncertain mechanism*	*Drugs with antidiuretic action*	*Other causes*
• Schizophrenia			Tricyclic antidepressants (e.g., amitriptyline, desipramine)				
• Shy-Drager syndrome • Subarachnoid hemorrhage • Subdural hematoma • Ventriculoatrial shunt obstruction • Wernicke encephalopathy							

Abbreviations: AVP, arginine vasopressin; ADH, antidiuretic hormone; HIV, human immunodeficiency virus; CNS, central nervous system; DDAVP, desmopressin

Table 7.2 Diagnostic criteria of syndrome of inappropriate antidiuretic hormone (SIADH) secretion

Essential features	*Supplemental features*
• Decreased effective serum osmolality (<275 mOsm/kg)	• Serum uric acid <4.0 mg/dL/<0.24 mmol/L
• Urinary osmolality >100 mOsm/kg during hypotonicity of the serum	• Serum urea 10.0 mg/dL/ <3.6 mmol/L, low normal serum creatinine
• Clinical euvolemia	• Fractional sodium excretion >1%, fractional urea excretion >55%
• Urinary sodium >40 mEq/L with normal dietary salt intake	• Failure to correct hyponatremia after 0.9% saline infusion
• Normal thyroid and adrenal function	• Correction of hyponatremia through fluid restriction
• No recent use of diuretics	• Abnormal water loading test (excretion <80% of a 20 mL/kg water load in 4 h)
	• Elevated vasopressin levels despite hypotonicity and clinical euvolemia

Table 7.3 Comparison between syndrome of inappropriate antidiuretic hormone (SIADH) secretion and cerebral salt wasting (CSW)

Biochemical marker	*SIADH*	*CSW*
Extracellular fluid volume	Normal to high	Low
Hematocrit	Normal	High
Serum albumin	Normal	High
Blood urea nitrogen (BUN)/creatinine	Low	High
Urinary sodium level	>40 mEq/L	>40 mEq/L
Serum uric acid level	Low	Low
Initial fractional excretion of urate	High	High
Fractional excretion of urate after correction	Normal	High
Urinary osmolality	High	High
Serum osmolality	Low	Low

More than 100 mOsm/kg other causes of hyponatremia in which water excretion is impaired.

- *Urine sodium concentration:* Less than 15 meq/L-effective volume depletion—diarrhea, vomiting.
  More than 20 meq/L-SIADH (euvolemia) or renal salt wasting (diuretics, renal disease or hypoaldosteronism).

TREATMENT OF HYPONATREMIA

Treatment of hyponatremia must be individualized considering the etiology, rate of development (acute vs chronic), severity and clinical signs and symptoms.

Flow chart 7.1 Approach to hyponatremia

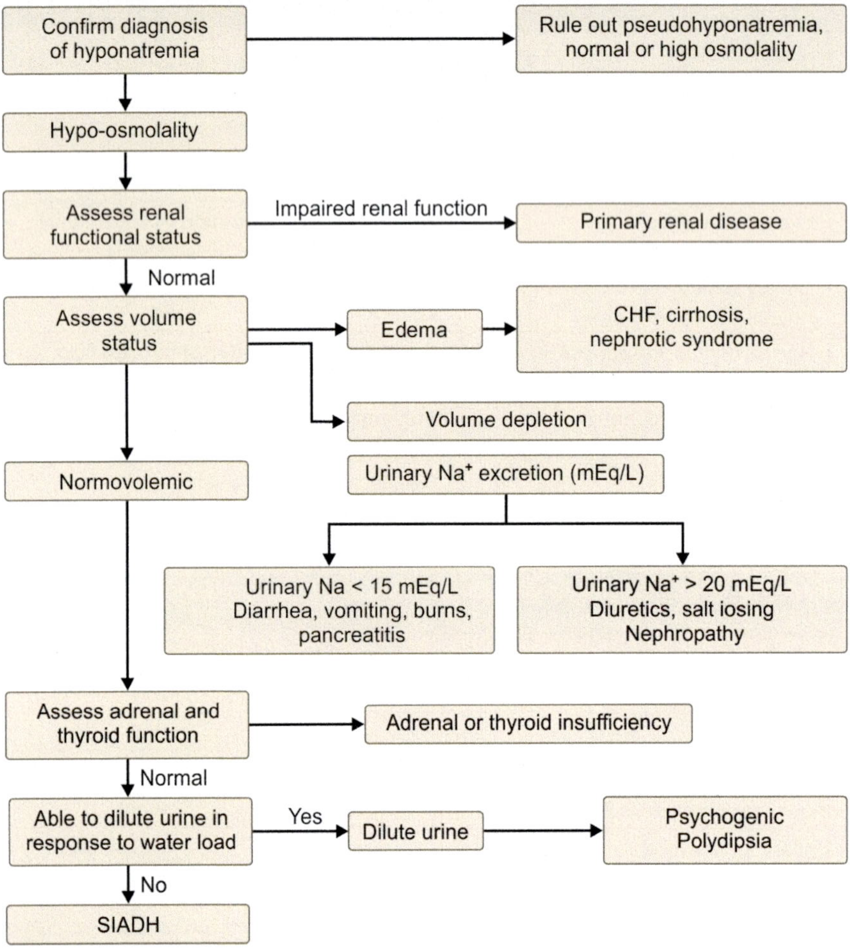

Abbreviations: SIADH, syndrome of inappropriate antidiuretic hormone secretion; CHF, congestive heart failure

Acute hyponatremic patients (hyponatremia developing within 48 hours) are at great risk for development of permanent neurologic sequelae from cerebral edema. Patients with chronic hyponatremia are at risk for osmotic demyelination if the hyponatremia is corrected too rapidly **(Flow chart 7.2)**.

Goals of therapy:

- To raise the plasma sodium concentration to a safe level.
- To replace sodium deficit.
- To correct underlying etiology.

In general, hyponatremia is corrected acutely by giving sodium to patients who are volume depleted and by restricting water intake in patients who are normovolemia or hypervolemic.

Flow chart 7.2 Algorithm for management of patient with hyponatremia

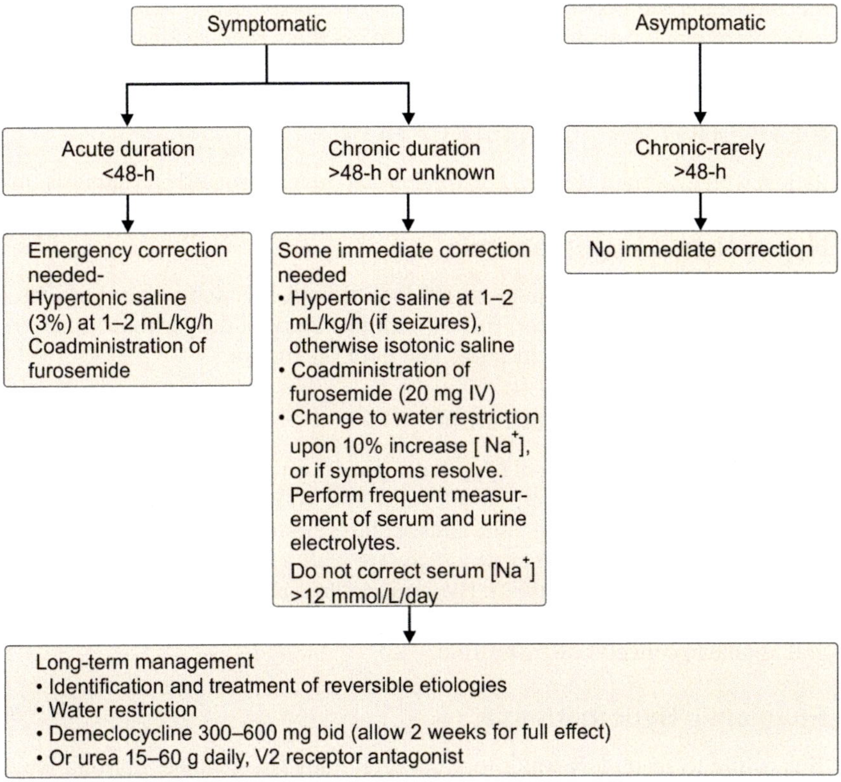

For acute symptomatic hyponatremia, serum sodium should be ideally corrected by 2 mmol/L/h until symptoms resolve.

For chronic hyponatremia, do not exceed a correction rate of 1.0–1.5 mmol/L in any given hour and not to increase the serum sodium by more than 12 mmol/L/24 h.

Fluid restriction is the first-line therapy in patients with chronic asymptomatic hyponatremia. If the patient remains unresponsive to fluid restriction, solute intake can be increased to facilitate an obligatory increase in excretion of solute and free water. Loop diuretics combined with high sodium intake (2–3 g of additional salt) are effective in the management of hyponatremia.

Vasopressin 2 (V2) receptor antagonist: Vaptans are novel oral V2 receptor antagonists that increase free water excretion without significantly altering electrolyte excretion. Vaptans are effective in the treatment of hyponatremia in euvolemic and hypervolemic patients. Tolvaptan is the drug, which is commonly used and is available at doses of 15–60 mg/day. Conivaptan, V2 and V1a receptor antagonist, is the only vaptan available for IV use.

HYPERNATREMIA

Hypernatremia is defined as plasma sodium concentration greater than 145 mEq/L.

It is usually due to water deficit and not due to sodium overload. The thirst mechanism is the first and most important defence mechanism in preventing hypernatremia. It usually does not occur unless there is nonavailability of water, impaired thirst or comatose-confused patient unable to drink water.

ETIOLOGY AND CLASSIFICATION

Patient with hypernatremia fall into *three broad categories* based on volume status.

Hypovolemic Hypernatremia

In these patients, there is a sustained loss of both Na^+ and water, but with a relatively greater loss of water. There are clinical signs of dehydration, including orthostatic hypotension, tachycardia and poor skin turgor.

Hypervolemic Hypernatremia

It is the least common form of hypernatremia. It results from the administration of hypertonic solutions such as 3% NaCl and $NaHCO_3$ for the treatment of metabolic acidosis, hyperkalemia, and cardiorespiratory arrest. It may also result from inadvertent dialysis against a dialysate with a high Na^+ concentration or from consumption of salt tablets. Hypernatremia is also increasingly recognized in hypoalbuminemic hospitalized patients with renal failure who are edematous and unable to concentrate their urine.

Euvolemic Hypernatremia

This is due to secondary water loss but total body Na^+ remains normal. Water loss can be renal or extrarenal. Renal water loss results either from a defect in vasopressin production or release (central diabetes insipidus) or from a failure of the collecting duct to respond to the hormone (nephrogenic diabetes insipidus). Extrarenal water loss occurs from the skin and respiratory tract in febrile or other hypermetabolic states and is associated with a high urine osmolality because the osmoreceptor-vasopressin-renal response is intact.

DIABETES INSIPIDUS

It is characterized by polyuria and polydipsia and is caused by defects in vasopressin action.

Central Diabetes Insipidus

Usually has an abrupt onset. Patient have a constant need to drink, have a predilection for cold water, and typically have nocturia. The plasma osmolality is usually more than 295 mOsm/kg **(Table 7.4)**.

Treatment of Central Diabetes Insipidus

In acute settings, when renal after losses are extensive, aqueous vasopressin (Pitressin) is useful. It should be used in caution in patients with underlying

Table 7.4 Etiology of central diabetes insipidus

Causes of central diabetes insipidus
Congenital
Autosomal dominant
Autosomal recessive
Acquired
Post-traumatic
Iatrogenic (postsurgical)
Tumors (metastatic from breast, craniopharyngioma, pinealoma)
Histiocytosis
Granuloma (tuberculosis, sarcoid)
Aneurysm
Meningitis
Encephalitis
Guillain-Barré syndrome
Idiopathic

Table 7.5 Treatment of central diabetes insipidus

Disease	*Drug*	*Dose*	*Interval*
Complete central diabetes insipidus	Desmopressin (DDAVP)	10–20 µg intranasally	12–24 h
	Desmopressin (DDAVP)	0.1–0.8 mg orally	Every 12 h
Partial central diabetes insipidus	Desmopressin (DDAVP)	10–20 µg intranasally	12–24 h
	Aqueous vasopressin	5–10 U subcutaneously	4–6 h
	Chlorpropamide	250–500 mg	24 h
	Clofibrate	500 mg	6 or 8 h
	Carbamazepine	400–600 mg	24 h

coronary artery disease and peripheral vascular disease because it may cause vascular spasm and prolonged vasoconstriction.

For chronic diabetes insipidus (DI), desmopressin acetate is the agent of choice. It has a long half-life. Desmopressin is administered at the dose of 10–20 mcg intranasal every 12–24 hours. It is tolerated well, safe in pregnancy, and resistant to degradation by circulating vasopressinase. In patients with partial DI, in addition to desmopressin, agents that potentiate the release of vasopressin may be used, including chlorpropamide, clofibrate, and carbamazepine **(Table 7.5)**.

Nephrogenic Diabetes Insipidus

- *Congenital*: Mutation in genes for aquaporins or vasopressin receptors.
- *Acquired nephrogenic DI*: It is more common than congenital nephrogenic DI but rarely as severe. In patients with acquired DI, the ability to elaborate

a maximal concentration of urine is impaired, but urine-concentrating mechanisms are partially preserved. Urine volumes are less than 3–4 L/day, which contrasts with much higher volumes seen in patients with congenital or central DI **(Table 7.6)**.

CLINICAL MANIFESTATION OF HYPERNATREMIA

Signs and symptoms mostly relate to the CNS and include altered mental status, lethargy, irritability, restlessness, seizures (usual in children), muscle twitching,

Table 7.6 Etiology of acquired nephrogenic diabetes insipidus
Chronic kidney disease
Hypokalemia
Hypercalcemia
Sickle cell disease
Protein malnutrition
Demeclocycline therapy
Lithium therapy
Pregnancy

Flow chart 7.3 Treatment of hypernatremia

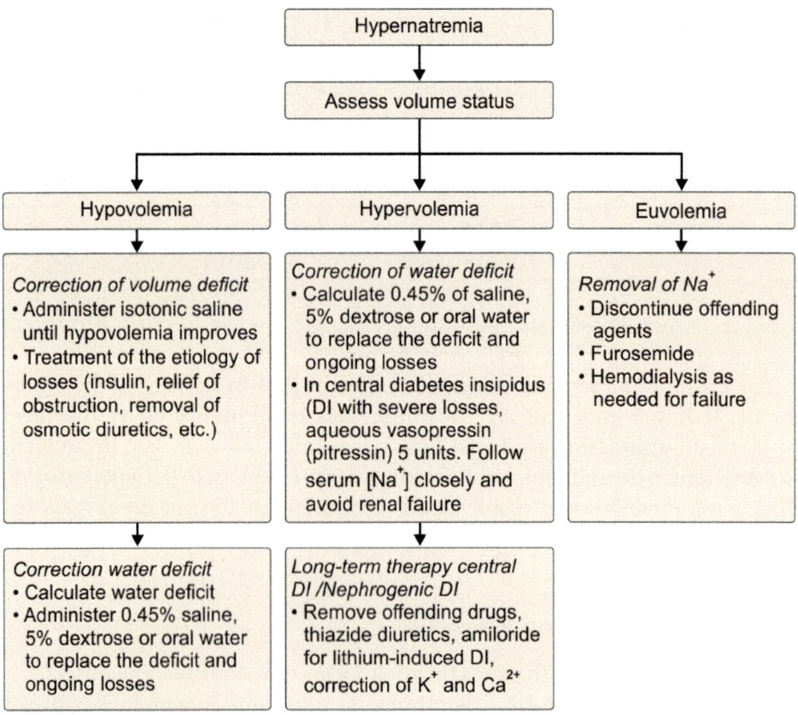

Abbreviation: DI, diabetes insipidus

hyperreflexia, and spasticity. Fever, nausea or vomiting, labored breathing, and intense thirst can also occur.

TREATMENT OF HYPERNATREMIA

Treatment of hypernatremia depends on the type of hypernatremia and rapidity of its development.

Treatment of hypernatremia has been summarized in **Flow chart 7.3**.

SUMMARY

- Abnormalities of sodium and water balance are frequently seen in hospitalized and OPD patients are frequently seen.
- It is important to pin down the exact etiology before formulating the treatment plan.
- Clinical examination along with lab findings are required for diagnosis.
- Rapid correction is usually undesirable unless the changes are acute and has effects on central nervous system.

Multiple Choice Questions

1. **The normal plasma osmolality is:**
   a. 275–290 mOsm/kg
   b. 290–310 mOsm/kg
   c. 260–275 mOsm/kg
   d. None of the above
2. **Pseudohyponatremia is seen in:**
   a. Surreptitious diuretic abuse
   b. Hypertriglyceridemia
   c. Nephritic syndrome
   d. Glucocorticoid deficiency
3. **Diagnostic criteria of SIADH includes all except:**
   a. Decreased serum osmolality <275 mOsm/kg
   b. Urine osmolality <50 mOsm/kg
   c. Failure to correct hyponatremia after 0.9% saline infusion
   d. Normal thyroid and adrenal function
4. **Euvolemic hyponatremia is seen in all except:**
   a. Glucocorticoid deficiency
   b. Hypothyroidism
   c. SIADH
   d. Cerebral salt wasting
5. **Cardinal principal of treatment of chronic hyponatremia include all except:**
   a. Correction rate not to exceed 1–1.5 mmol/hour
   b. Not to target serum sodium >12 mmol in 24 hours
   c. Use 3% saline infusion to achieve optimal resuscitation
   d. Not to correct beyond 125 mEq/L in 24 hours
6. **All the following statements on Vaptans are true except:**
   a. Contraindicated in hypovolemic hyponatremia
   b. Convaptan can be used intravenously
   c. Orally available drugs act on V_1 and V_2 receptors
   d. Increase free water clearance without salt excretion

7. One of the following conditions does not cause nephrogenic diabetes insipidus:
a. Hypokalemia
b. Demeclocycline toxicity
c. Hypocalcemia
d. Sickle cell disease

8. All the following can be used to treat partial central diabetes insipidus except:
a. Desmopressin
b. Chlorpropamide
c. Carbamazepine
d. Dexamethasone

9. Which one of the following statement is false?
a. Nephrogenic diabetes insipidus as well as central diabetes insipidus have euvolemic state
b. Hypervolemic hypernatremia is the least common type of hyponatremia
c. Hypovolemic hypernatremia is seen in patients with dehydration
d. Hypernatremia commonly occurs in conscious patients with intact thirst mechanism

10. In cerebral salt wasting fractional urate excretion after correction of hyponatremia is:
a. Remains high
b. Normalizes
c. Becomes very low
d. All of the above

Answers

1. a 2. b 3. b 4. d 5. c 6. c 7. c 8. d
9. d 10. a

SUGGESTED READING

1. Berl T, Parikh C. Disorders of water metabolism. In: Johnson RJ, Feehally J, Floege J (Eds). Comprehensive Clinical Nephrology, 5th edn. Philadelphia, PA: Elsevier/Saunders. 2015. pp. 94-110.
2. Bichet DG. Nephrogenic and central diabetes insipidus. In: Schrier RW, Coffman RM, Falk RJ, Molitoris BA, Neilson EG (Eds). Schrier's Diseases of the Kidney, 8th edn. Philadelphia. LWW. 2007. pp. 2249-69.
3. Eric E Simon (Ed). In: Hyponatremia evaluation and treatment, 1st edn. New York. Springer, 2013.
4. Slotki AN, Skorecki KL. Disorders of sodium balance. In: Skorecki KL, Chertow GM, Marsen MD, Taal MW, Alan SL (Eds). Brenner and Rector's The Kidney, 10th edn. Philadelphia, PA: Elsevier; 2016. pp. 390-459.
5. Verbalis JG. Disorders of water balance. In: Skorecki KL, Chertow GM, Marsen MD, Taal MW, Alan SL (Eds). Brenner and Rector's The Kidney, 10th edn. Philadelphia, PA: Elsevier; 2016. pp. 460-510.
6. Verbalis JG. The syndrome of inappropriate antidiuretic hormone secretion and other hypoosmolar disorders. In: Schrier RW, Coffman RM, Falk RJ, Molitoris BA, Neilson EG (Eds). Schrier's Diseases of the Kidney, 8th edn. Philadelphia. LWW; 2007. pp. 2214-48.

HYPOKALEMIA AND HYPERKALEMIA

Satish D, Gokulnath

INTRODUCTION

Potassium is the major intracellular cation in the body with more than 90% of total body potassium located in the intracellular compartment, mainly in muscle (60–75%). Only 1.4% of the total body K^+ is contained within the water space of the extracellular fluid, with the remainder of extracellular K^+ sequestered in bone. Its plasma concentration normally ranges from 3.5 to 5.2 mmol/L and is approximately 0.4 mmol/L greater in serum, because of K^+ release from cellular components during clot formation, whereas the intracellular concentration is estimated to be approximately 150 mmol/L.

Potassium uptake into the cell is mediated by Na^+ K^+-ATPase, a pump that couples the energy of ATP hydrolysis to the electrogenic extrusion of sodium and uptake of potassium, with a stoichiometry of three Na^+ to two K^+ ions for each ATP hydrolyzed **(Fig. 7.1)**. In steady-state conditions, the rate of active K^+ uptake through the pump is counterbalanced by passive K^+ losses through various leak pathways.

The transmembrane K^+ gradient largely determines the resting membrane potential of cells and alterations in the transcellular distribution of K^+ affect critical neuromuscular functions **(Table 7.7)**.

HYPOKALEMIA

Hypokalemia defined as serum potassium less than 3.5 mmol/L, can result either from a shift of K^+ into cells or from depletion of cellular K^+ stores. If serum potassium is less than 2.5 mmol/L, it is termed severe hypokalemia **(Table 7.8)**.

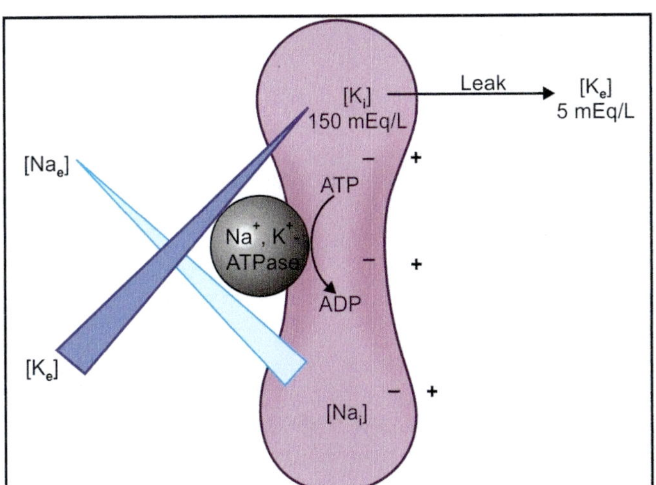

Figure 7.1 Potassium uptake by cells via Na^+ K^+-ATPase

Table 7.7 Factors that modify transcellular K^+ distribution

	Increase intracellular K^+ or decrease plasma K^+	*Decrease intracellular K^+/ Increase plasma K^+*
Acid-base status	Metabolic alkalosis	Metabolic and respiratory acidosis
	Respiratory alkalosis (chronic)	Acute respiratory alkalosis
	Increased plasma bicarbonate	
Hormones	Insulin	Glucagon
	β-Adrenergic agonists	Nonspecific beta-blockers α-Adrenergic stimulation
		Aldosterone
Others		Hyperosmolality For example, Mannitol, hyperglycemia
		Exercise

Table 7.8 Effects of hypokalemia

Cardiac	*Neuromuscular*	*Renal*	*Fluid -electrolytes*	*Endocrine*
Digitalis intoxication	Intestinal hypomotility Ileus	Impaired blood flow Decreased GFR	Polyuria	Low aldosterone
Ventricular arrhythmias Torsades de pointes	Muscular weakness Paralysis	Interstitial nephritis	Metabolic alkalosis	High renin
ECG changes: Flattening T-wave U-waves Prolonged QT ST depression	Rhabdomyolysis	Cyst formation	Increased ammon-iagenesis	Increased prostaglandins
		Polyuria	Chloride wasting	Glucose intolerance
		Increased ammoniagenesis	Hypercalciuria	Growth retardation
		Hypertension	Phosphaturia	

PATHOPHYSIOLOGY

Hypokalemia leads to increase in the K_i^+/K_e^+ ratio. The resultant hyperpolarization of the membrane increases the threshold for initiation, and interferes with the termination, of an action potential. Hence, a variety of neuromuscular functions can be impaired by hypokalemia. K^+ depletion also decreases the intracellular K^+ concentration with an attendant intracellular acidosis, and thereby interferes with both K^+ - and pH-dependent intracellular processes.

ETIOLOGY

Hypokalemia can be produced either by a transcellular shift of K^+ from the extra- to intracellular compartment (transcellular shift) or by actual K^+ depletion **(Table 7.9)**.

Approach to evaluation: The cause of hypokalemia is usually apparent from the history, and there are two major components to the diagnostic evaluation **(Flow chart 7.4)**:

1. *Assessment of urinary potassium excretion*: The best method for assessing renal potassium excretion is a 24-hour urine collection. However, the potassium concentration or, preferably, potassium-to-creatinine ratio on a spot urine

Table 7.9 Etiology of hypokalemia

Redistribution hypokalemia	*Actual K^+ depletion*	
	Extrarenal (Urine K <20 mmol/day)	*Renal (Urine K >20 mmol/day)*
Alkalosis	Inadequate intake	Renal tubular acidosis
Excessive insulin	Copious perspiration	Diabetic ketoacidosis
Drugs: • Adrenaline • Salbutamol • Terbutaline • Theophylline • Barium • Toluene • Chloroquine • Calcium-channel blockers	*Gastrointestinal losses:* • Diarrhea • Laxative abuse • Villous adenoma • Uretero sigmoidostomies	*Chloride depletion:* • Vomiting/gastric drainage • Diuretic therapy • Posthypercapneic state • Congenital chloride-wasting diarrhea • Certain secretory diarrheas • Sweat chloride losses as in cystic fibrosis • Inadequate chloride intake in infants
Hypokalemic periodic paralysis		Magnesium depletion
Thyrotoxicosis		*Genetic:* • Bartter's syndrome • Gitelman syndrome • Liddle syndrome
		Mineralocorticoid excess
		Glucocorticoid excess
		Drugs: • Diuretics • Sodium penicillin • Aminoglycosides
		Leukemia
		Interstitial nephritis

Flow chart 7.4 Diagnostic approach to hypokalemia

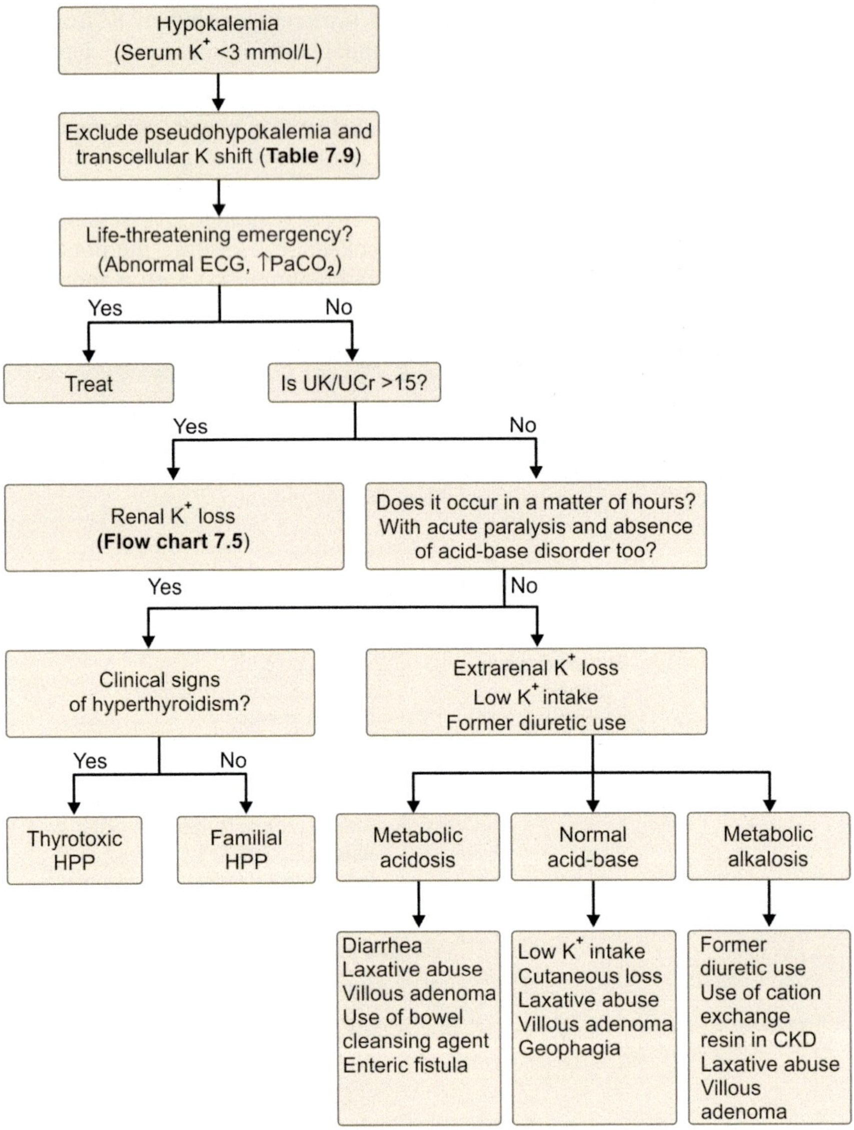

Abbreviations: HPP, hypokalmic periodic paralysis; ECG, electrocardiography; CKD, chronic kidney disease

are alternatives. Since creatinine is excreted at a near-constant rate, the urine potassium-to-creatinine ratio corrects for variations in urine volume. The urine potassium-to-creatinine ratio is usually less than 13 mEq/g creatinine (1.5 mEq/mmol creatinine) when hypokalemia is caused by transcellular potassium shifts, gastrointestinal losses, previous use of diuretics, or poor dietary intake. Higher values are seen with renal potassium wasting.

2. *Assessment of acid-base status.*

A few important points:

- Metabolic acidosis with a low rate of urinary potassium excretion is suggestive of lower gastrointestinal losses due to laxative abuse or a villous adenoma.
- Metabolic acidosis with urinary potassium wasting is most often due to diabetic ketoacidosis or to type 1 (distal) or type 2 (proximal) renal tubular acidosis **(Flow chart 7.5)**.
- Metabolic alkalosis with a low rate of urinary potassium excretion may be due to surreptitious vomiting (as in bulimic patients) or diuretic use.
- Metabolic alkalosis with urinary potassium wasting: with normotension **(Flow chart 7.6)** vs hypertension **(Flow chart 7.7)**.

TREATMENT

Although serum potassium is not an exact indicator of the total body K^+ deficit, a decrease (below 4 mEq/L) of 0.27 mEq/L is approximately equivalent to 100 mEq/L of K deficit (up to a total deficit of 500 mEq/L). Levels of <2.0 mEq/L may reflect deficit of >1000 mEq/L.

Goals

- Therapy is usually required only for replacement of K^+ deficits and not for hypokalemia that results from transcellular redistribution, because this is usually transitory.
- When feasible, K^+ should be given by the oral rather than intravenous route, slow rather than rapid K^+ replacement is preferable. Under most circumstances, administration of 40–120 mmol/day is adequate.

Flow chart 7.5 Diagnostic approach to hypokalemia due to renal loss

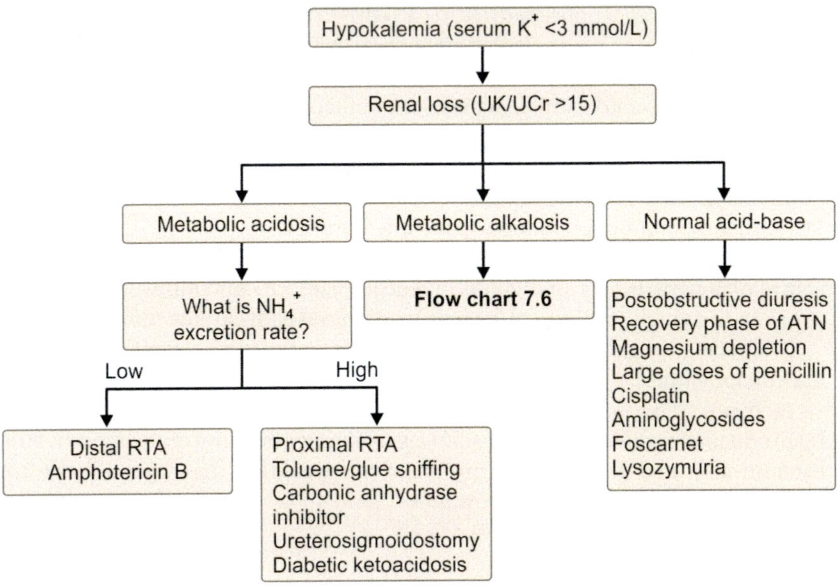

Abbreviations: RTA, renal tubular acidosis; ATN, acute tubular necrosis

Flow chart 7.6 Diagnostic approach to hypokalemia due to renal loss with metabolic alkalosis

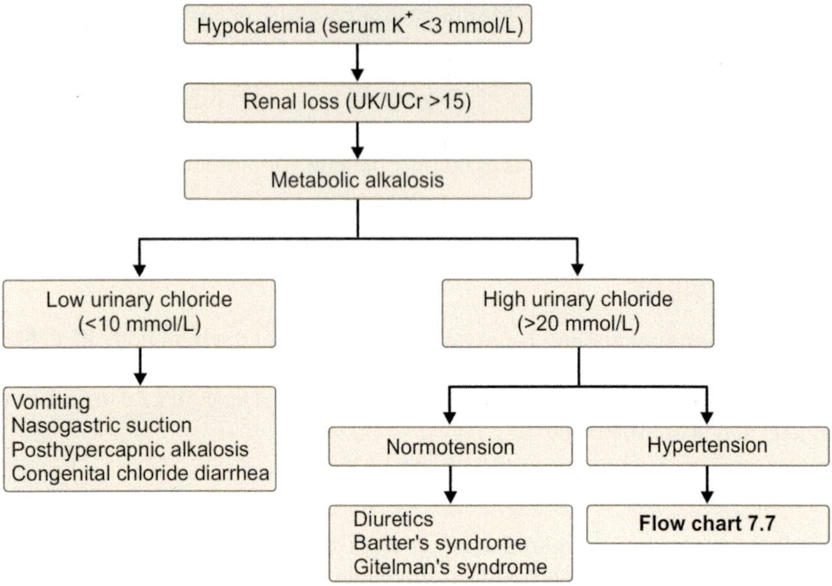

- Conservative approach to K^+ replacement since hyperkalemia from overzealous K^+ therapy is a life-threatening complication.
- Coexisting hypomagnesemia prevents correction of hypokalemia so it should be corrected as well.

The chloride salt of potassium (KCl) can correct any K^+ deficit and is an absolute requirement with chloride depletion such as with diuretic therapy or losses of upper gastrointestinal fluids. Bicarbonate or preparations containing bicarbonate precursors (gluconate, citrate, acetate) are indicated when a metabolic acidosis and K^+ deficit coexist. Similarly, phosphate compounds are useful when there is a concomitant phosphate deficit, as, for example, with diabetic ketoacidosis.

The K^+ sparing diuretics amiloride or triamterene are effective alternatives to KCl supplementation for patients receiving diuretics.

With life-threatening hypokalemic complications, such as paralysis, malignant ventricular arrhythmias, or digitalis intoxication, more rapid intravenous therapy (from 10 to as high as 40 mmol/h) may be required with cardiac monitoring.

β-blocking drugs may be useful in the treatment of hypokalemia due to drug like theophylline.

In hypokalemic periodic paralysis, treatment with acetazolamide, perhaps by producing chronic metabolic acidosis or, as suggested recently, by activating calcium-activated K^+ channels improves the weakness between attacks and reduces the incidence of paralytic attacks.

Flow chart 7.7 Diagnostic approach to hypokalemia due to renal loss with metabolic alkalosis and hypertension

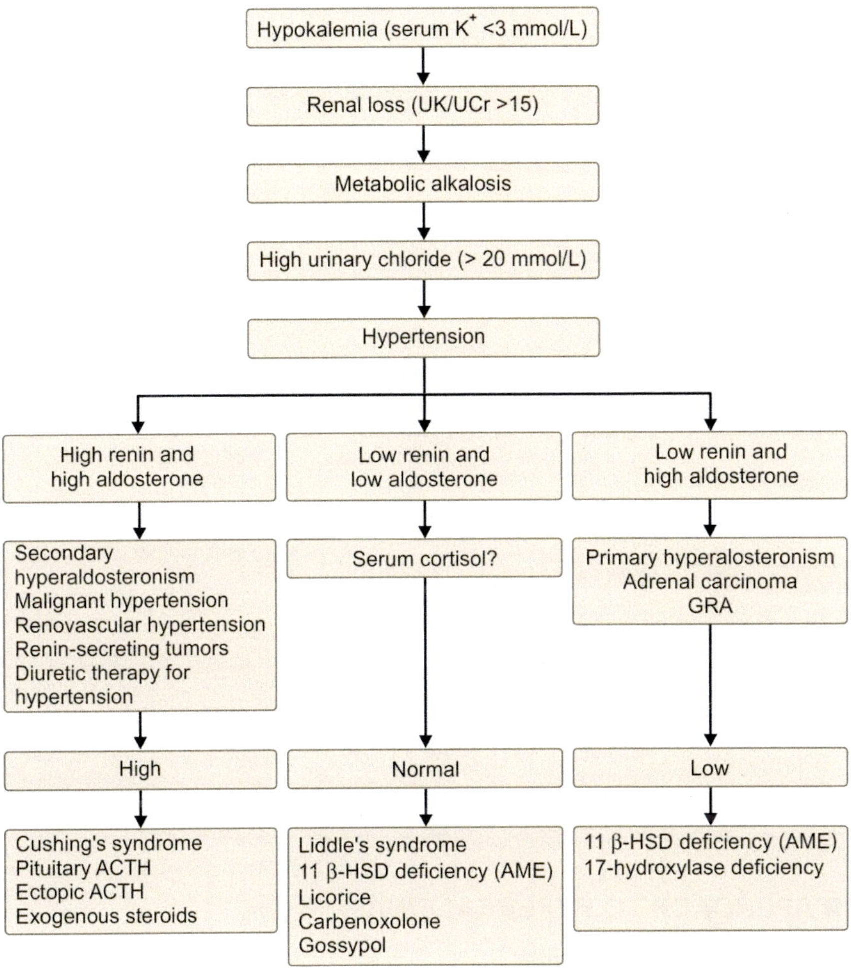

Abbreviations: ACTH, adrenocorticotropic hormone; HSD, hydroxysteroid dehydrogenase; AME, apparent mineralocorticoid excess

HYPERKALEMIA

When serum potassium is more than 5.5 mEq/L, it is termed hyperkalemia. Moderate hyperkalemia is when serum K >6 mEq/L and severe if serum K >7 mEq/L. It can result from a shift of K^+ from the intra- to extracellular fluid compartment or from excessive K^+ retention, which almost always implies a defect in the renal elimination of K^+. Several phenomena can spuriously elevate the serum K^+ (**Table 7.10**).

Table 7.10 Etiology of hyperkalemia

Spurious	*Redistribution*	*Renal*	
Ischemic blood drawing	Acidosis	Renal failure (severe)	Tubular dysfunction, e.g. obstructive uropathy, renal transplants, sickle-cell disease, lupus erythematosus, amyloidosis, and medullary sponge kidney
Hemolysis	Insulin deficiency	Aldosterone deficiency	Acquired disorders
Abnormal erythrocytes	Hyperosmolality	Addison's disease	Pseudohypoaldosteronism (Types I and II)
Thrombocytosis Leukocytosis	*Drugs*: β-Adrenergic blockade Digitalis Succinylcholine Arginine Fluoride Lithium	*Drugs*: PG synthase inhibitors ACE inhibitors Angiotensin II receptor blockers Heparin Cyclosporine Tacrolimus	K^+ -sparing drugs Spironolactone Amiloride/Triamterene Epithelial Na^+ channel blockers Trimethoprim Pentamidine Nafamostat mesilate
	Hyperkalaemic Periodic paralysis	HIV disease	
	Parathyroid hormone	Enzymatic defects Adrenogenital syndrome Aldosterone synthase Isolated aldosterone deficiency Hyporeninemic hypoaldosteronism	
	Exercise		
	Malignant hyperthermia		

APPROACH TO HYPERKALEMIA

Spurious Hyperkalemia

Tight or prolonged application of a tourniquet, especially if combined with exercise of the limb, can increase the K^+ concentration of the venous blood sample because of K^+ egress from muscle and its hemoconcentration. Severe leukocytosis (over 2×10^5 /mm^3) can result in sufficient egress of K^+ from white blood cells stored in the cold for spurious elevation of the K^+ determination.

Excessive Potassium Retention

Hyperkalemia can be produced by excessive K^+ intake, as in overzealous intravenous infusion, massive oral ingestion, or endogenous release from cell lysis during therapy of Burkitt lymphoma.

Defective urinary excretion of K^+ has three major causes: (a) renal failure-an inadequate number of functioning nephron units; (b) hypoaldosteronism; (c) defective tubular K^+ secretion.

The diagnostic evaluation of hyperkalemic patients without severe renal failure (GFR >20 mL/min) typically involves the measurement of plasma renin and aldosterone concentrations along with a determination of either fractional potassium excretion (FEK) or of the distal transtubular potassium gradient (TTKG).

FEK (urine-plasma ratio (U/P) of potassium divided by U/P creatinine) needs to be assessed in relation to GFR to determine whether renal secretion of potassium is impaired.

The TTKG, is determined by dividing U/P potassium concentration by U/P osmolality to correct for water abstraction by the medullary collecting duct. It provides an indirect measure of the K^+ concentration gradient and thereby of K^+ transport by the cortical collecting duct. In a hyperkalemic patient, a TTKG lesser than 8 implies an abnormal K^+ secretory response due to either hypoaldosteronism or a primary defect in tubular K^+ secretion. The accuracy of the TTKG is compromised during polyuria or excretion of dilute urine.

Renal Failure

Hyperkalemia poses a major, life-threatening risk to patients with renal failure. The risk of hyperkalemia is magnified in catabolic patients, in whom the daily increment in the plasma K^+ averages 0.7 mmol/L or more, in contrast to 0.3–0.5 mmol/L in noncatabolic patients with oliguric acute renal failure.

If K^+ intake is normal, chronic renal failure does not produce significant hyperkalemia until the GFR is less than 5 mL/min although milder elevations in K^+ may be present with less severe declines in GFR. K^+ balance is sustained because the remaining functional nephrons and the colon adapt their capacity to secrete K^+ in the same fashion as with a high K^+ diet. Upregulation of angiotensin II receptors may play a role in colon adaptation. Adaptation is detectable when the GFR is reduced to one-third of normal, is maximal at a GFR of less than 10 mL/min, and accounts for 10–20 mmol/day of the K^+ elimination.

Hypoaldosteronism

Hypoaldosteronism, especially when combined with a decrease in GFR or reduction in the delivery of salt and fluid to the distal nephron, can substantially impair urinary K^+ excretion. Diminished levels of aldosterone result from either a primary defect in the adrenal gland or from an abnormality in the renin-angiotensin II mechanism for stimulating aldosterone secretion.

Hyporeninemic hypoaldosteronism is characterized by low plasma renin activity unresponsive to Na^+ restriction or furosemide, low plasma and urinary aldosterone, hyperkalemia, and hyperchloremic metabolic acidosis (type IV renal tubular acidosis). Fractional K^+ excretion is low for the existing GFR, TTKG is low, and the response to kaliuretic stimuli is blunted. Mineralocorticoid replacement with fludrocortisone (0.2 mg/day) for 2 weeks usually corrects the plasma K^+ to normal.

Defective Tubular Secretion

In tubule interstitial renal diseases, have normal aldosterone and plasma renin activity and primary defect in the K^+ secretory function of the distal nephron. In contrast to patients with hyporeninemic hypoaldosteronism, the hyperkalemia is unresponsive to mineralocorticoid replacement therapy. Furthermore, the hyperchloremic metabolic acidosis is usually accompanied by an inability to lower the urine pH appropriately, which, in combination with hyperkalemic suppression of ammoniagenesis, and contribute to the acidosis.

All K^+ -sparing diuretics directly impair K^+ secretion by the distal nephron. Spironolactone, a specific aldosterone antagonist, impairs mineralocorticoid-dependent K^+ secretion. Amiloride and triamterene both block the apical Na^+ channel, impede electrogenic Na^+ reabsorption, decrease the transtubular voltage gradient, and thereby reduce both proton and potassium secretion.

CLINICAL MANIFESTATIONS

Hyperkalemia depolarizes excitable tissues by decreasing the K_i^+/K_e^+ ratio and impairs recovery of an action potential by increasing the K^+ conductance. This can result in life-threatening cardiac events **(Table 7.11)**.

TREATMENT

Treatment of hyperkalemia is dictated by the magnitude of the elevation in the plasma K^+, its electrocardiographic manifestations **(Table 7.12)**, and the likelihood of progressive worsening. As it is a life-threatening abnormality, it is wise to err in the direction of overly vigorous management. Prompt and intensive treatment is indicated if the serum K^+ concentration exceeds 6.5 mmol/L, if QRS prolongation is present on the electrocardiogram, or if it seems likely that the condition will rapidly worsen.

Table 7.11 Manifestations of hyperkalemia

Cardiac	*Fluid and electrolytes*	*Endocrine*	*Hemodynamic*
Impaired conduction	Decreased ammonia production	High aldosterone Low renin	Decreased blood pressure Decreased stroke
Ventricular fibrillation	Metabolic acidosis	Increased insulin and glucagon	
Pacemaker dysfunction	Natriuresis	Increased prostaglandin F 2α excretion Increased kallikrein excretion	*Muscle*: Flaccid paralysis

Table 7.12 Progressive ECG changes in hyperkalemia

Serum K > 5.5 mEq/L	*Serum K >6 mEq/L*	*Serum K >7 mEq/L*	*Serum K >9 mEq/L*
• Tall peaking T-waves-earliest change	• P-wave widens and flattens, eventually disappears • PR segment lengthens	• Prolonged QRS interval Bizarre QRS morphology • Sinus bradycardia • High-grade AV block • Conduction block (bundle branch blocks, fascicular blocks) • Sine wave appearance (a preterminal rhythm)	• Asystole • Ventricular fibrillation

Table 7.13 Therapy for hyperkalemia

Drug	*Dose*	*Onset of action*
Calcium gluconate	10% solution, 10–30 mL	Few minutes
Glucose and insulin	*Glucose*: 25–50 g/hour Regular insulin 5 units IV	15–30 min
Salbutamol	Nebulization	15–30 min
Sodium polystyrene	Enema 50–100 g	60 min
	Oral 40 g (with sorbitol)	120 min

The therapies used are outlined in **Table 7.13**. Initial steps are designed to counteract cardiac toxicity directly and to shift K^+ into the intracellular compartment. Definitive therapy requires removal of excessive potassium from the body.

Calcium counteracts the effect of hyperkalemia on cardiac conduction. It can be given as the gluconate or chloride salt, and acts almost immediately. Insulin, which must be given in combination with glucose to avoid hypoglycemia, rapidly promotes cellular uptake of K^+. Sodium bicarbonate has been traditionally viewed as useful in promoting cellular uptake of K^+; and there is conflicting evidence whether it can act in a synergistic fashion with insulin.

β-Adrenergic agonists, which also induce cellular K^+ uptake, are useful for the therapy of hyperkalemia. The one shortcoming is that some patients with renal failure are refractory to the K^+ lowering effects of β-agonists. An advantage is their effectiveness by inhalational as well as intravenous routes of administration.

Potassium elimination from the body is usually accomplished by use of the *cation-exchange resin* sodium polystyrene sulfonate. By retention enema each gram removes approximately 0.5 mmol of K^+, whereas oral administration in combination with sorbitol removes approximately 1.0 mmol/g. Colonic necrosis has been described in several postoperative uremic patients subjected to sodium polystyrene sulfonate and sorbitol enemas.

When cation-exchange resin therapy is insufficient or not feasible, dialysis may be required. *Hemodialysis* is substantially more effective than peritoneal dialysis for the purposes of K^+ removal.

Therapy for hyporeninemic hypoaldosteronism includes the avoidance of drugs that can cause hyperkalemia, and appropriate dietary K^+ restriction. Measures to increase urinary excretion of K^+, such as the use of thiazide or furosemide diuretics, can be useful. Mineralocorticoid replacement effectively treats the hyperkalemia, but Na^+ retention and worsening hypertension are potentially unacceptable side-effects.

SUMMARY

- Disorders of potassium balance are frequently seen in medicine and nephrology clinics
- These disorders may be life-threatening and require immediate attention and correction
- Hypokalemia may be corrected slowly and orally depending upon the severity
- The appropriate correction in hyperkalemia must be fast enough to prevent any cardiac complications.

Multiple Choice Questions

1. **Potassium is a major intracellular cat ion and total intracellular potassium concentration is:**
   a. 140 mmol/L b. 150 mmol/L
   c. 145 mmol/L d. 160 mmol/L

2. **ECG changes seen in hypokalemia are all except:**
   a. Flattening T-wave b. U-waves
   c. Prolonged QT d. Tenting T-wave

3. **Hypokalemia with normotensive metabolic alkalosis is seen in:**
   a. Bartter's syndrome b. Cushing's syndrome
   c. ACTH secretion tumors d. Liddle syndrome

4. **Hypokalemia with hyper-reninemic hyperaldosteronism is a feature of all except:**
   a. Primary hyperaldosteronism b. Secondary hyperaldosteronism
   c. Cushing's syndrome d. Ectopic ACTH production

5. **Earliest ECG abnormality evident in hypokalemia is:**
   a. U-wave b. Tall T-wave
   c. Prolonged QRS d. Flattening P-wave

6. **All the following ECG changes are seen in hyperkalemia except:**
   a. Sinus bradycardia b. Asystole
   c. Ventricular fibrillation d. ST depression

7. **In management of patients with acute hyperkalemia, which should be administered first?**
   a. IV Sodium bicarbonate b. IV Magnesium
   c. IV Calcium gluconate d. IV Dextrose

8. **All the following drugs cause hyperkalemia except:**
   a. Beta blockers b. Heparin
   c. Aminoglycosides d. Spironolactone

9. **Spurious hyperkalemia is classically seen in:**
   a. Hemolysis b. Acidosis
   c. Parathyroid hormone excess d. Exercise

10. **Which of the following medication used in hyperkalemia does not directly affect serum potassium:**
    a. Sodium polystyrene b. Insulin
    c. Dextrose d. Calcium

Answers

1. b 2. d 3. a 4. a 5. a 6. d 7. c 8. c
9. a 10. d

SUGGESTED READING

1. Mount DB, Zandi-Nejad K. Disorders of potassium balance. In: Taal MW, Chertow GM, Marsden PA, et al (Eds). Brenner and Rector's The Kidney, 9th edn. Philadelphia, PA: Elsevier Saunders; 2012. pp. 640-72.
2. Perazella MA, Rastegar A. Disorders of potassium and acid-base metabolism in association with renal disease. In: Schrier RW, Coffman RM, Falk RJ, Molitoris BA, Neilson EG (Eds). Schrier's diseases of the kidney, 8th edn. Philadelphia. LWW; 2007. pp. 2270-94.
3. Weiner ID, Linas SL, Wingo CS. Disorders of potassium metabolism. In: Johnson RJ, Feehally J, Floege J (Eds). Comprehensive Clinical Nephrology, 5th edn. Philadelphia, PA: Elsevier/Saunders; 2015. pp. 111-23.

HYPOCALCEMIA AND HYPERCALCEMIA

Manisha Sahay

INTRODUCTION

Calcium disturbances are commonly encountered in day-to-day practice. Hypocalcemia is commonly due to intracellular shifts or due to vitamin D deficiency while hypercalcemia is most often due to hyperparathyroidism or malignancies. This chapter deals with the practical approach to evaluation of hypocalcemia and hypercalcemia.

REGULATION OF CALCIUM BALANCE

Calcium (Ca^{2+}) is the most abundant mineral in the body. A normal adult ingests 1000 mg of Ca^{2+} per day, of which 400–500 mg is absorbed. However, 300 mg of calcium from digestive secretions is lost in the stool, resulting in the net absorption of only 100–200 mg. In the steady state, this quantity of calcium is excreted in the urine. Approximately 500 mg of calcium is removed from the bones daily and replaced by an equal amount **(Fig. 7.2)**.

Calcium distribution: More than 99% of calcium is stored as hydroxyapatite in bones. The total calcium concentration in the plasma is 4.5–5.1 mEq/L (9–10.2 mg/dL). Fifty percent of plasma calcium is ionized, 40% is bound to proteins (90% to albumin), and 10% circulates bound to anions (e.g. phosphate, carbonate, citrate, lactate, sulfate) **(Fig. 7.2)**. Total calcium level includes the ionized fraction and the bound fraction. The normal range for ionized calcium is 4–5 mg/dL.

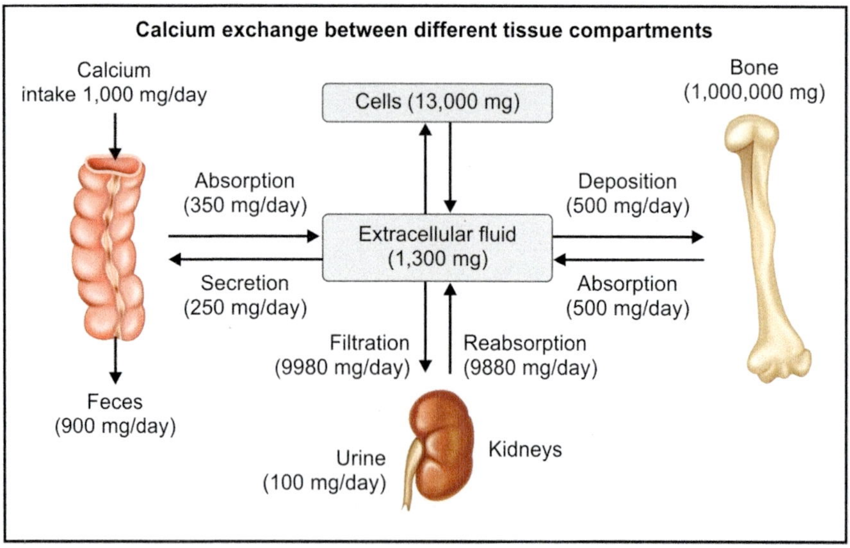

Figure 7.2 Distribution of calcium

Calcium absorption and transport: Calcium is absorbed across the intestinal epithelial cell's brush border membrane and is immediately bound to calbindin, a vitamin D-dependent calcium-binding protein. Calbindin transfers the calcium directly into the epithelial cell's endoplasmic reticulum, through which the calcium is transferred to the basal membrane on the opposite side of the cell, without entering its cytosol. TRPV6 and calcium pumps (PMCA1) actively transport calcium into the body. Active transport of calcium occurs in the duodenum when calcium intake is low; and through passive paracellular transport in the jejunum and ileum when calcium intake is high, independently of vitamin D level **(Fig. 7.3)**.

Renal handling of calcium: Filtered calcium is reabsorbed along most segments of the nephron **(Fig. 7.4)**. Most filtered calcium is reabsorbed passively in the proximal tubule down the favorable electrochemical gradients created by sodium and water reabsorption.

The filtered sodium chloride enters the cells in the thick ascending limb of the loop of Henle via $Na^+K^+2Cl^-$ cotransporters in the luminal membrane. Most of the potassium reabsorbed by the cotransporter leaks back into the lumen (through ROMK) to drive further inward sodium chloride transport. Movement of potassium into the lumen plus the movement of reabsorbed chloride (via a chloride channel) out of the basolateral surface of the cells makes the tubular lumen positive which drives the passive reabsorption of cations (sodium, calcium and magnesium) via the paracellular pathway (paracellin) **(Fig. 7.5)**. The high serum calcium itself also contributes to the calciuresis, acting via the calcium-sensing receptor **(Fig 7.6)**. In contrast, calcium transport is actively regulated in the distal nephron, i.e. in the cortical thick ascending limb of the loop of Henle (cTAL) as well as in the distal convoluted tubule (DCT) and adjacent connecting segment **(Figs 7.7A and B)**.

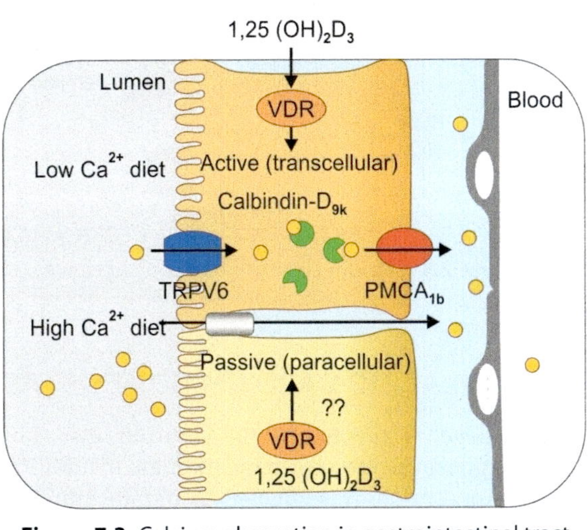

Figure 7.3 Calcium absorption in gastrointestinal tract

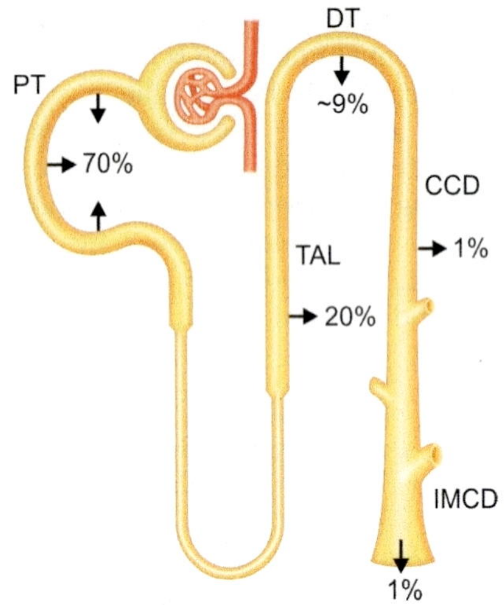

Figure 7.4 Renal handling of calcium

Abbreviations: PT, proximal tubule; DT, distal tubule; TAL, thick ascending limb of Henle's loop; CCD, cortical collecting duct; IMCD, inner medullary collecting duct

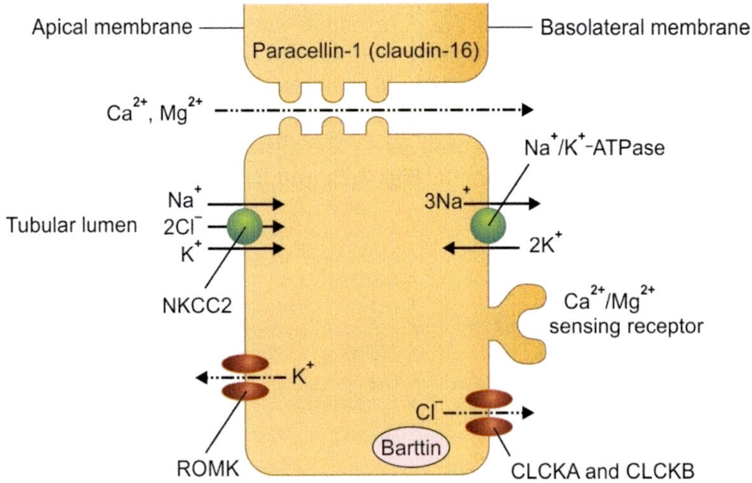

Figure 7.5 Calcium absorption of Loop of Henle

■ FACTORS REGULATING CALCIUM HOMEOSTASIS

The ionized calcium level is affected by the albumin level, blood pH, serum phosphate, serum magnesium and serum bicarbonate in addition to factors that affect total calcium. Total calcium is affected by parathormone (PTH), vitamin D, hepatic and renal function, and serum phosphate and magnesium levels. The maintenance of calcium homeostasis involves changes in intestinal, bone and renal function.

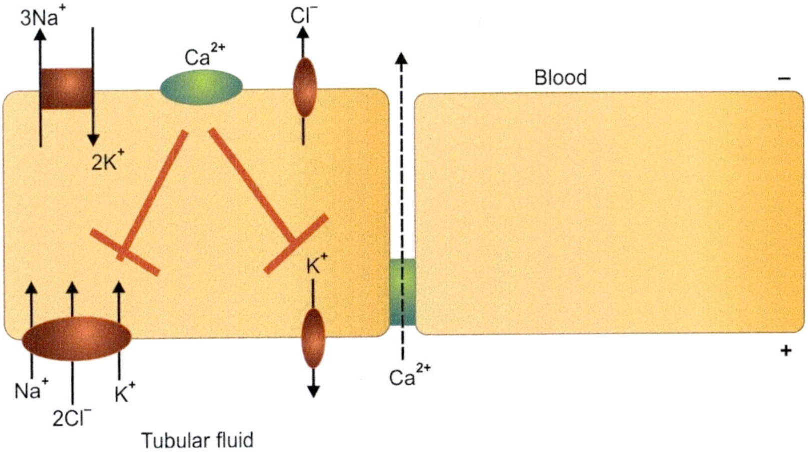

Figure 7.6 Calcium sensing receptor

Parathormone

Intact parathormone (PTH) is 84-amino acid polypeptide and is biologically active form of the hormone. During hypocalcemia, PTH 1-84 is secreted. The classical PTH/PTHrP receptor, PTH1R is expressed in bone and kidney. The PTH1R binds intact PTH and PTH-related protein (PTHrP) and releases calcium from bones and decreases calcium excretion from the kidneys.

Regulation of Parathormone

- Calcitriol-parathyroid cells contain vitamin D receptors, and the PTH gene contains a vitamin D-response element. Calcitriol, by binding to the vitamin D receptor, inhibits PTH gene expression and, therefore, PTH synthesis. Calcitriol also inhibits parathyroid-cell proliferation.
- Calcium, magnesium, aluminum and strontium bind to the CaSR on chief cells of parathyroid. Hypercalcemia inhibits PTH secretion.
- Hyperphosphatemia stimulates PTH secretion independent of the serum concentrations of calcium and calcitriol. Also hyperphosphatemia decreases serum calcium.

Actions of Parathormone

In normal subjects, a decrease in serum ionized calcium of as little as 0.1 mg/dL results in a large increase in serum PTH concentration within minutes; and vice versa. 7 PTH acts to increase the plasma Ca^{2+} concentration in four ways:

1. It enhances intestinal Ca^{2+} and phosphate absorption by promoting the formation within the kidney of calcitriol (1,25 dihydroxycholecalciferol).
2. PTH acts on bone in presence of calcitriol to release calcium in two phases: The immediate effect of PTH is to mobilize calcium from skeletal stores that are readily available. Later, PTH stimulates release of calcium by activation of bone resorption. The osteoblasts, but not osteoclasts, express PTH receptors. Osteoblasts increase osteoclast activity and number through interaction of

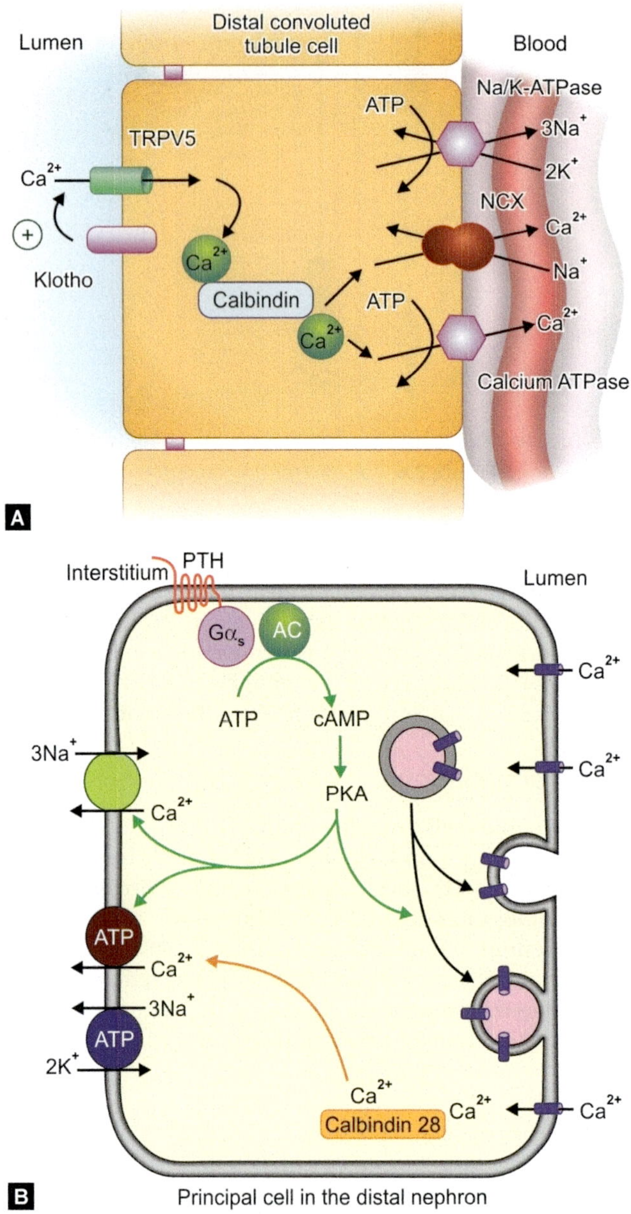

Figures 7.7A and B (A) Calcium absorption in distal tubule; (B) Regulation of calcium absorption in distal tubule by PTH

RANK (Receptor activator for nuclear factor k) on osteoclasts and RANKL on osteoblasts. Osteoprotegerin (OPG) binds to RANKL on osteoblast/stromal cells, blocks the RANKL-RANK interaction between osteoblast/stromal cells and osteoclast precursors. This has the effect of inhibiting the differentiation of the osteoclast precursor into a mature osteoclast.

3. *Renal actions of PTH*: It augments active renal Ca^{2+} reabsorption. The stimulatory effect of PTH on Ca^{2+} reabsorption occurs via adenyl cyclase primarily in the early cortical distal nephron, particularly the distal tubule and connecting segment and lesser extent in proximal tubule. Calcitriol and PTH both are needed for calcium resorption in renal tubules. If one is given in presence of deficiency of other the plasma calcium cannot be normalized.
4. PTH stimulates the synthesis of 1-alpha hydroxylase in the proximal tubules and decreases the activity of a 24-hydroxylase that inactivates calcitriol.

Vitamin D

Vitamin D_3 (cholecalciferol) is a steroid, which is present in the diet and also can be synthesized in the skin from 7-dehydrocholesterol in the presence of ultraviolet light. The hepatic enzyme 25-hydroxylase leads to the formation of 25-hydroxyvitamin D or calcidiol. Calcidiol produced by the liver enters the circulation and travels to the kidney, bound to vitamin D binding protein. In the kidney, tubular cells contain two enzymes (1-alpha-hydroxylase and 24-alpha-hydroxylase) that can further hydroxylate calcidiol, producing 1,25 dihydroxyvitamin D (calcitriol), the most active form of vitamin D, or 24,25-dihydroxyvitamin D, an inactive metabolite. The proximal tubule is the most important site of calcitriol synthesis. Calcitriol can also be synthesized in activated macrophages. The formation of calcitriol is stimulated by PTH and hypophosphatemia. The hepatic production of calcidiol is substrate-dependent and is not hormonally regulated. Hypercalcemia impairs and hypocalcemia promotes PTH-induced calcitriol production. Excessive stimulation is prevented by the rise in plasma Ca^{2+} itself and by negative feedback regulation of the 1-alpha- hydroxylase via binding of calcitriol to the vitamin D receptor. Calcitriol is degraded in part by being hydroxylated at the 24-position by a 24-hydroxylase. The activity of the 24-hydroxylase gene is increased by calcitriol (which therefore promotes its own inactivation) and reduced by PTH. The main action of calcitriol is to enhance the availability of both calcium and phosphate for new bone formation. This is primarily achieved by increases in bone resorption, intestinal absorption, and renal tubular Ca^{2+} reabsorption. Some of the bone and renal actions of calcitriol are mediated by PTH. Calcitriol also regulates the plasma Ca^{2+} concentration by binding to receptors in the parathyroid gland, leading to a diminution in further PTH production and release.

Calcitonin

Lowers calcium by targeting bone, renal, and GI losses.

Calcium-sensing Receptor

The calcium-sensing receptor (CaSR) is expressed in the chief cells of parathyroid glands, kidneys, bone marrow, osteoclasts and osteoblasts and others. CaSR senses small changes in the serum ionized calcium concentration and then brings about changes in the function of parathyroid glands and kidneys, to normalize serum calcium concentration. This receptor is also activated by magnesium. In kidney CaSR is located on the basolateral aspect of Loop of Henle. CaSR acts by inhibiting the apical K channel. When calcium intake is increased, there is increase in calcium excretion.

Role of calcium in body: Ionized calcium is the necessary plasma fraction for normal physiologic processes. Calcium is critical for normal cell function, neural transmission, membrane stability, bone structure, blood coagulation and intracellular signaling.

HYPOCALCEMIA

DEFINITION

Hypocalcemia is defined as a total serum calcium concentration of less than 8.5 mg/dL.

ETIOLOGY

The causes of hypocalcemia can be:

- Decreased calcium intake and absorption
- Increased renal excretion
- Low levels of regulatory hormone—hypoparathyroidism or vitamin D deficiency or resistance
- Intracellular shifts
- Altered binding to albumin/phosphates or chelates and other miscellaneous causes **(Table 7.14)**.

Drugs causing hypocalcemia are listed in **Table 7.15**. Acute hypocalcemia is commonly due to intracellular shifts, i.e. acute kidney injury or rhabdomyolysis. Chronic hypocalcemia may be due to parathyroid or vitamin D disorders.

SYMPTOMS AND SIGNS

In children, there may be no symptoms or they may present with lethargy, poor feeding, vomiting and abdominal distension. There may be seizures and laryngospasm. Patients may show cyanosis, tremulousness, apnea, tetany and signs of nerve irritability, such as the Chvostek sign (tapping of facial nerve branches leads to facial twitches), carpopedal spasm, Trousseau sign (carpal spasm in response to forearm ischemia caused by inflation of sphygmomanometer cuff) and stridor. Depression may occur. Chronic hypocalcemia may be associated with cataracts, brittle nails with transverse grooves, dry skin, absent or reduced axillary and pubic hair.

DIAGNOSIS

Diagnostic approach is shown in **Flow chart 7.8**.

Serum calcium should be done to document hypocalcemia. Hypocalcemia may be false due to low serum albumin. For each unit decrease of albumin from 4 g/dL–0.8 mg/dl should be added to the measured calcium. Another method is to measure ionized calcium level directly. Other situations in which the assessment of serum calcium may be inappropriately low include recent use of certain gadolinium contrast agents and contamination of blood samples by EDTA.

Table 7.14 Etiology of hypocalcemia

Decrease Ca absorption Low dietary intake Excess dietary zinc or Mg	Calcium complexes with these
Increased calcium excretion CaSR-activating mutation (Autosomal dominant hypocalcemia) Acquired mutation CaSR	– Activation of CaSR inhibits PTH – Idiopathic hypoparathyroidism
Parathyroid-related hypocalcemia	
Hereditary hypoparathyroidism isolated	AD,AR,XL
Autoimmune parathyroiditis /Poly Glandular autoimmune syndrome I Autosomal polyendocrinopathy candidiasis, ectodermal dystrophy DiGeorge syndrome, Kenny Caffey syndrome, Kearns-Sayre's syndrome (22q deletion) CHARGE syndrome, VATER syndrome, Velocardiofacial syndrome, GDM, Retinoic acid exposure fetus	CaSR antibody Parathyroid aplasia
Infiltrative lesions	Sarcoid Wilson Hemosiderosis
Postsurgical	
Hypoparathyroidism 1a 1b 1c 2 McCune Albright syndrome (round face, short neck and short metacarpals)	– Gs α mutation, AHO phenotype, Ch 20 – ↓CAMP, mutation in receptor, Gs α N, No AHO – Gs α N – Downstream CAMP defective – End organ resistance
Inhibits PTH Hypomagnesemia	Inhibit PTH
Vitamin D deficiency Inadequate sunlight exposure, malabsorption, liver diseases	Less Ca absorption and more renal loss
Vitamin D dependency1, Vitamin D dependency 2	
Hyperphosphatemia Sodium phosphate enema, TPN, Rhabdomyolysis, Renal failure	High P binds to calcium
Decreased bone resorption Drugs	
Chelates Citrate in blood transfusion, in liver disease, Foscarnet, EDTA, Gadolinium, Ethylene glycol, Pancreatitis	Chelate calcium
Hypomagnesemia and hypokalemia	End organ resistance
Hypoalbuminemia Sepsis, nephrotic syndrome, cirrhosis	Reduced total calcium, ionized normal
Miscellaneous Rhabdomyolysis, toxic shock syndrome, Hydrofluoric acid, osteoblastic metastasis, Alkalosis Hungry bone syndrome on vitamin D Rx, tumor lysis syndrome, acute hyperphosphatemia	Multiple mechanisms

Table 7.15 Drugs causing hypocalcemia

Mechanism of hypocalcemia	*Drugs*
Impair absorption	PPI H_2 blockers
Chelate calcium from blood	Fluoride, citrate, ethylene glycol, phosphate enemas, gadolinium, EDTA, foscarnet
Inhibit PTH	Magnesium, cinacalcet, alcohol, aluminum
Vitamin D metabolism	Phenytoin, phenobarbitone, carbamazepine, 5 Fluorouracil and leucovorin, INH, Rifampicin
PTH resistance	
Inhibit bone resorption	Estrogens, calcitonin, bisphosphonates Denosumab

Flow chart 7.8 Approach to hypocalcemia

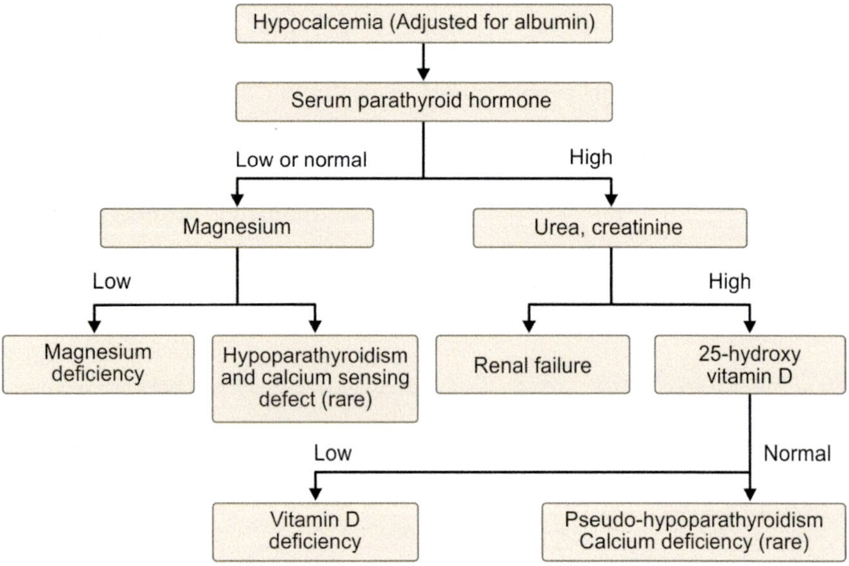

Blood tests: Serum magnesium, serum electrolytes including bicarbonate, glucose, phosphorus and serum alkaline phosphatase levels should be measured.

- *Low magnesium* may be associated with hypoparathyroidism.
- *Low calcium and high phosphorus* levels are seen in hypoparathyroidism while most other diseases have low calcium associated with a low phosphorus level.
- Low *bicarbonate levels* and acidosis may be associated with Fanconi syndrome and renal tubular acidosis.
- *Alkaline phosphate* is high in osteomalacia.

Urine tests: Urine should be evaluated for pH, glucose, and protein. *Urine calcium, magnesium, phosphorus, and creatinine* levels should be assessed in patients with suspected renal tubular defects and renal failure **(Table 7.16)**. A urine calcium-to-creatinine ratio of more than 0.3 on a spot sample in presence of hypocalcemia suggests renal loss. 24 hours urinary calcium excretion to look for renal losses can be done instead of spot urine calcium creatinine ratio.

Other tests: PTH levels are indicated if hypocalcemia persists in the presence of normal magnesium and normal or elevated phosphate levels especially if the cause of hypocalcemia is not obvious.

Vitamin D metabolite (25-hydroxyvitamin D) levels may be assessed if PTH is abnormal to eliminate uncommon causes of hypocalcemia (e.g. malabsorption, disorders of vitamin D metabolism). Evidence of rickets may be seen in patients.

Electrocardiography shows prolongation of corrected QT interval. CT scan shows basal ganglia calcification in 20% cases of idiopathic hyperparathyroidism. Karyotyping helps in identification of genetic defects.

MANAGEMENT

Acute Hypocalcemia

Most hypocalcemic emergencies are mild and require only supportive treatment and further laboratory evaluation. Severe hypocalcemia may result in seizures, tetany, refractory hypotension, or arrhythmias that require a more aggressive approach **(Flow chart 7.9)**.

Calcium and magnesium are the only medications necessary to treat hypocalcemic emergencies. IV treatment is indicated in patients having seizures, those who are critically ill, and those who are planning to have surgery. In patients with concurrent acidemia, hypocalcemia should be corrected first. If acidemia is corrected first, ionized calcium levels decrease. Solutions available are:

Table 7.16 Lab diagnosis of hypocalcemia

	S. Ph	*U Ca*	*25 Vit. D*	*1,25 Vit. D*	*Mg*	*PTH*
Parathyroid-related hypocalcemia	↑ ↓U Ph	↑	N	N	N/↓	↓
Pseudohypoparathyroidism	↑ and ↓U Ph	↑	N	N	N	↑
CaSR Activating mutation (Autosomal dominant hypocalcemia)	↑	↑	N	N	N	↓
Vitamin D deficiency	↓	↓	↓	↓	N	↑
Vitamin D dependency 1 Vitamin D dependency 2	↓ ↓	↓	↑ ↑	↓ ↑	N	
Chronic kidney disease	↑ and ↓U Ph	Variable	↓	↓	N	↑

Abbreviations: U Ca, urinary calcium; S Ph, serum phosphorus; U Ph, Urinary phosphorus; Vit., vitamin

Flow chart 7.9 Management of acute hypocalcemia

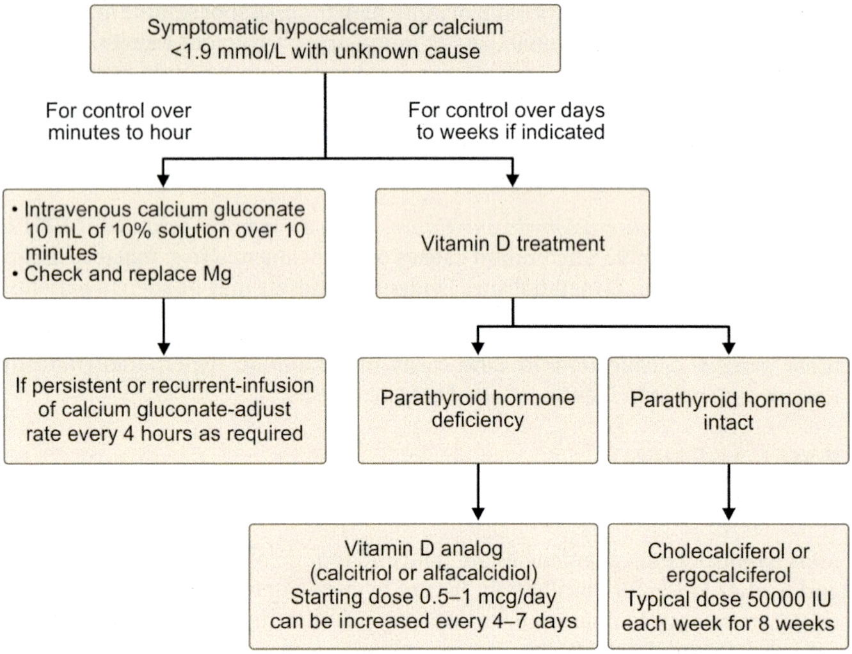

- *Calcium gluconate 10%* (100 mg/mL) IV solution contains 9.8 mg/mL (0.45 mEq/mL) elemental calcium; calcium gluconate 10 mL IV is given as bolus diluted in 50 mL of 5% dextrose or isotonic saline.
- *Calcium chloride 10%* (100 mg/mL) contains 27 mg/mL (1.4 mEq/mL) of elemental calcium. Calcium chloride is avoided as it leads to skin necrosis in accidental extravasation.

Measure serum calcium every 4–6 hours to maintain serum calcium levels at 8–9 mg/dL. Identify and treat the cause of hypocalcemia and taper the infusion.

Patients with cardiac arrhythmias or patients on digoxin therapy need continuous electrocardiographic (ECG) monitoring during calcium replacement because calcium potentiates digitalis toxicity.

Patients with postparathyroidectomy hungry bone disease, especially those with osteitis fibrosa cystica, can present with a dramatic picture of hypocalcemia. Treatment with calcium and vitamin D for 1–2 days prior to parathyroid surgery may help prevent the development of severe hypocalcemia.

Hypocalcemia due to acute respiratory alkalosis can be corrected by using a rebreathing bag.

Magnesium administration is necessary to correct any hypomagnesemia (serum magnesium <0.75 mmol/L). Magnesium can be given as magnesium oxide 250–500 mg every 6 hours or intramuscular magnesium sulfate 4–8 mmol per day or IV, i.e. 12 mL of 50% magnesium sulfate in 1 L in 5% dextrose over 4 hours.

Once patient is stable start oral calcium and vitamin D treatment early and evaluate for the cause of hypocalcemia.

Chronic Hypocalcemia

Treatment of chronic hypocalcemia depends on the cause of the disorder. In chronic hypocalcemia oral calcium carbonate is the calcium supplement of choice and provides 40% elemental calcium. Calcium chloride, lactate and gluconate provide 36, 12 and 8% of elemental calcium respectively. The daily dose required is 2–4 g of elemental calcium and should be given in between meals.

Treatment of specific cause is important.

In patients with hypoparathyroidism treatment with calcium leads to increased calcium excretion in urine. Hence, concomitant thiazides and adequate water intake is required to prevent nephrocalcinosis. Thiazides reduce calcium excretion. A minimum daily intake of 400 IU of vitamin D is recommended. Calcitriol (active vitamin D) is the therapy of choice in cases of acquired hypoparathyroidism as hypoparathyroidism impairs the conversion of vitamin D to the active form. Administration of recombinant PTH in hypocalcemia refractory to calcitriol and calcium supplementation is effective.

Nutritional vitamin D deficiency is treated with calcium and vitamin D, i.e. cholecalciferol. Calcitriol may be used, but it has the disadvantages of a higher price and the possibility of producing hypervitaminosis D with hypercalcemia.

In renal failure, administration of phosphate-lowering agents may be necessary as hypocalcemia is associated with hyperphosphatemia. A diet high in calcium and low in phosphate is required. Renal failure patients should be given a low-solute, low-phosphate diet.

Those patients on hemodialysis who have hypocalcemia, especially those who have undergone parathyroidectomy may have considerable difficulty in maintaining calcium levels. For these patients oral calcium supplements should be provided. They must be given between meals; otherwise, they will primarily act as phosphate binders. Active vitamin D (calcitriol) enhances the absorption of calcium. Finally, the calcium in the dialysate bath can be increased.

Prognosis: Higher mortality rates have been reported in patients with hypocalcemia than in normocalcemic patients in ICU settings.

HYPERCALCEMIA

DEFINITION

The reference range of serum calcium levels is 8.7–10.4 mg/dL. Hypercalcemia is defined as serum calcium greater than 10.4 mg/dL. Hypercalcemic crisis is defined as marked elevation of serum calcium more than 14 mg/dL and is associated with acute signs and symptoms of hypercalcemia, i.e. oliguria, somnolence and coma.

ETIOLOGY

Malignancy and primary hyperparathyroidism account for 90% of the cases of hypercalcemia **(Table 7.17)**.

Table 7.17 Causes of hypercalcemia

Increased intake	
Hyperparathyroidism	Primary-Adenoma (80%), hyperplasia (15%), cancer (5%) Tertiary Ectopic- PTH Lithium -CaSR Neonatal severe homozygous mutation in CaSR, AR MEN I (Wermer) Autosomal dominant and MEN II
Malignancy	• PTHrP-related (80%)—bronchogenic, renal, thyroid, pheochromocytoma • Osteolytic metastasis (15%)—breast cancer • Hematopoietic—leukemia, lymphoma, multiple myeloma
Vitamin D	Intoxication, Granulomatous diseases—Sarcoidosis, TB, Wegener's, Crohn's
CaSR mutations Familial hypocalciuric hypercalcemia	CaSR in kidney inactivated, more calcium absorbed. CaSR in parathyroid inactivated—Increased PTH (high Mg) due to CaSR inactivation; autosomal dominant
Transcellular shifts—Immobilization, Rhabdomyolysis	Release of calcium from bones and muscles
PTH receptor mutation	Continuous activation of PTH receptor
Non-parathyroid endocrinopathies	Hyperthyroidism, adrenal insufficiency, pheochromocytoma, acromegaly
Increased bone turnover	Vitamin A, Thiazides
Drugs	PPI, Theophylline, GH, Hepatitis B vaccine, Mn
Renal failure	Secondary hyperparathyroidism Milk-alkali syndrome Aluminum intoxication
Miscellaneous	
Congenital lactase deficiency	High calcium absorption in presence of nonhydrolyzed lactose
William syndrome	Increased sensitivity to Vit D, deletion of Elastin gene in Ch 7
Down syndrome	Genetically increased GI absorption via paracellular route
Jansen metaphyseal dysplasia (Pseudohyperparathyroidism)	Due to PTH receptor mutations
Primary hyperoxaluria	Pathogenesis unclear
Congenital hypothyoidism	
Idiopathic infantile	PTHrP defects
Hypophosphatasia	Deficiency of tissue non specific alkaline phosphatase
Chronic liver disease, SLE, AIDS	

SYMPTOMS AND SIGNS

Hypercalcemia has nonspecific symptoms especially if it is mild or gradual in onset. Patient may present with symptoms or signs of underlying disorder. Initial symptoms may be fatigue, excess sleep, etc. Gastrointestinal symptoms may result from pancreatitis. Renal symptoms include stones, nephrocalcinosis, etc. Increased calcium levels may cause polydipsia and nocturia. Neuropsychiatric manifestations may be seen. Hypertension and bradycardia may be noted with coving of ST and long QT. Long-standing hypercalcemia may cause band keratopathy and soft tissue calcification.

Hypercalcemia caused by hyperparathyroidism is remembered by the mnemonic "Stones, bones, abdominal moans, and psychic groans." Hypercalcemia of malignancy may lack many of the features commonly associated with hypercalcemia caused by hyperparathyroidism. In addition, the symptoms of elevated calcium level may overlap with the symptoms of malignancy.

LABORATORY DIAGNOSIS

Serum calcium: Corrected total calcium should be calculated. Patients with hyperalbuminemia due to severe dehydration and adults with multiple myeloma have high total calcium. Alternatively, in patients with hypoalbuminemia due to chronic illness or malnutrition, total serum calcium concentration may be normal when serum ionized calcium is elevated. However, if the corrected serum calcium level still is not accurate, the free calcium ion activity (i.e. ionized calcium level) should be measured.

After a diagnosis of hypercalcemia is established, the next step is to determine the cause. Initial testing is directed at malignancy, hyperparathyroidism and hyperthyroidism, which are the most common causes of hypercalcemia. Primary hyperparathyroidism is associated with borderline or mild hypercalcemia and values above 13 mg/dL are unusual while they are more common in patients with malignancy-associated hypercalcemia. High *creatinine* is found in patients with hypercalcemia and is nonspecific. *Serum phosphate* levels may be low or normal in primary hyperparathyroidism and humoral hypercalcemia of malignancy. Serum phosphate concentration is normal or elevated in granulomatous diseases, vitamin D intoxication, immobilization, thyrotoxicosis, milk-alkali syndrome and metastatic bone disease. Serum phosphate is variable in familial hypocalciuric hypercalcemia (FHH). *Serum chloride levels* usually are higher than 102 mEq/L in hyperparathyroidism. *Urinary calcium excretion* calculation of the Ca/Cr clearance ratio, which is equivalent to the fractional excretion of calcium, is preferable to measuring 24-hour excretion of calcium. Ca/Cr clearance ratio = [24-hour urine Ca × serum Cr] ÷ [Serum Ca × 24-hour urine Cr] is usually raised or high normal in hyperparathyroidism (250–300 mg/day) and hypercalcemia of malignancy. In contrast, relative hypocalciuria (less than 100 mg/day) is seen in milk-alkali syndrome, thiazide diuretics, and FHH in which the fractional excretion of calcium is often less than 1%.

Hyperparathyroidism should be excluded first as it is simpler to test for. The measurement of *circulating PTH* in the serum is the most direct and sensitive measure. A nonsuppressed PTH level in the presence of hypercalcemia suggests a diagnosis of primary hyperparathyroidism (FHH, however, cannot be ruled out at this stage). In a patient with hypercalcemia, the serum PTH level should be lower than 10 pg/mL. A definitive diagnosis of hyperparathyroidism is confirmed by a PTH level higher than 50 pg/mL. Cervical ultrasound and sestamibi scan are done to look for parathyroid adenoma.

If PTH is low or normal, *PTH-related peptide (PTHrP)* should be measured for malignancy. A low anion gap may indicate multiple myeloma. Serum and urinary protein electrophoresis should be checked for possible multiple myeloma.

Serum concentrations of the *vitamin D metabolites,* 25-hydroxyvitamin D and 1,25-dihydroxyvitamin D should be measured if there is no obvious malignancy and neither PTH nor PTHrP levels are elevated. An elevated serum concentration of 25-hydroxyvitamin D [25 (OH) D) >150 ng/mL indicates intoxication. Measurement of calcitriol is useful in diagnosing hypercalcemia secondary to a granulomatous disease such as sarcoidosis. In the absence of malignancy or increased PTHrP, unsuspected stimulation of bone resorption (as with thyrotoxicosis, immobilization, or vitamin A toxicity) and unrecognized calcium intake in the face of renal insufficiency (as in the milk-alkali syndrome) are the most likely. *Serum TSH and vitamin A* levels should also be done.

Imaging studies: If laboratory evidence of primary hyperparathyroidism is present, CT scan of the head, MRI, ultrasound, or nuclear parathyroid scans may be helpful. Excess PTH also can result in subperiosteal resorption, leading to osteitis fibrosa cystica with bone cysts and brown tumors of the long bones.

TREATMENT

- *Hydration with IV saline*: The initial step is *hydration with saline* to maintain a urine output of 100 mL/hour. Hydration is ineffective in patients with kidney failure or CHF and dialysis may be necessary to correct hypercalcemia in these patients.
- *Loop diuretics*: It may be used after correction of hydration to increase calcium excretion (100 mg can be given every other hour). These are particularly indicated if patient has renal failure or heart failure and is at risk of developing overload with saline. Thiazide diuretics should be avoided because they increase the reabsorption of calcium.
- Use of *IV phosphate* is very effective in lowering serum calcium levels by a precipitation phenomenon.
- *Corticosteroids* are useful for treating hypercalcemia caused by vitamin D toxicity, certain malignancies (e.g. multiple myeloma, lymphoma), sarcoidosis, and other granulomatous diseases.
- *Calcitonin* has the most rapid onset of action of anticalcemic agents but has short duration of action and other more potent but slower-acting agents should be started in patients with severe hypercalcemia. Calcitonin is indicated only if serum calcium is more than 14 mg/dL and patient is symptomatic.
- *Bisphosphonates* act by binding to hydroxyapatite in bone matrix and prevent bone resorption over the next 24–48 hours and by shortening the life span of osteoclasts and inhibit osteoclast activity for up to a month. In addition these inhibit calcitriol synthesis. Current available drugs include clodronate (1600–3200 mg oral) etidronate, tiludronate, pamidronate (15-90 mg over 1-3 days IV every month), alendronate (10 mg oral daily), zoledronate, risedronate, ibandronate and neridronic acid. IV preparations are given over at least over 2 hour in NS or 5% D. All patients with cancer-associated hypercalcemia should receive treatment with bisphosphonates. Bisphosphonates are relatively contraindicated in renal failure. Denosumab is an option for

patients with hypercalcemia that is refractory to zoledronic acid or in whom bisphosphonates are contraindicated due to severe renal impairment.

- *Other measures—Gallium nitrate*—reduces bone resorption and has slow onset of action. *Plicamycin (Mithramycin)* acts on osteoclasts or block action of PTH; the onset of action is within 24–48 hours. Dose is 25 mcg/kg. It is not recommended for long-term use due to side effects. *Treatment of cause*—For those patients with *malignancy* as the cause of their hypercalcemia, a cure may not be possible. Patients with primary *hyperparathyroidism* who present with symptoms of severe or moderate elevations of calcium levels should be referred for parathyroidectomy while those with with mild-to-moderate elevations of calcium are treated medically. *Calcimimetic drugs* are useful for the treatment of patients with primary or secondary hyperparathyroidism. A long-acting calcimimetic drug, *cinacalcet,* is available for the treatment of secondary hyperparathyroidism associated with renal failure, and for hypercalcemia in parathyroid cancer. Calcimimetics may prove useful in the treatment of neonatal severe primary hyperparathyroidism, FHH, and forms of hyperparathyroidism other than primary hyperparathyroidism. *Non-hypercalcemic vitamin D analogs,* oxacalcitriol, paricalcitol and 1-alpha-hydroxy vitamin D_2 inhibit PTH synthesis and secretion to a greater extent than they stimulate intestinal calcium absorption or bone resorption. Such analogs are available for use in patients with chronic renal failure and secondary hyperparathyroidism.

Mortality/morbidity-prognosis of hypercalcemia associated with malignancy is poor.

SUMMARY

- Calcium disorders, both hypocalcemia as well as hypercalcemia are common and if untreated especially in acute settings may be life-threatening.
- A proper approach to diagnosis helps in management and reduces morbidity and mortality.

Multiple Choice Questions

An infant presents with tetany. On examination there are widened wrists and wide open anterior fontanelle. His lab investigations reveal serum calcium of 7 mg/dL, serum phosphorus of 4 mg/dL, serum albumin of 4 g/dL, hemoglobin 13 g%. Arterial blood gas (ABG) is normal. X-ray of the wrists reveals cupping and fraying of the lower end of ulna.

1. **Which of the diagnosis is likely?**
   a. Vitamin D-dependent rickets
   b. Vitamin D-resistant rickets
   c. Distal renal tubular acidosis
   d. Proximal renal tubular acidosis
2. **What further tests are needed to confirm the diagnosis?**
   a. Acid load test
   b. Serum vitamin D levels
   c. Abdominal CT to look for nephrocalcinosis
   d. Urine fractional excretion of phosphorus

3. **How would you treat this child?**
   a. Joulies solution
   b. Bicarbonate solution
   c. Calcitriol
   d. PTH injections

A 60-year-old male presents with dehydration and polyuria. On evaluation he was found to have serum calcium of 11 mg/dL. Serum albumin was 3 g/dL. Serum phosphorus was 2.2 mg/dL, alkaline phosphate was normal, and serum creatinine was 1.8 mg/dL. Imaging showed fracture of the left 7th rib. Ultrasound showed bulky kidneys. Hemoglobin was found to be 8.2 g/dL. He was taking calcium supplements and vitamin D 200 IU per day since 1 year.

4. **What is the most likely diagnosis?**
   a. Multiple myeloma
   b. Hyperparathyroidism
   c. Acute kidney injury
   d. Vitamin D intoxication

5. **All the following tests will be useful for diagnosis except:**
   a. Serum electrophoresis
   b. Skull X-ray
   c. Bone marrow biopsy
   d. Serum PTH levels

6. **All can be used to treat this patient if the serum calcium is 15 mg/dL except:**
   a. Hydration
   b. Steroids
   c. Alkalinization of urine
   d. Thiazide diuretics.

A female patient, 41 years old, was admitted with history of four spontaneous fractures (foot, clavicle, upper arm, forearm). She complained about gastric problems for many years accompanied by minor loss of weight. She also reported poor appetite, nausea and vomiting every day during the last several months, constipation (up to 10 days), regular urination. Menstrual cycles were irregular. Three years before she had a maxillofacial operation which was performed because of cystic changes. She had difficulty in walking, numbness, and dull pain and soon she was confined to bed. On examination, extremities were painful on palpation and movement, fractures were conservatively treated by plaster fixation.

Laboratory analyses: Showed Hb 11.6 g%, AP 605 IU/L, serum calcium 10 mg/dL, serum albumin of 2.8 g/dL, K 3.8 mEq/L and serum P 1.8 mg/dL. X-rays showed multiple lytic lesions in the bone. Scintigraphy of the parathyroid glands showed intensive accumulation of radiopharmaceutical material next to the thyroid gland and laterally down under the lower pole of the left lobule of thyroid gland, which most probably correspond to increased and hyperactive parathyroid gland (PTH : 1346 pg/mL). There was calciuresis of 1000 mg/day. USG of kidneys showed a few small stones, other findings were normal. X-ray skull showed signs of diffused osteoporosis and numerous cystic lesions.

7. **What is the most likely cause of hypercalcemia?**
   a. Multiple myeloma
   b. Hyperparathyroidism
   c. Humoral hypercalcemia of malignancy
   c. Vitamin D intoxication

8. **Which of the following statements is correct?**
   a. A combination of hypercalcemia with hypophosphatemia suggests primary hyperparathyroidism

b. A combination of hypercalcemia and hyperphosphatemia suggests secondary hyperparathyroidism due to renal failure
c. Humoral hypercalcemia of malignancy is characterized by high levels of iPTH hormone
d. Tertiary hyperparathyroidism is characterized by hypocalcemia and hypophosphatemia

A 48-year-old woman presented with an acute episode of carpopedal spasm of bilateral hands noted at midnight while she was sleeping. There was no significant history preceding this episode. Family history was unremarkable. On lab evaluation hypocalcemia was found with a high normal serum phosphorus. Serum Magnesium was normal. GFR was found to be 90 mL/min. PTH was found to be 20 pg/mL. There were no features of any other glandular disease.

9. Which of the following statements is correct?
a. Hypocalcemia with high normal phosphorus suggests vitamin D deficiency
b. Hypocalcemia and hyperphosphatemia suggest chronic kidney disease
c. Low intact PTH levels suggest hypoparathyroidism
d. Pseudohypoparathyroidism is associated with low levels of PTH

10. All can be used for treatment of this condition except:
a. Calcium
b. Calcitriol
c. Recombinant PTH
d. Cinacalcet

Answers

1. a 2. b 3. c 4. a 5. d 6. d 7. b 8. a
9. c 10. d

SUGGESTED READING

1. Berenson JR. Treatment of hypercalcemia of malignancy with bisphosphonates. Semin Oncol. 2002;29:12.
2. Brenner and Rector. The Kidney, 8th edn 2008. Diseases of the Kidney and Urinary Tract Ed.
3. Burtis WJ, Wu TL, Insogna KL, Stewart AF. Humoral hypercalcemia of malignancy. Ann Intern Med. 1988;108:454.
4. Cooper MS, Gittoes NJ. Diagnosis and management of hypocalcaemia. BMJ. 2008;336(7656):1298-302.
5. Desai TK, Carlson RW, Geheb MA. Prevalence and clinical implications of hypocalcemia in acutely ill patients in a medical intensive care setting. Am J Med. 1988;84(2):209-14.
6. Endres DB, Villanueva R, Sharp CF Jr, Singer FR. Immunochemiluminometric and immunoradiometric determinations of intact and total immunoreactive parathyrin: performance in the differential diagnosis of hypercalcemia and hypoparathyroidism. Clin Chem. 1991;37:162.
7. Forsythe RM, Wessel CB, Billiar TR, Angus DC, Rosengart MR. Parenteral calcium for intensive care unit patients. Cochrane Database Syst Rev. 2008;(4):CD006163.
8. Hannan FM, Thakker RV. Investigating hypocalcaemia. BMJ. 2013;346:f2213.

9. Hebert SC. Extracellular calcium-sensing receptor: implications for calcium and magnesium handling in the kidney. Kidney Int. 1996;50:2129.
10. Hoenderop JG, Nilius B, Bindels RJ. Calcium absorption across epithelia. Physiol Rev. 2005;85:373.
11. Hofer AM, Brown EM. Extracellular calcium sensing and signalling. Nat Rev Mol Cell Biol. 2003;4(7):530-8.
12. Hosking DJ, Cowley A, Bucknall CA. Rehydration in the treatment of severe hypercalcaemia. QJ Med. 1981;50:473.
13. Jurgen Floege, Richard J Johnson, John Feehally. Comprehensive Clinical Nephrology. 4th edition; 2011.
14. Kimball S, Vieth R. Self-prescribed high-dose vitamin D_3: effects on biochemical parameters in two men. Ann Clin Biochem. 2008;45:106.
15. Kremer R, Shustik C, Tabak T, et al. Parathyroid-hormone-related peptide in hematologic malignancies. Am J Med. 1996;100:406.
16. Kumar R, Tebben PJ, Thompson JR. Vitamin D and the kidney. Arch Biochem Biophys. 2012;523:77.
17. Kurokawa K. Calcium-regulating hormones and the kidney. Kidney Int. 1987; 32:760.
18. Lafferty FW. Differential diagnosis of hypercalcemia. J Bone Miner Res. 1991;6 (Suppl 2):S51.
19. Maier JD, Levine SN. Hypercalcemia in the Intensive Care Unit: A Review of Pathophysiology, Diagnosis, and Modern Therapy. J Intensive Care Med. 2015; 30:235.
20. Mannstadt M, Clarke BL, Vokes T, Brandi ML, Ranganath L, Fraser WD, et al. Efficacy and safety of recombinant human parathyroid hormone (1-84) in hypoparathyroidism (REPLACE): a double-blind, placebo-controlled, randomised, phase 3 study. Lancet Diabetes Endocrinol. 2013;1(4):275-83.
21. Mantovani G. Clinical review: Pseudohypoparathyroidism: diagnosis and treatment. J Clin Endocrinol Metab. 2011;96:3020.
22. Mundy GR, Guise TA. Hormonal control of calcium homeostasis. Clin Chem. 1999;45(8 Pt 2):1347-52.
23. Robert W. Schrier Publ Lippincott Williams & Wilkins, 2007.
24. Rosol TJ, Capen CC. Mechanisms of cancer-induced hypercalcemia. Lab Invest. 1992;67:680.
25. Russell CF, Edis AJ. Surgery for primary hyperparathyroidism: experience with 500 consecutive cases and evaluation of the role of surgery in the asymptomatic patient. Br J Surg. 1982;69(5):244-7.[Medline].
26. Schimatschek HF, Rempis R. Prevalence of hypomagnesemia in an unselected German population of 16000 individuals. Magnes Res. 2001;14:283-90.
27. Shoback D. Clinical practice. Hypoparathyroidism. N Engl J Med. 2008;359(4):391-403.
28. Silver J, Yalcindag C, Sela-Brown A, Kilav R, Naveh-Many T. Regulation of the parathyroid hormone gene by vitamin D, calcium and phosphate. Kidney Int Suppl. 1999;73:S2-7.
29. Suki WN, Yium JJ, Von Minden M, et al. Acute treatment of hypercalcemia with furosemide. N Engl J Med. 1970;283:836.
30. Wisneski LA. Salmon calcitonin in the acute management of hypercalcemia. Calcif Tissue Int. 1990;(46 Suppl):S26.
31. Yu AS. Claudins and the kidney. J Am Soc Nephrol. 2015;26:11.
32. Zivin JR, Gooley T, Zager RA, Ryan MJ. Hypocalcemia: a pervasive metabolic abnormality in the critically ill. Am J Kidney Dis. 2001;37(4):689-98

HYPOPHOSPHATEMIA AND HYPERPHOSPHATEMIA

Manisha Sahay

INTRODUCTION

Hypophosphatemia and hyperphosphatemia are seen in day-to-day practice. Hypophosphatemia is commonly due to inadequate dietary intake, intracellular shifts or due to excess renal losses. Hyperphosphatemia is due to impaired renal excretion or excess phosphate load. The impaired renal excretion may be due to either hypoparathyroidism or renal failure. A correct approach to evaluation helps in appropriate diagnosis and treatment.

PHOSPHORUS METABOLISM

Phosphate is one of the major components of the skeleton, providing mineral strength to bone. Phosphate is a component of DNA and RNA. Phosphate functions as a buffer in bone, serum and urine. Phosphate homeostasis is a highly regulated process.

About 85% of phosphorus is in the bone as part of the mineralized extracellular matrix. Most intracellular phosphate is either complexed or bound to proteins or lipids. Plasma phosphorus consists of phospholipids, ester phosphates, and inorganic phosphates. The latter are completely ionized, circulating primarily as HPO_4^{2-} or $H_2PO_4^-$ in a ratio of 4:1 at a plasma pH of 7.40 as the ionization constant of acid (pK) of phosphate is 6.8. Renal excretion of excess phosphate is responsible for maintenance of serum phosphate. Serum phosphate concentration varies with age, time of day, fasting state, and season. Serum phosphate concentration is higher in children than adults; the reference range is 4–7 mg/dL in children compared with 3–4.5 mg/dL in adults. Highest phosphate level occurs near noon. A normal diet provides approximately 1000 mg of phosphate, two thirds of which is absorbed, predominantly in the proximal small intestine **(Fig. 7.8)**. Nuts, legumes, dairy products and non-vegetarian diet are rich in phosphorus.

The kidney exerts a major influence on phosphate balance. The filtered load of phosphorus is approximately 4–8 g/day. Only 5–20% of the filtered phosphorus is normally excreted, with most being reabsorbed in the proximal tubule. Renal phosphate transport occurs in the proximal tubule (60–70% of the filtered load being reabsorbed) and in the distal tubule (10–15 percent of the filtered load being reabsorbed) **(Fig. 7.9)**. Phosphate is generally absorbed along with sodium.

Phosphate transporters: There are three types of phosphate cotransporters. Type 2a transporters are expressed in the apical membranes of kidney proximal tubules and absorb the majority of filtered phosphate **(Fig. 7.10)**. The expression of these cotransporters is increased by low dietary phosphate intake, vitamin D and several growth factors and decreased by high dietary phosphate intake, PTH and dopamine. Phosphate absorption in the remainder of the nephron is mediated by type 1 or 3 sodium phosphate cotransporters, which are not regulated. Type 2b transporters are similar to type 2a transporters. They are

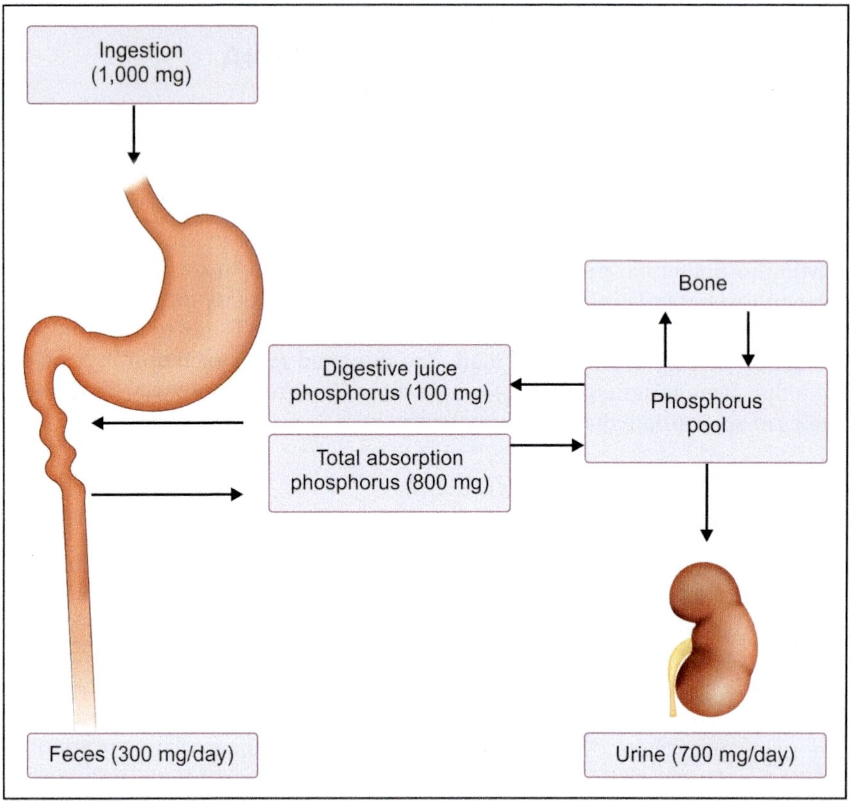

Figure 7.8 Distribution of phosphorus in the body

expressed in the small intestine and are also up regulated under conditions of dietary phosphate deprivation. Type 2c transporters are expressed exclusively on the S1 segment of the proximal tubule and together with Type 2a transporters are essential for normal phosphate homeostasis. Type 2c transporters are also regulated by diet and PTH.

PHOSPHATE HOMEOSTASIS

Physiologic regulators of renal tubular phosphate reabsorption include the following:

- *Serum phosphate concentration*: Mild phosphate depletion and low dietary intake stimulate phosphate reabsorption in the proximal tubule.
  Hyperphosphatemia decreases phosphorus absorption. High serum phosphate has dual effects on P absorption.
  1. It inhibits 1-alpha hydroxylase in the proximal tubule.
  2. It stimulates the secretion of paratharmone (PTH), which increases the activity of 1-alpha hydroxylase.

  The result is generally a neutral effect on intestinal phosphate absorption. With normal renal function, the transient increase in PTH and

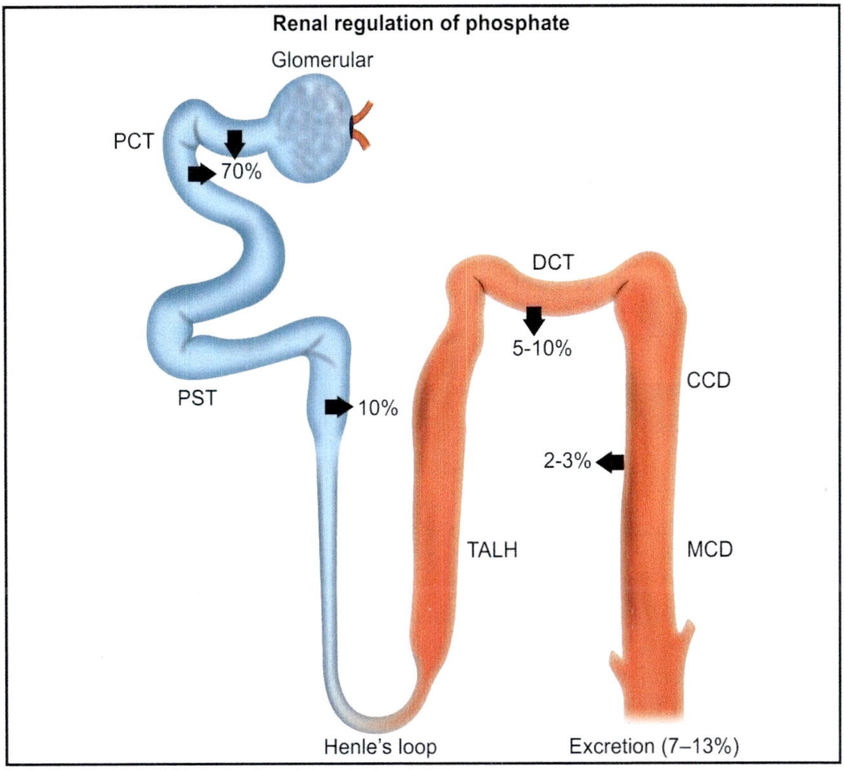

Figure 7.9 Renal handling of phosphorus

Abbreviations: TALH, thick-ascending limb of the loop of Henle; MCD, medullary collecting duct; CCD, cortical collecting duct; PCT, proximal convoluted tubule; PST, proximal straight tubule; DCT, distal convoluted tubule

decrease in vitamin D serve to inhibit renal and intestinal absorption of phosphate, resulting in resolution of the hyperphosphatemia. In contrast, under conditions of renal failure, sustained hyperphosphatemia results in sustained hyperparathyroidism and exacerbates hyperphosphatemia.

- Parathyroid hormone (*PTH)* increases phosphate excretion by diminishing activity of sodium-phosphate cotransporters in the proximal and distal tubule and increases the activity of 1-alpha hydroxylase, stimulates fibroblast growth factor (FGF) and promotes bone resorption **(Fig. 7.10)**.
- *High vitamin D levels* enhance renal proximal tubule phosphate absorption in the kidney. It also acts on Type 2b transporters in the gut and enhance P absorption in the intestine. Vitamin D levels fall after a phosphate load and thus protect against hyperphosphatemia. Niacin inhibits Type 2b receptors and has been used for treatment of hyperphosphatemia.

  A gastrointestinal sensor of dietary phosphate may lead to direct enhancement of renal phosphate excretion by an unknown mechanism.
- *Phosphatonins*: Phosphatonins are fibroblast growth factor 23 (FGF-23), frizzled-related protein-4 (FRP4) and matrix extracellular phosphoglycoprotein (*MEPE*) which regulate P metabolism. Phosphatonins are under the

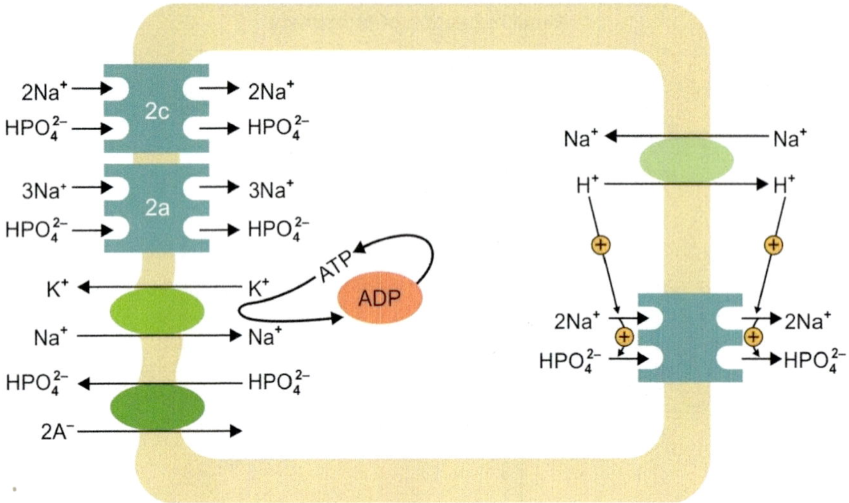

Figure 7.10 Phosphorus handling in the proximal tubule

control of *PHEX* gene (Phosphate-regulating gene with homologies to endopeptidases on the X chromosome). *PHEX*-gene product is a neutral endopeptidase, which regulates P metabolism. It is responsible for the catabolism of *FGF23*, which has a phosphaturic role. *FGF23* is produced in bone. *FGF23* levels rise with decreasing creatinine clearance rates and increasing plasma phosphorus levels. FGF also inhibits calcitriol synthesis. *Klotho*, a transmembrane protein, is an essential cofactor for the effects of *FGF23* on renal proximal tubule cells. *FGF23* is cleared by the kidney. sFRP-4 decreases phosphate reabsorption by sodium-phosphate cotransporters and also inhibits calcitriol synthesis such as FGF. FGF plays a role in pathogenesis of many hereditary and some acquired causes of hypophosphatemia.

- *Other hormones*: Stanniocalcins (STC1) stimulates phosphate reabsorption in the small intestine and renal proximal tubules and STC2 inhibits the promoter activity of the type 2 sodium phosphate cotransporter. Insulin like growth factor (IGF) also influences P metabolism.

HYPOPHOSPHATEMIA

Hypophosphatemia is defined as a serum concentration of P less than 3 mg/dL in adults and less than 4 mg/dL in children.

SIGNS AND SYMPTOMS OF HYPOPHOSPHATEMIA

The manifestations depend upon the rate of development and severity and chronicity of the phosphate depletion. Symptoms appear at plasma phosphate concentration of less than 1.0 mg/dL.

- Prolonged hypophosphatemia inhibits distal tubular reabsorption of calcium and magnesium and causes hypercalciuria. The initial response of bone to hypophosphatemia is increased resorption with release of bone calcium with hypercalciuria. This occurs as phosphate depletion induces a rise in the synthesis of calcitriol. More prolonged hypophosphatemia leads to *rickets* and *osteomalacia* due to decreased bone mineralization.

- Intracellular phosphate depletion causes fall of red cell 2,3-DPG (diphosphoglycerate) levels, reducing oxygen release at the tissue level and fall of intracellular ATP. Severe hypophosphatemia may cause *central pontine myelinolysis*.
- Heart failure, impaired myocardial contractility and arrhythmias may occur when the plasma phosphate concentration falls to 1.0 mg/dL.
- Hypophosphatemia causes *proximal myopathy* of skeletal muscles and *ileus* involving smooth muscles. Respiratory failure may occur. Rhabdomyolysis is common in alcoholics, and in patients on total parenteral nutrition without phosphate supplementation. Rhabdomyolysis with release of phosphate from the damaged muscle cells protects against the development of other hypophosphatemic symptoms.
- Hematological abnormalities include hemolysis (Serum phosphate < 0.5 mg/dL), reduced phagocytosis and granulocyte chemotaxis, defective clot retraction and thrombocytopenia.
- Metabolic encephalopathy and insulin resistance may occur.

CAUSES OF HYPOPHOSPHATEMIA

Hypophosphatemia may be due to inadequate intake or excess renal loss. Other causes include hyperparathyroidism, vitamin D deficiency or transcellular shifts. Up to 5% of hospitalized patients may have low serum phosphate concentrations (less than 2.5 mg/dL). Profound hypophosphatemia (less than 1.0 mg/dL) is much less common. Poor intake and transcellular shifts are important causes of hypophosphatemia **(Table 7.18)**. In DKA, the serum P may be high (with consequent phosphaturia) despite severe P depletion due to shift of phosphate from intracellular to extracellular compartment. Postoperative period, sepsis and refeeding are other important causes of hypophosphatemia due to transcellular shifts. Genetic causes such as hypophosphatemic rickets or vitamin D-dependent rickets (VDDR) are rare **(Table 7.19)**. Hypophosphatemia is common in critically ill patients due to multiple factors **(Table 7.20)**.

DIAGNOSIS AND TREATMENT

A comprehensive physical examination should identify consequences of hypophosphatemia and clues to an underlying cause. Special focus should be on the musculoskeletal examination, looking for signs of weakness, pathological fractures or pseudofractures, and skeletal deformities. Bone pain may be present, but severe muscle pain may indicate rhabdomyolysis. In children, rachitic features should be noted, and in adults, rachitic features suggest chronic hypophosphatemia since childhood. Short stature with increased upper to lower segment ratio also suggests previous childhood rickets, even without leg deformities. Decreased range of motion at the spine, hips, and other large joints can indicate calcified entheses, a common feature in adults with X-linked hypophosphatemia (XLH). Facial asymmetry or deformation of long bones may be signs of underlying FD. Maxillary bones are common sites of FD, whereas the

Table 7.18 Causes of hypophosphatemia

	Basic defect
Redistribution	
Refeeding after starvation	P enters cell with glucose
Anorexia	P depletion
Alcoholism	P depletion, poor intake
Respiratory alkalosis	Intracellular shift
Diabetic ketoacidosis	shift
Nonketotic hyperglycemia	shift
Hungry bone syndrome Cinacalcet use	After parathyroidectomy thyroidectomy
Decreased intestinal absorption	
• Decreased intake • Malabsorption • Antacids • Al, Mg, calcium • Vitamin D deficiency	Less P absorption Chelate P Less P absorption in GIT
Renal losses	
• Hyperparathyroidism – Primary – Secondary with Vitamin D deficiency/ VDDR • Hypophosphatemic rickets • Fanconi syndrome • McCune-Albright syndrome	– Excess PTH – Vitamin D deficiency with ↑PTH – Renal loss – Proximal tubule dysfunction – α-subunit of G-protein
Tumor induced hypophosphatemia	
• Mesenchymal tumor • Focal dysplasia **Post-transplant** **Diuretics, bicarbonate**	FGF ↑ MEPE↑ FRP↑ FGF ↑
Miscellaneous	
• Osmotic diuretics • Acetazolamide • Metolazone • Volume expansion • Imatinib	– Glycosuria with phosphaturia – Carbonic anhydrase inhibition – Carbonic anhydrase inhibition – Na absorption↓ ?

Abbreviations: VDDR, vitamin D-dependent rickets; PTH, parathyroid hormone; FGF, fibroblast growth factor; MEPE, matrix extracellular phosphoglycoprote; FRP, frizzled-released protein; Na, sodium

sinuses are a common location for tumors causing tumor-induced osteomalacia (TIO). If TIO is suspected, a thorough examination for palpable soft tissue masses should be performed. Hepatomegaly may suggest either an underlying tumor or chronic alcoholism. Skin findings such as café-au-lait macules focal dysplasia (FD and McCune Albright syndrome) and linear sebaceous nevi should be noted.

Table 7.19 Genetic causes of hypophosphatemia

Type	*Mutation*	*Effect on FGF*
Autosomal dominant hypophosphatemic rickets	FGF gain of function mutation	High FGF
X-linked dominant hypophosphatemic rickets	PHEX gene mutation	High levels of FGF
Autosomal recessive hypophosphatemic rickets	Dentin matrix protein mutation	DMP inhibits FGF
Hereditary hypophosphatemic rickets with hypercalciuria (HHRH)	NaP 2c mutation	Non-FGF mediated
Fanconi's syndrome	NaP 2a mutation	Non-FGF mediated
Dent disease	Cl CN5 mutation	Non-FGF mediated
Vitamin D dependent rickets	Type 1–1 hydroxylase deficiency Type 2-end organ resistance to vitamin D	
Distal renal tubular acidosis		

Abbreviations: PHEX, phosphate regulating endopeptidase homologous X-linked

Table 7.20 Hypophosphatemia in critically ill

Substance	*Reabsorption*
• Drugs – Diuretics – Catecholamines – Insulin/glucose	
• Refeeding	
• Trauma	
• Respiratory or metabolic alkalosis	
• Sepsis	
• Burns	
• Postoperative state, especially cardiac, liver, abdominal surgery	
• Fluid therapy	
• Renal replacement therapy	

Lab evaluation: True hypophosphatemia should be differentiated from spurious hypophosphatemia, which is caused by interference of paraproteins with the phosphate assay. The diagnosis of true hypophosphatemia may be evident from the history.

The evaluation of cause of true hypophosphatemia requires a step-wise approach.

- *Renal losses of phosphorus* are measured **(Table 7.21)**. *Phosphate excretion* can be measured either from a 24-hour urine collection or by calculation of the fractional excretion of filtered phosphate ($FEPO_4$) from a random urine

Table 7.21 Lab diagnosis of hypophosphatemia

	Serum Ca	*PTH*	*Urine P*	*Vitamin D*
Redistribution Refeeding after starvation	N	N	N	N
Anorexia	N	N	N	N/low
Alcoholism	N	N	N	N
Respiratory alkalosis	N/low	N	N	N
Diabetic ketoacidosis	N/low	N	N	N/low
Non-ketotic hyperglycemia	N	N	N	N
Hungry bone syndrome Cinacalcet use	Low	Low	Low	
Decreased intestinal absorption Decreased intake Malabsorption Antacids Al, Mg, calcium Vitamin D deficiency	 N/↓ ↑ ↓	 N N ↑	 N N ↑	 N N ↓
Renal losses Hyperparathyroidism • Primary • Secondary with vitamin D deficiency/ VDDR Hypophosphatemic rickets Fanconi syndrome McCune-Albright syndrome	 ↑ ↓ N N N	 ↑ ↑ 	 ↑ ↑ ↑ ↑ ↑	 ↓ ↓↓
Tumor-induced hypophosphatemia Mesenchymal tumor	N		↑	N/↓
Post-transplant diuretics/bicarbonate			↑	
Miscellaneous Osmotic diuretics Acetazolamide Metalazone Volume expansion Imatinib	N	N	↑	N

specimen: $FEPO_4 = [UPO_4 \times PCr \times 100] \div [PPO_4 \times UCr]$, where U and P refer to the urine and plasma concentrations of phosphate (PO_4) and creatinine (Cr). The 24-hour collection is preferable as there is diurnal variation in P excretion.

- Daily phosphate excretion should be less than 100 mg and the fractional excretion of phosphate should <5% (normal value is 5–20%), if hypophosphatemia is due to non-renal causes.
- Inappropriately high phosphate excretion, i.e. above 100 mg/day or a fractional excretion of phosphate above 5% is due either to hyperparathyroidism or to a renal tubular defect. Renal tubular defect can

be isolated or generalized (Fanconi syndrome). In Fanconi's syndrome, urinalysis shows the presence of amino acids (proteinuria) and glucose (renal glycosuria). Uric acid levels are low, often less than 2 mg/dL. Mild nonanion gap metabolic acidosis may be seen.

- *PTH levels*: If renal losses are high a PTH level is done.
  - A high PTH level in the presence of high calcium and low phosphate levels is very suggestive of primary hyperparathyroidism.
  - If the PTH level is high and the calcium and phosphate levels are low, secondary hyperparathyroidism is probable, due to intestinal malabsorption.
- Hypophosphatemia and urinary phosphate wasting without hypercalcemia should prompt an evaluation for *vitamin D deficiency.*
- Low *magnesium* indicates a poor diet intake and associated low *potassium* may be seen in alcoholism or DKA.

Serum lactate, complete blood count (CBC), and *serum ammonia* level, may be useful in sepsis and hepatic encephalopathy, which can cause respiratory alkalosis with hypophosphatemia. Routine measurement of FGF levels is not indicated.

TREATMENT

Most mildly hypophosphatemic patients do not require therapy except for treating the underlying cause.

Vitamin D deficiency should be treated with *vitamin D* supplementation 800 units/day. The treatment of symptomatic patients varies with the severity of the hypophosphatemia:

Phosphate supplementation: Oral is preferred rather than intravenous phosphate therapy. In asymptomatic patients with a serum phosphate less than 2.0 mg/dL, *oral phosphate* therapy can be given. Oral dosing varies between 1 mmol/kg of elemental phosphorous to 1.3 mmol/kg in 3–4 divided doses over a 24-hour period with less dose in renal failure. Commonly used oral phosphate supplements include 250 mg (8 mmol) of sodium or potassium phosphate per tablet. *Intravenous phosphate* is given, if the serum phosphate is less than 1.0 mg/dL, and switch to oral replacement when the serum phosphate exceeds 1.5 mg/dL. Stop phosphate repletion when the serum phosphate is greater than or equal to 2.0 mg/dL. Sodium phosphate is preferred for intravenous therapy. For intravenous treatment, the dose is 0.32–1.0 mmol/kg at 7.5 mmol per hour depending on level of serum phosphorus (1 mL IV solution contains 3 mmol of P). If hypophosphatemia persists, additional doses are given. The serum phosphate concentration should be monitored every 6 hours when intravenous phosphate is given.

In hypophosphatemia due to persistent urinary phosphate loss *dipyridamole* is administered.

Foods that are high in phosphate include dairy items, meats, and beans. Cow's milk, an excellent and accessible source of phosphate, contains 1 mg/mL.

Surgical care: Patients with primary hyperparathyroidism benefit from parathyroidectomy. For patients in whom parathyroidectomy is not feasible, calcium mimetic agents can be used. Patients with oncogenic osteomalacia are cured by excision of the tumor causing the phosphate wasting and relative vitamin D deficiency.

Morbidity and mortality: Though hypophosphatemic patients have a higher mortality, it remains unclear whether hypophosphatemia actually contributes to mortality, or merely is a marker for severity of illness. Whether correction of hypophosphatemia reduces mortality, is currently unknown.

HYPERPHOSPHATEMIA

EPIDEMIOLOGY

Hyperphosphatemia is rare in the general population; however, in patients with renal failure, the rate of hyperphosphatemia is as high as 70%. The normally higher level of serum phosphate in neonates, infants and patients (sometimes >6 mg/dL) must be considered when making a diagnosis of hyperphosphatemia.

ETIOLOGY

The main causes include excess ingestion, less renal excretion or altered intracellular distribution. In addition, alteration in regulatory mechanisms, i.e. hyperparathyroidism, vitamin D intoxication may also contribute to hyperphosphatemia **(Tables 7.22 and 7.23)**. Mutations of CaSR and PTH genes constitute some of the important genetic causes **(Table 7.24)**. Overall the most common cause of acute hyperphosphatemia is acute phosphate load while that of chronic hyperphosphatemia is renal failure and hypoparathyroidism.

Acute phosphorus load sufficient to overwhelm renal excretion can be either endogenous or exogenous. Phosphate enemas or any cause of marked tissue breakdown can lead to release of intracellular phosphate into the extracellular fluid. Examples of marked tissue breakdown include tumor lysis syndrome, muscle necrosis (rhabdomyolysis), and, rarely, marked hemolysis or transfusion of stored blood.

Tumor lysis syndrome: Tumor lysis syndrome is most often caused by cytotoxic therapy (but can occasionally occur spontaneously) in patients with a large burden of a tumor characterized by rapid cell turnover, such as lymphomas (particularly Burkitt's lymphoma and non-Hodgkin lymphoma) and certain leukemias. In addition to release of phosphate, this syndrome is also associated with the release of potassium, purines (which can be metabolized to uric acid), and cell proteins (which can be metabolized to urea). Thus, hyperkalemia, hyperuricemia (which may lead to acute renal failure), and azotemia are other common metabolic complications.

Familial-isolated hypoparathyroidism is caused by mutations to one of several different genes. Heterozygous mutations of the CaSR gene on chromosome 3 can cause autosomal dominant or sporadic hypoparathyroidism. Mutations of the parathyroid hormone (PTH) gene can cause both autosomal dominant and recessive hypoparathyroidism. Individuals with GMC2 (glial cells missing, Drosophilia homologue B) gene located on the short arm of chromosome 6

Table 7.22 Causes of hyperphosphatemia

Artefactual or spurious • Hemolysis • Hyperbilirubinemia • Hypergammaglobulinemia • Drugs **(Table 7.23)**
High dietary intake and increased absorption • Phosphate IV • Phosphate enemas (Acute Phosphate nephropathy) • Infants fed cow milk • Drugs **(Table 7.23)**
Vitamin D intoxication
Hypoparathyroidism, Pseudohypoparathyroidism
Internal redistribution • Tumor lysis syndrome • Rhabdomyolysis • Lactic acidosis • Diabetic ketoacidosis
Decreased phosphate excretion • Renal failure • Acromegaly (increase renal absorption) • Idiopathic childhood nephritic syndrome • Familial tumoral calcinosis • Drugs **(Table 7.23)**

Table 7.23 Drugs causing hyperphosphatemia

Mechanism	*Drugs*
Artefactual hyperphosphatemia	• Recombinant tissue plasminogen activator • Liposomal amphotericin • Heparin
Drugs which provide P load	• Fleet phosphosoda • Fosphenytoin
Drugs which increase absorption	Vitamin D intoxication
Drugs which decrease P excretion	• Growth hormone • Bisphosphonates • Dipyridamole

may have extremely low activity of parathyroid hormone. X-linked recessive hypoparathyroidism is caused mutations of a gene located on the long arm (q) of the X chromosome.

Familial tumoral calcinosis: Familial tumoral calcinosis is a rare autosomal recessive disorder characterized by hyperphosphatemia due to an increase in proximal tubular phosphate reabsorption, often in association with increased serum calcitriol concentrations. *GALNT3* gene encodes a glycosyltransferase that prevents the degradation of *FGF23*. Inactivating mutations in either the *GALNT3*

Table 7.24 Genetic causes of hyperphosphatemia

	FGF 23	*TRP*	*1,25 di OH D*	*PTH*	*Ca*	*U Ca*	*Mutant gene*
Tumoral calcinosis	High intact, C terminal	High	N/high	High	↑	↑	FGF excess as GALNT mutation reduces glycosyl transferase which degrades FGF, Klotho
Isolated hypoparathyrodism	N or high	High	Low normal	High	↓	↑	CaSR PTH gene
Pseudohypopara-thyroidism	N/ high	High	Low normal	Low	↓	↓	

or *FGF23* genes lead to deficiency of circulating intact *FGF23*. *FGF23* requires Klotho to bind to its receptor; therefore, a deficiency in klotho could lead to a state of *FGF23* end-organ resistance. The gold standard for diagnosis is genetic sequencing from whole blood samples. Serum calcium and PTH are within the normal range. The combination of hyperphosphatemia and normocalcemia results in a high calcium-phosphate product and calcium-phosphate deposition in the skin and subcutaneous tissues. Dietary restriction and phosphate binders and increasing urinary phosphate excretion by chronic administration of acetazolamide may be beneficial.

SIGNS AND SYMPTOMS

Irrespective of the cause, hyperphosphatemia produces similar signs and symptoms. An individual can ingest a large phosphate load without exhibiting frank hyperphosphatemia. Also, hyperphosphatemia can occur without a true increase in total body phosphate. Most patients with hyperphosphatemia are asymptomatic. Some patients have hypocalcemic symptoms, bone and joint pain, pruritus, or rash. More commonly, symptoms are related to the cause. Acute phosphate nephropathy presents with renal failure.

LABORATORY STUDIES

Spurious causes, i.e. hemolysis, high bilirubin, hyperproteinemia and hyperlipidemia should be excluded first. Improper sampling and prolonged clotting may also increase the serum phosphorus level.

Measurement of serum *calcium, magnesium, blood urea nitrogen (BUN), and creatinine* should be done in all cases of hyperphosphatemia.

Twenty-four hour urine phosphorus excretion should be checked. Normal is 800 mg in an adult. *Fractional excretion of phosphorus* should be calculated. Normal value is >15% in hyperphosphatemia. $FEPO_4 = [UPO_4 \times PCr \times 100] \div [PPO_4 \times UCr]$. Intact PTH should be measured.

Serum vitamin D levels should be estimated once renal failure and hyperparathyroidism are ruled out. Hyperphosphatemia with hypercalcemia suggests vitamin D intoxication.

Renal ultrasound, bone densitometry, electron beam CT for vascular calcification can be done as needed. Radiography is not necessary for the work-up of hyperphosphatemia, but it may reveal evidence of metastatic calcifications (e.g. bilateral, symmetrical calcifications of the basal ganglia; periarticular calcifications around large joints; soft tissue calcifications at pressure point areas).

Lab parameters in different causes of hyperphosphatemia:

- *Renal failure*: Patients with renal failure have high levels of intact PTH, low serum calcium and high serum creatinine. Urine phosphate excretion is low (Fe P <15%).
- *Hypoparathyroidism*: Patients with hypoparathyroidism have low levels of intact PTH, low serum calcium and normal renal function. Urine phosphate excretion is low. Most cases of pseudohypoparathyroidism are diagnosed based on clinical grounds, i.e. characteristic physical features of Albright hereditary osteodystrophy (e.g. short phalanges, short stature, obesity, round face, mental retardation) accompanied by low calcium levels, high phosphate levels, and positive findings from the family history. Biochemical investigations are like those with hypoparathyroidism but these patients have high PTH and 24-hour urine measurement for cyclic adenosine monophosphate shows abnormally low levels.
- *Vitamin D intoxication*: Intoxication. High serum calcium and high phosphate levels are observed with vitamin D intoxication. Patients with vitamin D intoxication show low PTH and high 25 and 1,25 vitamin D.
- *Milk-alkali syndrome:* Patients have high calcium and high serum phosphate but show low PTH and vitamin D.
- Unusual disorders, such as laxative abuse, tumor lysis or rhabdomyolysis should be considered. In tumor lysis or rhabdomyolysis, the fractional renal excretion exceeds 15%.

TREATMENT

If the cause of hyperphosphatemia can be determined, then specific treatment can be provided.

- *Hyperphosphatemia due to renal failure*: Patients with chronic kidney disease should avoid foods high in phosphate, such as dairy products and dark colas. Most patients require phosphate binders to inhibit gastrointestinal absorption of phosphate. The various phosphate binders available include calcium-containing binders, sevelamer and lanthanum carbonate. Niacin is also used as a phosphate binder. An alternative therapy to remove phosphorus in renal failure patients is dialysis. Parathyroidectomy is indicated in patients with renal failure who have tertiary hyperparathyroidism complicated by hypercalcemia, hyperphosphatemia, and severe bone disease. The agents commonly used to control secondary hyperparathyroidism are vitamin D metabolites and the calcium-sensing receptor agonists, e.g. alfacalcidol and paricalcitol.
- *Hyperphosphatemia for patients with normal renal function,* e.g. hyperphosphatemia associated with tumor lysis syndrome is treated by volume repletion with saline coupled with forced diuresis with a loop diuretic such as furosemide.

- *Hypoparathyroidism-associated hyperphosphatemia*: Calcium and vitamin D are prescribed for treatment of hypocalcemia. Recombinant PTH injections can be considered. Surgery may be required for removal of large calcium phosphate deposits.

Patients with hyperphosphatemia due to administration of liposomal amphotericin B who continue to require antifungal therapy may be switched to the formulation amphotericin B lipid complex, which contains less inorganic phosphate.

Mortality/morbidity: The short-term complications of hyperphosphatemia include acute hypocalcemia with tetany, acute deposition of calcium/phosphate complexes into joints or other soft-tissues and acute renal failure. Acute phosphate loads may also cause endothelial cell dysfunction.

Chronic hyperphosphatemia leads to the PTH and vitamin D derangements and result in abnormal bone architecture, increased vascular calcifications, papular rash, uremic pruritus, ischemic ulcers, restricted joint movements, rupture of tendons and band-shaped keratopathy. Chronic hyperphosphatemia increases the risk of cardiovascular deaths in chronic kidney disease (CKD).

SUMMARY

- Hypophosphatemia may be spurious or true hypophosphatemia. True hypophosphatemia may be due to decreased intestinal uptake increased renal losses or transcellular shifts.
- Usually, the cause is evident from history. If history and clinical examination are not conclusive urine phosphorus excretion can help in the diagnosis.
- Mild hypophosphatemia may be asymptomatic and correction of underlying cause is sufficient. In severe hypophosphatemia, intravenous phosphorus repletion is required.
- Acute hyperphosphatemia, on the other hand, is due to acute phosphate loads or transcellular shifts. Chronic hyperphosphatemia may be due to renal failure or hypoparathyroidism. Severe hyperphosphatemia needs saline diuresis or dialysis especially in the setting of renal failure. Phosphate binders are helpful in chronic hyperphosphatemia.
- Appropriate diagnosis and treatment reduces morbidity and mortality.

Multiple Choice Questions

A 1-year-old child presents with photosensitivity and rickets. ABG showing metabolic acidosis with a pH of 7.3 and bicarbonate of 18 mEq/L, urine pH of 5.1, glycosuria, urine phosphate of 820 mg per, day serum creatinine of 0.5 mg/dL, K 3.5 mEq/L, Na 135 mEq/L, serum calcium 7.8 mg/dL, serum phosphorus of 2 mg/dL. Serum creatinine is 0.6 m/dL. Imaging shows cupping and fraying of the lower end of ulna.

1. **What do you think is the likely diagnosis?**
   a. Distal renal tubular acidosis
   b. Fanconi's syndrome
   c. X linked hypophosphatemic rickets
   d. Vitamin D dependent rickets

2. **Which of the following statements is correct for the above patient?**
   a. Acid-load test will help to differentiate proximal and distal RTA
   b. Acid-load test is not needed, urine pH is sufficiently low, i.e. <5.5 and this rules out distal RTA
   c. Arginine hydrochloride should be used for the acidification test
   d. Ammonium hydrochloride should be used for acid-load test

3. **Which of the following statements is incorrect?**
   a. cystinosis should be checked for by slit-lamp examination
   b. A normal slit-lamp examination of cornea rules out cystinosis
   c. Bicarbonate supplementation is needed in this child
   d. Joulies solution can be used to correct hypophosphatemia

A 79-year-old man with a history of progressive bone pain was admitted for evaluation 3 years ago. The patient reported that the pain began in both the feet and gradually spread to the rest of the body over a 2-year period. Further assessment revealed multiple stress fractures in the feet. Bone mineral density test indicated osteopenia. Results of several serum protein electrophoreses were normal. His medical history suggested no pertinent etiologic factors. Physical examination revealed no clinically significant findings except unsteady gait. His serum phosphate concentrations declined from 2.5–1.8 mg/dL over the 2 years before admission. The patient's phosphate concentration reached a nadir of 1.2 mg/dL at admission. His serum alkaline phosphatase was 600 IU/mL. Other notable abnormalities included Serum calcium 8.8 mg/dL, parathyroid hormone (PTH) 79 pg/mL, and increased 24-hour urine phosphate and calcium excretion ie 1400 mg P and 300 mg calcium per day. Other routine biochemical parameters [including ionized calcium, thyroid-stimulating hormone, and free thyroxine (T_4)] were normal. The patient underwent a whole-body scan showing multiple bone lesions.

4. **Which of the following statements is incorrect?**
   a. X-ray, a computer axial tomography (CAT), and MRI of the lungs, abdomen, and pelvis should be done
   b. Most common cause of chronic hypohosphatemia may be a soft tissue tumor
   c. FGF23 may be elevated
   d. Treatment with oral phosphorus supplementation will be sufficient

5. **Which of the following statements is least likely?**
   a. Tumor-induced osteomalacia
   b. X-linked hypophosphatemic rickets (XHR)
   c. Autosomal dominant hypophosphatemic rickets (ADHR)
   d. Hyperparathyroidism

6. **Which of the following about the above case scenario is incorrect?**
   a. A negative family history can be useful in distinguishing tumor induced osteomalacia from XHR and ADHR
   b. Genetic testing for PHEX can be used to conclusively diagnose XHR
   c. Testing for the FGF23 gene will identify patients with ADHR
   d. TIO is only due to benign mesenchymal tumors

7. **All of the following are true about options for treatment of TIO except:**
   a. Resection of the tumor is the ideal treatment
   b. If the tumor cannot be located, treatment with calcitriol and phosphorus is instituted

c. Tumors which secrete somatostatin receptors may respond to treatment with octreotide
d. Cinacalcet is contraindicated in treatment of TIO

A patient under treatment of acute lymphatic leukemia presents with serum creatinine of 2 mg/dL, normal-sized kidneys, serum calcium of 7 mg/dL, serum phosphorus of 9 mg/dL, serum uric acid of 10 mg/dL

8. Which of the following statements is incorrect and unlikely to cause above?
a. Tumor lysis syndrome
b. Chronic kidney disease
c. Rapidly progressive renal failure
d. High uric acid may be due to gout in this patient

9. Tumor lysis syndrome is characterized by all except:
a. It can occur spontaneously without chemotherapy
b. Steroids can cause tumor lysis syndrome
c. Hyperkalemia may be seen
d. Urine uric acid/creatinine ratio may be high

10. All the statements are correct for tumor lysis syndrome except:
a. Saline diuresis is the treatment of choice
b. Mannitol is recommended for treatment
c. Allopurinol is recommended for prophylaxis
d. Rasburicase may prevent tumor lysis syndrome

Answers

1. b 2. b 3. b 4. d 5. d 6. d 7. d 8. d
9. c 10. b

SUGGESTED READING

1. Araya K, Fukumoto S, Backenroth R, et al. A novel mutation in fibroblast growth factor 23 gene as a cause of tumoral calcinosis. J Clin Endocrinol Metab. 2005; 90:5523.
2. Arrambide K, Toto RD. Tumor lysis syndrome. Semin Nephrol. 1993;13:273.
3. Assadi F, Hypophosphatemia: an evidence-based problem-solving approach to clinical cases. Iran J Kidney Dis. 2010;4(3):195-201.
4. Bijvoet OL. Relation of plasma phosphate concentration to renal tubular reabsorption of phosphate. Clin Sci. 1969;37:23-36.
5. Bollerslev J, Rejnmark L, Marcocci C, Shoback DM, Sitges-Serra A, van Biesen W, et al. European Society of Endocrinology Clinical Guideline: Treatment of chronic hypoparathyroidism in adults. Eur J Endocrinol. 2015;173(2):G1-20.
6. Brame LA, White KE, Econs MJ. Renal phosphate wasting disorders: clinical features and pathogenesis. Semin Nephrol. 2004;24:39-47.
7. Brenner and Rector. Diseases of the Kidney and Urinary Tract Ed. The Kidney, 8th edn; 2008.
8. Felsenfeld AJ, Levine BS. Approach to treatment of hypophosphatemia. Am J Kidney Dis. 2012;60(4):655-61.
9. Friedlander G. Autocrine/paracrine control of renal phosphate transport. Kidney Int Suppl. 1998;65:S18-23.

10. Gaasbeek A, Meinders AE. Hypophosphatemia: an update on its etiology and treatment. Am J Med. 2005;118:1094-101.
11. Geersel DA, Bindels AJ, Kuiper MA, Roos AN, Spronk PE, Schultz MJ. Treatment of hypophosphatemia in the intensive care unit: a review. Critical Care. 2010, 14:R147.
12. Grossman RA, Hamilton RW, Morse BM, et al. Nontraumatic rhabdomyolysis and acute renal failure. N Engl J Med. 1974;291:807.
13. Imel EA, Michael J Econs. Approach to the hypophosphatemic Patient. Clin Endocrinol Metab. 2012;97(3):696-706.
14. Improving Global Outcomes (KDIGO) CKD-MBD Work Group. Kidney Disease. KDIGO clinical practice guideline for the diagnosis, evaluation, prevention, and treatment of chronic kidney disease-mineral and bone disorder (CKD-MBD). Kidney Int Suppl. 2009;S1.
15. Jurgen Floege, Richard J Johnson, John Feehally (Eds). Comprehensive Clinical Nephrology, 4th Edition 2011.
16. Kestenbaum B, Sampson JN, Rudser KD, et al. Serum phosphate levels and mortality risk among people with chronic kidney disease. J Am Soc Nephrol. 2005;16:520-8.
17. Kurosu H, Ogawa Y, Miyoshi M, et al. Regulation of fibroblast growth factor-23 signaling by klotho. J Biol Chem. 2006;281:6120.
18. Larner AJ. Pseudohyperphosphatemia. Clin Biochem. 1995;28:391
19. Lederer E. Regulation of serum phosphate. J Physiol. 2014;592:3985.
20. Lederer E. Renal phosphate transporters. Curr Opin Nephrol Hypertens. 2014; 23:502.
21. Markowitz GS, Nasr SH, Klein P, et al. Renal failure due to acute nephrocalcinosis following oral sodium phosphate bowel cleansing. Hum Pathol. 2004;35:675.
22. Markowitz GS, Stokes MB, Radhakrishnan J, D'Agati VD. Acute phosphate nephropathy following oral sodium phosphate bowel purgative: an under-recognized cause of chronic renal failure. J Am Soc Nephrol. 2005;16:3389-96.
23. Murer H, Hernando N, Forster L, Biber J. Molecular mechanisms in proximal tubular and small intestinal phosphate reabsorption (plenary lecture). Mol Membr Biol. 2001;18:3-11.
24. Prie D, Friedlander G. Genetic disorders of renal phosphate transport. N Engl J Med. 2010;362:2399-2409.
25. Robert W Schrier. Publ. Lippincott Williams & Wilkins, 2007.
26. Shaikh A, Berndt T, Kumar R. Regulation of phosphate homeostasis by the phosphatonins and other novel mediators. Pediatr Nephrol. 2008;23:1203-10.
27. Shimada T, Muto T, Urakawa I, et al. Mutant FGF-23 responsible for autosomal dominant hypophosphatemic rickets is resistant to proteolytic cleavage and causes hypophosphatemia in vivo. Endocrinology. 2002;143:3179-82.
28. Slatopolsky E, Brown A, Dusso A. Calcium, phosphorus and vitamin D disorders in uremia. Contrib Nephrol. 2005;149:261-71.
29. Weiss-Guillet E-M, Takala J, Jakob SM. Diagnosis and management of electrolyte emergencies. Best Pract Res Clin Endocrinol Metab. 2003;17:623-51.
30. Wolf M. Update on fibroblast growth factor 23 in chronic kidney disease. Kidney Int. 2012;82:737-47.

CHAPTER

8 Acid-base Disorders

Mysore Keshavmurthy Phanish

INTRODUCTION

A basic and clear understanding of acid-base disorders and interpretation of acid-base gas (ABG) is essential for all the health care professionals dealing with critically ill patients. This chapter aims to provide a clear understanding of this vital and complex subject and a practical approach to the interpretation of an ABG. Detailed physiology and the description of numerous complex transporters within the nephron that regulate acid-base balance is not the purpose of this chapter and the reader is referred to many available textbooks and reviews for this.

The regulation of pH within a narrow range of around 7.4 is achieved by controlling the ratio of CO_2 (acid) and HCO_3^- (base) in the plasma. Fundamentally, acid is a hydrogen ion (H^+) donor and base is an H^+ acceptor. The relation between the H^+ concentration and the pH is logarithmic, pH= -log (H^+). Higher the H^+ ions in a solution lower the pH. Acid (H^+) ions are constantly added to the plasma and for the body to maintain physiological plasma pH (in other words, regulate the amount of H^+ ions to around 40 mEq/L), following processes take place:

- Buffering of the acid by extracellular and intracellular buffers
- Ventilation to control the level of $PaCO_2$
- Renal bicarbonate reclamation and H^+ excretion.

Buffers are weak acids or bases that regulate the pH by taking up or releasing H^+. Two important buffers to remember are bicarbonate (HCO_3^-) and phosphate. HCO_3^-/H_2CO_3 is a major extracellular buffering system.

Equation 1: $H_2O+CO_2 \leftrightarrow H_2CO_3 \leftrightarrow H^+ + HCO_3^-$

As you can see from this equation, if you add CO_2 (hypoventilation or respiratory failure) equation is driven to right resulting in more HCO_3 production. Metabolism of food generates acid (H^+) which reacts with HCO_3^- to produce CO_2 (equation 1) and the CO_2 generated is exhaled by the lungs. In this process, HCO_3^- is used up which is then replenished by the reabsorption (reclamation) of filtered bicarbonate by the proximal tubule and generation of additional bicarbonate. If more acid (i.e. H^+ ions) is added, more carbonic acid (H_2CO_3) is produced which in turn breaks down to CO_2 and H_2O. CO_2 is then cleared by the lungs and HCO_3^- consumed in this reaction and is regenerated (reclaimed) by the kidneys.

Therefore, in order to maintain a physiological plasma pH, kidneys control the HCO_3^- level and lungs control the CO_2 level with an intricate interdependency of these two organs. Oxygen that we breathe in is used in aerobic metabolism of carbohydrates and lipids and the end products of this are H_2O and CO_2. In hypoxic conditions, metabolism is predominantly anaerobic resulting in the production of lactic acid. Metabolic acid production is balanced by acid excretion. CO_2 produced by oxidative metabolism is excreted by the lungs. CO_2 is a volatile acid as shown in the equation above; it combines with H_2O to produce H^+ and HCO_3^-. If the lungs are unable to excrete the CO_2 produced, more H^+ are produced leading to acidosis, which would be termed respiratory acidosis. When a person hyperventilates, more CO_2 is eliminated resulting in a reduction in H^+ ions and consequent alkalosis. Metabolism of dietary proteins (and phosphate) produces nonvolatile acids such as sulphuric and phosphoric acids that are excreted by the kidneys. The amount of acid produced in this manner is usually 1 mmol/kg body wt of H^+ ions per day. The main extracellular buffer, as described above, is bicarbonate and the main intracellular buffers are sodium, phosphate and proteins. The buffering activity of Phosphate (HPO_4^{2-}) is shown in following equation:

$$HPO_4^{2-} + H^+ \leftrightarrow H_2PO_4$$

As you can see from this equation, addition of acid (H^+) to extracellular fluid results in conversion of monohydrogen phosphate (HPO_4^{2-}) to dihydrogen phosphate (H_2PO_4) hereby buffering the H^+ ions.

ACID HANDLING BY THE KIDNEY AND THE ROLE OF KIDNEY IN THE REGULATION OF PLASMA pH

The kidneys play a key role in the acid-base balance. Acid is excreted by the kidneys by urinary loss of H^+ ions associated with a buffer or by the excretion of H^+ ions as ammonium ions. Bicarbonate is freely filtered in the glomerulus, most of which (90%) is reabsorbed in the proximal tubule to maintain normal plasma bicarbonate concentration and the plasma pH. The proximal tubule cells excrete H^+ ions in exchange of HCO_3^- ions. When the secreted H^+ ions interact with bicarbonate in the filtrate, the end result is bicarbonate reabsorption **(Fig. 8.1)**. When secreted H^+ ions interact with a urinary buffer (mainly phosphate or NH_3) the end result is the excretion of acid. When buffered acid excretion occurs, the new bicarbonate generated in the renal cells by carbonic anhydrase is added to the blood. Titrable acidity is the amount of H^+ that is buffered by filtered weak acids (predominantly HPO_4^{2-}). Most important buffer for the secreted H^+ ions in tubule lumen is *ammonia* (NH_3) and this occurs via the reaction:

$$NH_3 + H^+ \leftrightarrow NH_4^+$$

The proximal tubule cells metabolize glutamine to produce ammonia, glucose (gluconeogenesis) and bicarbonate **(Fig. 8.2)**. The bicarbonate enters the blood and the NH_4^+ ions which carry H^+ ions are carried down the lumen to thick ascending limb of loop of Henle where they are reabsorbed in to the medullary interstitium. In the interstitum, NH_4^+ is broken down to NH_3 and H^+, NH_3 then passively diffuses in to the collecting duct, H^+ is secreted in to the collecting duct lumen by H^+ ATPase and reacts with NH_3 to produce NH_4^+ which is excreted in the urine. Therefore, final excretion of NH_4^+ in the urine requires H^+ secretion by the distal convoluted tubule and collecting duct via H^+- ATPase.

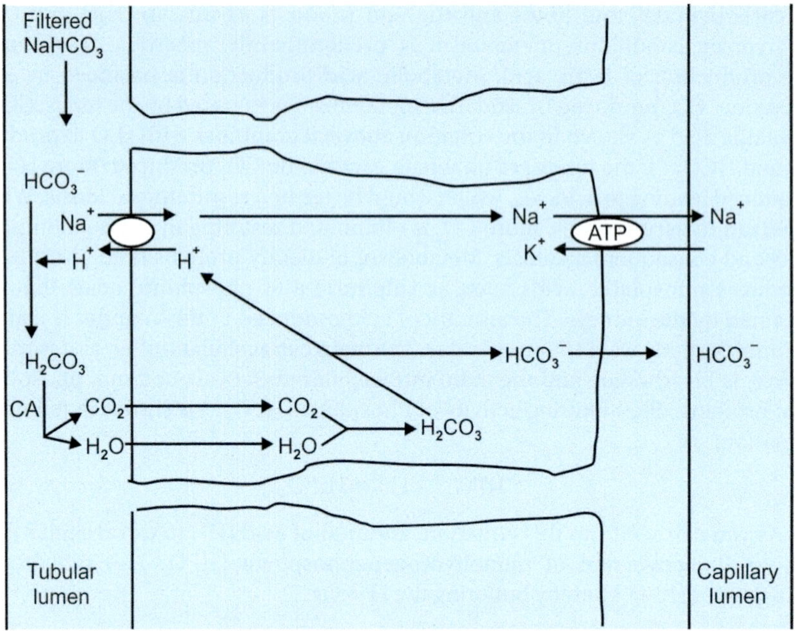

Figure 8.1 Bicarbonate reabsorption in the proximal tubule. Left side of the figure depicts the tubule lumen and the right side capillary lumen. The H^+ secreted into the lumen combines with filtered HCO_3^- to form carbonic acid (H_2CO_3) which is converted to CO_2 and H_2O by the enzyme carbonic anhydrase present in brush border of the cells. CO_2 then enters the cells, reacts with H_2O inside the cell to produce H_2CO_3, which then releases HCO_3^- to be reabsorbed into the capillary blood

COMPENSATORY MECHANISMS

Kidneys compensate for the acid-base disturbances generated by respiratory disorders and vice-versa. Compensation is generally not complete and never there is an over compensation.

In the presence of respiratory acidosis the kidneys compensate for the fall in pH by excreting H^+ ions and retaining HCO_3^- ions. This results in a rise in HCO_3^- concentration and the pH. This compensatory mechanism takes few days to complete and generally not adequate to normalize the pH and does not over compensate (i.e. the pH will not become alkalotic). In acute respiratory acidosis, excess CO_2 modifies the carbonic anhydrase reaction such that HCO_3^- production is increased. In chronic respiratory acidosis, there is increased HCO_3^- absorption in the proximal and distal tubules. In respiratory alkalosis, the kidneys compensate for the increase in pH by retaining H^+ ions and excreting HCO_3^- ions.

In metabolic acidosis, plasma concentrations of bicarbonate are low. Acidosis stimulates glutamine metabolism in the proximal tubule which produces NH_4^+ for urinary excretion and generates new bicarbonate. Acidosis also increases H^+ secretion and simultaneous increase in bicarbonate reabsorption in both the proximal (predominantly) and distal tubule. In proximal tubule, this happens

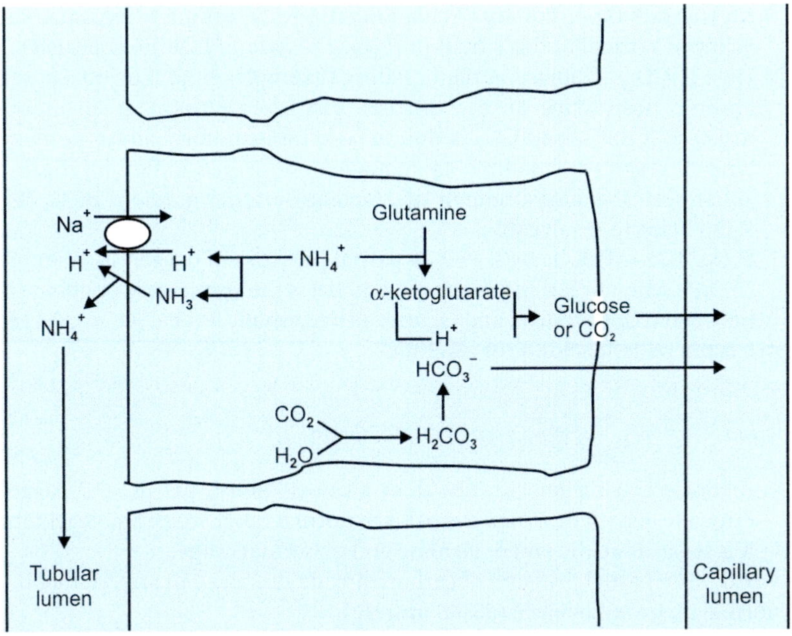

Figure 8.2 NH_4^+ is produced by the deamination of glutamine in proximal tubule. In this process, HCO_3^- enters the plasma and NH_4^+ enters the tubular lumen. A large portion of this NH_4^+ secreted into the lumen of proximal tubule cells is reabsorbed by the thick ascending limb of loop of Henle and accumulates in the medullary interstitium (not shown in this figure). The ammonia (NH_3) released from NH_4^+ in the interstitium then enters the collecting duct tubule cells and is secreted in to the lumen where it combines with H^+ ions secreted by the H^+ ATPase to form NH_4^+ which is then excreted

through an increase in apical Na/H exchangers and increased activity of the basolateral Na/3HCO_3 co-transporters. Respiratory compensation for metabolic acidosis is an increase in pulmonary ventilation through stimulation of central chemoreceptors in the medulla and peripheral chemoreceptors in the carotid and aortic bodies.

PRACTICAL INTERPRETATION OF ABG: A STEP-WISE APPROACH

- Is there hypoxia?
  - *PaO_2*: The partial pressure of Oxygen dissolved in arterial blood. The normal range is 10.5–13.5 kPa (70–100 mm Hg). PaO_2 of <12 kPa (<90 mm Hg) is generally considered hypoxia. With increasing age, PaO_2 can fall and following equation gives a reasonable estimate of PaO_2 in persons over the age of 40.
  - PaO_2=104 - (age × 0.27) mm Hg
  - SaO_2: The arterial oxygen saturation, normal range is >95%.
  - Type 1 respiratory failure is due to lung or pulmonary vascular disease (e.g. pneumonia and pulmonary embolism), which results in ventilation-perfusion (V/Q) mismatch. In this situation, O_2 delivered to alveoli is not

transferred to pulmonary circulation efficiently leading to hypoxia. $PaCO_2$ is low or normal in this situation. Type 2 respiratory failure (Low PaO_2 and High $PaCO_2$) is due to ventilator failure (Examples-opioid overdose, severe chronic obstructive airway disease, brainstem stroke). It is important to know if the raised CO_2 is due to type 2 respiratory failure or a severe type 1 respiratory failure as management would differ in these two situations. The measurement of Alveolar—arterial gradient of O_2 (P_AO_2-P_aO_2) helps to resolve this.

- $P_AO_2 = P_IO_2 - (PaCO_2/0.8)]$ PiO_2 is partial pressure of oxygen in inspired air (21 kPa when breathing room air) and 0.8 is the respiratory quotient (ratio between CO_2 produced and O_2 utilized). Normally, P_AO_2-P_aO_2 is <2–4 kPa.

- *pH*: Is the patient acidotic or alkalotic?

	Normal	Acidosis	Alkalosis
pH	7.35–7.45	<7.35	>7.45

  - Acidosis is a bigger concern than alkalosis and a pH of <7.2 suggest a critically ill patient. When the pH is in normal range make a note whether if it is towards acidic end or alkaline end of normal range.

- *$PaCO_2$*: The partial pressure of carbon dioxide dissolved in arterial blood. The normal range is 4.6–6 kPa (35–45 mm Hg).

	Normal	Respiratory acidosis	Respiratory alkalosis
$PaCO_2$	4.6–6 kPa (35–45 mm Hg)	>6 kPa (>45 mm Hg)	<4.6 kPa (<35 mm Hg)

  - Is the $PaCO_2$ contributing to or compensating for (or attempting to compensate for) change in the pH? For example, if pH is acidotic and $PaCO_2$ is low, it suggests that the primary problem is metabolic acidosis and that lungs are trying to compensate by increasing CO_2 elimination.

- *Bicarbonate*: Normal range of serum/plasma bicarbonate is 22–26 mEq/l. ABG reports often report standard and actual bicarbonate values. Actual bicarbonate ($aHCO_3^-$) is the measured value of bicarbonate from the actual blood sample and this is very dependent on $PaCO_2$. It will be high if $PaCO_2$ is high and vice-versa. One should look at the standard bicarbonate ($sHCO_3^-$) value and not actual value for the purpose of interpretation of acid-base disturbance. Standard bicarbonate concentration is the bicarbonate value corrected for a normal $PaCO_2$; i.e. it is what bicarbonate concentration would have been if the $PaCO_2$ was normal. Therefore, $sHCO_3^-$ concentration is the derived bicarbonate concentration after eliminating respiratory changes and reflects only metabolic changes.
  - Base excess reflects the amount of base that needs to be removed to bring the pH back to normal when pCO_2 is corrected to 5.4 kPa or 40 mm Hg. In acidosis, there is a deficiency of base and a base excess (BE) of -4 should really be called base deficit of 4.

	Normal	Metabolic acidosis	Metabolic alkalosis
Std HCO_3^-	22–26 mmol/L	<22 mmol/L	>26 mmol/L
BE	–2 to +2 mmol/L	> –2 mmol/L	>2 mmol/L

- Next step would be to assess respiratory and metabolic compensations. Look at pH, $PaCO_2$ and BE/$sHCO_3$.

Acidosis	pH <7.35 Acidosis	↑ $PaCO_2$ Respiratory	↔ BE/ $sHCO_3^-$ No metabolic compensation
	pH<7.35 Acidosis	↑ $PaCO_2$ Respiratory	↑ BE/ ↑ $sHCO_3^-$ with metabolic (renal) compensation
	pH<7.35 Acidosis	↔ $PaCO_2$ No respiratory compensation	↓ BE/ ↓ $sHCO_3^-$ Metabolic
	pH <7. 35 Acidosis	↓ $PaCO_2$ Respiratory compensation	↓ BE/ ↓ $sHCO_3^-$ Metabolic
Alkalosis	pH >7. 45 Alkalosis	↓ $PaCO_2$ Respiratory	↔ BE/ $sHCO_3^-$ No renal compensation
	pH >7.45 Alkalosis	↓ $PaCO_2$ Respiratory	↓ BE/$sHCO_3^-$ Renal compensation
	pH >7. 45 Alkalosis	↔ $PaCO_2$ No Respiratory compensation	↑ BE/ $sHCO_3^-$ Metabolic
	pH >7. 45 Alkalosis	↑ $PaCO_2$ Respiratory compensation	↑ BE/ $sHCO_3^-$ Metabolic

In clinical practice, mixed acid-base disturbances are common. For example, a patient with severe COPD, pneumonia and sepsis leading to AKI may have combined metabolic and respiratory acidosis. Renal physicians often encounter metabolic acidosis in their clinical practice and these patients are often critically ill. There are direct clinical consequences of metabolic acidosis (in addition to problems caused by the underlying etiology of acidosis such as sepsis). These include:

- Hypotension–due to impaired myocardial contractility and reduced peripheral resistance.
- Hyperkalemia due to potassium shift out of the cells.
- Leukocytosis
- Chronic metabolic acidosis results in loss of bone calcium due to buffering of the acid and increased urinary calcium excretion.

How do we approach a patient with metabolic acidosis? Clinical assessment remains paramount to make sense of laboratory investigations including blood gas analysis. For example, a patient who attends out-patient clinic with renal stones and metabolic acidosis is likely to have renal tubular acidosis while a septic patient in the ward will have metabolic acidosis secondary to renal failure or lactate accumulation.

Once metabolic acidosis is confirmed on blood gas analysis, check anion gap. Is it elevated or normal? Elevated anion gap means an acid has been gained or bicarbonate has been lost.

The anion gap (AG) is the difference between the measured cations (Na^+ and K^+) and measured anions (Cl^- and HCO_3^-) in plasma. The electroneutrality in the plasma is maintained by unmeasured anions, mainly the proteins (albumin) and phosphate. Normal anion gap is 6–15 mmol/L. In metabolic acidosis, increased anion gap occurs if an acid is added to the body such as ketoacids or lactic acid. The acid then releases H^+ ions, which use up the bicarbonate. Normal anion gap occurs when there is bicarbonate loss. This results in a compensatory increase in plasma chloride concentration (increased renal absorption of chloride) resulting in normal anion gap.

$$\text{Anion gap} = \{(Na+K)-(Cl+HCO_3)\}$$

- Causes of normal AG metabolic acidosis are:
  - *GI tract bicarbonate loss*: Bicarbonate loss from the gut occurs due to diarrhea, enterocutaneous fistulae, pancreatic drains, ileal conduits, ureterosigmoidostomy (bowel mucosa exchanges chloride in the urine for bicarbonate), pancreatic transplantation with bladder anastomosis (uncommon these days as most of the pancreatic anastomosis are enteric).
  - *Renal bicarbonate loss*: Renal tubular acidosis.
- Increased AG metabolic acidosis: This occurs when there is addition of acid to plasma.
  - *Lactic acid*: This is an end-product of anaerobic metabolism. When there is adequate oxygenation of the tissues, lactate is metabolized to bicarbonate in the liver. In tissue hypoxia, impaired oxidative metabolism and liver disease the lactate accumulates. Lactic acidosis occurs in sick patients who are in shock, septic and increased lactic acid is a marker of poor tissue perfusion. Poor liver perfusion impairs the ability of liver to metabolise lactate to bicarbonate contributing to lactate accumulation.
  - *Dibaetic ketoacidosis (DKA):* The ketoacids, acetoacetic acid and β hydroxybutyric acid accumulate during DKA. The absence of insulin increases their production and inhibits their catabolism. Excess alcohol intake coupled with malnutrition is another cause of ketoacid accumulation.
  - *Methanol and ethylene glycol:* These toxic alcohols cause high AG acidosis and also cause an increase in osmolal gap. Osmolal gap is a difference between the measured osmolality and calculated osmolality [(2 × Na) + glucose + urea] where the units are in mmol/L). Alcohol dehydrogenase metabolizes both methanol and ethylene glycol in to toxic metabolites and the treatment is dialysis and ethanol to saturate the alcohol dehydrogenase enzyme. Methanol causes abdominal pain, headaches, vomiting, visual disturbances (including blindness) while ethylene glycol causes similar symptoms and acute kidney injury.
  - *Salicylic acid:* An overdose with Aspirin (salicylic acid) results in increased ventilation causing respiratory alkalosis and it directly causes metabolic acidosis.
  - *Impaired acid excretion:* Acute or chronic renal failure leads to retention of phosphates and sulphates (and phosphoric and sulphuric acids respectively), coupled with reduced ability to reabsorb bicarbonate from the proximal tubule and to excrete H^+ ions at the level of distal nephron. Initially, accumulated acid is buffered by bicarbonate and later by the bone buffers.

MANAGEMENT OF METABOLIC ACIDOSIS

Treat the underlying disorder. There is a temptation to give intravenous bicarbonate for the management of acute metabolic acidosis in clinical practice and this should be resisted for the following reason:

Acute intravenous administration of bicarbonate leads to production of CO_2, which then diffuses in to the cells and lowers intracellular pH. My advice would be to give IV bicarbonate in patients who are acidotic and volume depleted, in particular, if there is GI tract bicarbonate loss (hyperchloremic normal anion gap acidosis). It is preferable to avoid IV bicarbonate in patients who have high anion gap acidosis in particular in oligo-anuric patients with fluid overload. When used, it should be used as an isotonic solution (1.4% or 1.26%) and not as hypetonic (8.4%) solution as the latter will both cause rapid rise in serum sodium and potentially could worsen intracellular acidosis as described above. Treatment of underlying condition will lead to metabolism of acids such as lactate and ketones (e.g. correction of sepsis and hypovolemia in case of lactic acidosis and insulin with IV fluids in case of ketoacidosis). In acidosis associated with AKI (acute kidney injury), if there is no reversible factor such as dehydration and obstruction, dialysis or hemofiltration are required to correct metabolic acidosis.

If IV bicarbonate is used, dose (in mEq) can be calculated as follows:

HCO_3^- required =
- 0.2 × weight (kg) × base deficit

  or
- 0.5 × weight (kg) × [25-serum HCO_3^- (mEq/L)].

RENAL TUBULAR ACIDOSIS

Defective acidification of the urine results in normal anion gap hyperchloremic acidosis termed renal tubular acidosis (RTA). Various types of RTA are shown in **Table 8.1**. Proximal tubular acidosis is an uncommon disorder arising from defective proximal tubular reabsorption of bicarbonate. Distal tubular acidosis is due to defective H^+ secretion and is more common.

Table 8.1 Renal tubular acidosis

	Type 1 (Distal)	*Type 2 (Proximal)*	*Type 4*
Hyperchloremic normal AG acidosis	Yes	Yes	Yes
Minimum urine pH	>5.5	<5.5 (can be >5.5 in early stages)	<5.5
Plasma potassium	Low	Low	High
Renal stones	Yes	No	No
Defect	Reduced H^+ excretion in distal tubule	Defective HCO_3 reabsorption in proximal tubule	Defective cation exchange in distal tubule either due to pump defect or low renin

Suspect renal tubular acidosis in patients with:

- Normal anion gap metabolic acidosis with normal or mildly impaired renal function (In other words, preserved glomerular filtration).
- Random urinary pH of >5.5 despite the presence of metabolic acidosis.
- Multiple or recurrent kidney stones.

Proximal Renal Tubular Acidosis (Type 2)

Proximal RTA occurs due to a failure of bicarbonate reabsorption and H^+ secretion by the proximal tubule. It can occur as an isolated defect or a generalized defect whereby absorption of other solutes such as glucose and phosphate is impaired in addition to the acidification defect (Fanconi's syndrome). This is seen in disorders that cause proximal tubule cell damage such as cystinosis, myeloma light chains, amyloidosis, medullary cystic disease and perhaps more commonly recovering acute tubular necrosis (ATN). When proximal tubule bicarbonate reabsorption fails, urinary bicarbonate loss occurs as the capacity of the distal tubule to reabsorb bicarbonate is limited. Plasma bicarbonate levels fall with a consequent fall in bicarbonate levels in the glomerular ultrafiltrate, which eventually becomes low enough for the distal nephron to reabsorb completely. Therefore, acidosis is never severe (plasma bicarbonate levels are generally >15 mmol/L). Upon acid loading (e.g. with ammonium chloride, urinary pH can drop to less than 5.5. Associated electrolyte abnormalities are hyperchloremia and hypokalemia. Hypokalemia is a result of aldosterone secretion in response to volume depletion resulting from sodium and bicarbonate loss. Treatment is with sodium bicarbonate and potassium supplements. Bicarbonate requirement is generally large (up to 10 mmol/kg/day). In those patients with phosphate loss, phosphate and vitamin D supplements are needed. 1 g sodium bicarbonate tablet contains 12 mEq (mmol) each of sodium and bicarbonate.

Distal Renal Tubular Acidosis (Type 1)

Distal renal tubular acidosis results from impaired H^+ secretion in the distal convoluted tubule and collecting ducts. The acidosis is severe, bone buffers are mobilized leading to rickets in children and osteomalacia in adults, growth retardation in children, hypercalciuria, renal stone formation and nephrocalcinosis. Distal RTA can occur in primary form as an inherited defect due to mutations (autosomal dominant or recessive) of the basolateral anion exchanger or apical proton pump. Secondary distal RTA can occur in autoimmune disorders (most commonly described in Sjögren's syndrome). It is also seen in renal diseases that affect medulla predominantly such as pyelonephritis, obstructive uropathy, medullary sponge kidney and drugs such as amphotericin B. Diagnosis can be made by giving an acid load in the form of ammonium chloride (NH_4Cl). While this is the gold standard, NH_4Cl is not palatable, tolerated poorly by patients often leading to vomiting. A practical alternative to ammonium chloride test is frusemide test. This test is a very useful screening test for patients with renal stones to exclude distal renal tubular acidosis. The principle of the test is that frusemide increases distal delivery of sodium ions, which get reabsorbed in distal nephron in exchange for H^+ ions resulting in acidic urinary pH.

Frusemide test: Ideally patient should fast overnight (allowed to drink water). Discontinue spiranolactone or amiloride for 4 weeks before the test. Obtain a baseline urine sample for pH.

- 9 am- Administer Frusemide 40 mg orally.
- 9.30 am–1 pm: collect urine samples every 30 minutes for 4 hours and analyze for pH.

A normal response is lowering of urine pH to <5.5 by 4 hours. If pH remains above 5.5, it is suggestive of distal RTA. Addition of *fludrocortisone* to enhance principal cell Na^+ absorption and intercalated cell H^+ secretion makes the test more sensitive and specific. In this *frusemide + fludrocortisone test*, 1 mg fludrocortisone is given along with 40 mg frusemide followed by urine sample collections as described above. In the absence of distal RTA, pH will drop to <5.5 by 3–4 hours while patients with distal RTA fail to acidify the urine and pH remains above 5.5.

Classic distal RTA is associated with hypokalemia that occurs due to K^+ secretion instead of H^+ during sodium absorption in distal nephron.

Hyperkalemic distal RTA (Type 4 RTA)—Here both K^+ and H^+ secretion are reduced. This occurs either because of voltage defect or hypoaldesteronism.

- *The voltage defect*: This occurs due to defective distal tubule Na^+ reabsorption resulting in more Na^+ in tubular lumen and therefore, less negative luminal charge. As tubular secretion of K^+ and H^+ are dependent on negative luminal charge, secretion of these ions decreases, leading to hyperkalemia and acidosis.
- *Hyporeninemic hypoaldosteronism*: Aldosterone stimulates Na^+ absorption, K^+ secretion and H^+ (acid) secretion in distal tubule and collecting duct. Low aldosterone levels can occur due to adrenal failure, low renin levels or drugs inhibiting the renin-angiotensin-aldosterone axis (ACE inhibitors and angiotensin II receptor antagonists). Diabetic nephropathy is a common cause of defective renin production leading to low aldosterone levels and type 4 RTA. Calcineurin inhibitors (Ciclosporine A and tacrolimus) are the other common cause of type 4 RTA leading to commonly observed hyperkalemia and mild metabolic acidosis following kidney transplantation.

SUMMARY

- A thorough understanding of basics of acid-base balance is important when treating critically ill patients.
- Kidneys and lungs coordinate with each other to maintain the acid-base balance and homeostasis. Renal response is usually slower.
- Kidneys excrete the acid load and generate HCO_3^- to replenish the buffer.
- Renal dysfunction can lead to abnormalities of acid-base balance.

Multiple Choice Questions

1a. A 25-year-old man with recurrent renal stones but otherwise well has a plasma bicarbonate of 10 mmol/L and a urine pH of 6.5. What is the probable diagnosis?
a. Proximal renal tubular acidosis
b. Distal renal tubular acidosis
c. Infection with urea splitting organisms (proteus)
d. Cystinuria

1b. What are the four groups of relevant investigations you would like to do?

1c. If this patient had an abdominal surgery with a stoma bag draining urine, what would that surgery be?

2a. A 65-year-old man is admitted generally ill, hypotensive and drowsy. The ABG reveals $PaCO_2$ 20 mm Hg, pH 7.12 and HCO_3^- 6 mmol/L and anion gap of 29. What is the blood gas interpretation?
a. Respiratory acidosis
b. Metabolic acidosis
c. Normal anion gap metabolic acidosis
d. High anion gap metabolic acidosis

2b. Blood results showed creatinine of 450 μmol/L (5 mg/dL), leukocytosis and raised CRP with normal sized unobstructed kidneys on ultrasound scan. What is the likely diagnosis?

2c. He is oliguric and fluid overloaded. What are the four most important therapeutic measures that you need to undertake?

3a. A 50-year-old smoker presented with sepsis and hypotension. The ABG showed PaO_2 of 70 mm Hg, $PaCO_2$ of 55 mm Hg, pH 7.35 and HCO_3^- 18 mmol/L. What is the blood gas interpretation?

3b. What is the probable diagnosis?

4. A 65-year-old woman presented with nephrotic syndrome and a κ/λ free light chain ratio of 20. Plasma bicarbonate levels were reduced at 15 mmol/L with normal creatinine levels. What is the probable diagnosis?

Answers

1a. Answer is b (Distal RTA). Renal stones are not a feature of proximal RTA. Infection with urea splitting organisms result in an increase in urinary ammonium with an increase in urinary pH which then promotes calcium phosphate crystallization and the ammonium crystallizes with phosphate and magnesium. This results in staghorn calculi (magnesium ammonium phosphate and calcium phosphate). Both this and cystinuria are not associated with metabolic acidosis unless there is sepsis and/or renal failure.

1b. Four relevant groups of investigations would be: 1. Renal function tests, electrolytes (Na and K), serum chloride, serum calcium levels. 2. Ultrasound kidneys. 3. 24-hour urinary calcium, citrate and oxalate excretion. 4. Urinary acidification test- Frusemide/Fludrocortisone test.

1c. The surgery would be a urinary diversion such as ureterosigmoidostomy or an ileal conduit.

2a. Answer is d—High anion gap metabolic acidosis.

2b. Acute kidney injury (AKI), secondary to sepsis is the most likely diagnosis. Differential diagnosis includes rapidly progressive renal failure (due to crescentic glomerulonephritis/small vessel vasculitis) and multiple myeloma.

2c. As he is oliguric and fluid overloaded, intravenous bicarbonate to correct acidosis is likely to cause more harm. Most appropriate therapeutic measures are oxygen, IV antibiotics, IV Frusemide and renal replacement therapy (Hemodialysis or CVVH/CVVHDF).

3a. Hypoxia with combined respiratory and metabolic acidosis.

3b. Probable diagnosis is chronic obstructive airway disease with type 2 respiratory failure (causing respiratory acidosis), pneumonia, sepsis, AKI causing metabolic acidosis.

4. Proximal renal tubular acidosis secondary to free light chain induced damage to proximal tubules.

SUGGESTED READING

1. Burns KD, Levine DZ. Acid-base balance. In: R Wilkinson, Rex L Jamison (Eds). Nephrology, Chapman and Hall, London; 1997.pp.117-33.
2. Cogan MG, Rector FC Jnr. Acid-base disorders. In: BM Brenner, FC. Rector (Eds). The Kidney, Saunders, Philadelphia; 1991 .pp. 737-804.
3. Chris O'Callaghan, Barry M Brenner. The Kidney at a Glance. Blackwell Science.
4. Principles of Renal Physiology. Christopher J. Lote. Kluwer Academic Publishers.

CHAPTER

9 Urinary Tract Infection

KC Prakash, V Ramasubramanian

INTRODUCTION

Urinary tract infection (UTI) is defined as invasion of microorganisms in the urinary tract and causing, in most of the cases, inflammation. It is one of the most common bacterial infections plaguing mankind. It can have a wide spectrum, varying between asymptomatic bacteriuria to prostatitis and pyelonephritis.

UTI TERMINOLOGY

Table 9.1 shows definition of various types of UTI. These definitions are important so as to establish whether the infection is true and requires treatment or not. It also guides whether corrective measure other than antibiotics are required. It also gives us a clue to whether long-term antibiotics are required (antibiotic prophylaxis).

Table 9.1 Terminology defining different types of urinary tract infections

Contamination	Organisms are introduced during collection or processing of urine culture.
Uncomplicated UTI	There are no structural or neurological problems that could be attributed to predisposition towards infection. Acute uncomplicated urinary infection rarely occurs in men and occurs generally in women between 20–50 years of age.
Complicated UTI	This is seen with structural or neurological disease or associated with co-morbid conditions such as diabetes mellitus or immunocompromised patients or in the presence of a urinary catheter.
Recurrent UTI	More than three symptomatic infections within 12 months after treatment with appropriate antibiotics based on urine culture.
Relapsing UTI	Infection by the same organism within two weeks after stopping an appropriate treatment.
Reinfection	Urinary infection caused by different organisms at anytime. This is seen in patients with comorbid conditions which make them susceptible to infection, such as diabetes or other immunocompromised states.
Persistent UTI	Infections present despite appropriate treatment. This is seen in patients with indwelling urinary catheters or neurogenic bladder or in transplant patients due to immunosuppressive state or due to medications such as mycophenolate mofetil.

Asymptomatic bacteriuria is the presence of significant bacterial growth in urine without any symptoms, usually detected during routine investigations. Asymptomatic bacteriuria is not considered significant and not treated except in the following situations: pregnant women, children with vesicoureteric reflux, patients undergoing genitourinary instrumentation or surgery and in transplant patients.

UTI CLASSIFICATION

Upper urinary tract infection can present as *acute pyelonephritis, renal abscess* or *perirenal abscess.*

Lower urinary tract infection can present as *cystitis, urethritis* in both sexes or *prostatitis* in males. *Acute urethral syndrome* seen in women occurs with dysuria and frequency, resembling cystitis. Urine cultures are either sterile or have low colony counts. This could be due to urethritis probably caused by *Chlamydia trachomatis* infection.

EPIDEMIOLOGY

UTI is more common in females than in males except at the extremes of age, when the incidence is higher in males. This is because of various anatomical reasons as follows:

- The short urethra in females coupled with the proximity to the anus makes it easier for bacteria from the perineum to ascend into the bladder and initiate an infection in young women.
- The infection is more prevalent in male infants due to a greater frequency of congenital anomalies such as vesicoureteric reflux, posterior urethral valve and spinal cord problems.
- In elderly men, prostatic hypertrophy leading to urinary outflow obstruction increases the risk of UTI.

At least three quarters of women develop one UTI in their entire lifetime. Sexual intercourse also plays a role in the occurrence of UTI. About a quarter of women, who have had one episode of UTI, will have recurrent episodes, either because of relapse or re-infection. The incidence of asymptomatic bacteriuria varies from 5 to 10% in pregnant women, much higher than in non-pregnant population. If untreated, a significant number will develop pyelonephritis later in pregnancy. This can be associated with premature births and increased perinatal mortality. The rate of asymptomatic bacteriuria is also higher in diabetic women. The causes are multifactorial including poor bladder function, obstruction to urinary flow, incomplete voiding and poor sugar control.

ETIOLOGY

In community-acquired infection, UTI is the second most common infectious disease caused by various organisms. *Escherichia coli* is the infective agent in 95% of all cases; others like *Klebsiella pneumoniae, Proteus mirabilis, Enterococcus faecalis, Acinetobacter* and *Staphylococcal saprophyticus* contributing to less than 5%. The etiologic agents in community and hospital-acquired infection differ. In hospitalized patients, the incidence of *E. coli* causing UTI accounts for 50% while

Klebsiella, Proteus, Enterobacter, and *Pseudomonas* contribute for 40% and the remaining by gram-positive organisms. Insignificant growth of bacteria in urine with true infection can be seen in patients who were on prior antibiotic therapy or having polyuria or having obstructed system or suffering from infection due to slow growing organisms. Apart from bacteria, fungi, *Mycobacterium tuberculosis* or virus can also cause urinary infections.

PATHOGENESIS

Urinary tract is always sterile in normal individuals, resistant to invasion by microorganisms, despite distal urethra getting colonized by bacteria from the colon. The major defense mechanism against infection is the total emptying of bladder, which has a flushing effect and prevents bacteria from colonizing the bladder. Other defense mechanisms maintaining infection free urinary system are urinary acidification, competent vesicoureteric junction, and other bladder mucosal and immunological factors.

In 95% of cases the microorganisms gain entry and ascend through the urethra and then into the urinary bladder. The colonization of the vaginal introitus is the prelude to UTI. Sexual intercourse causes alterations in the normal vaginal microflora, and is strongly associated with risk of UTI. In post-menopausal women, vaginal colonization of gram-negative bacteria due to disappearance of normally predominant lactobacilli from the vaginal microflora, predispose to UTI. If the individual has vesicoureteric reflux the microorganism may gain entry into the pelvis and then into the kidneys causing acute pyelonephritis. Repeated infection in kidneys can cause scars and lead to chronic pyelonephritis and chronic kidney disease. Less than 5% of cases of UTI result from blood-borne infection, the source being bacterial endocarditis, tuberculosis or intra- abdominal abscesses. Rarely, the microorganism can spread directly from the intestine to the bladder through fistulous communication as in Crohn's disease or malignancy. These patients will have polymicrobial infection with pneumaturia. **Table 9.2** shows various factors that increase the risk of UTI.

CLINICAL PRESENTATION

The clinical presentation of UTI ranges from asymptomatic bacteriuria to symptomatic cystitis to acute pyelonephritis. The symptoms may not always correlate with site of infection. The common symptoms have been shown in **Table 9.3**, while various symptoms in children have been mentioned in **Table 9.4**.

Acute onset of fever, shaking chills and loin pain, with or without symptoms of cystitis, is indicative of pyelonephritis. These patients may have costovertebral tenderness on examination. Bacteremia may complicate acute pyelonephritis, leading to septic shock and disseminated intravascular coagulation, especially with an obstructed urinary system. When diabetic patients present with features of acute pyelonephritis with severe shock, papillary necrosis leading to ureteric obstruction has to be suspected. Relief of the obstructed system is imperative to prevent recurrent attacks and progressive renal failure.

Renal and perirenal abscess are complications arising from hematogenous dissemination of bacteria, especially *Staphylococcus aureus* or due to gram-negative infections in an obstructed urinary system. Patients may present with

Table 9.2 Various factors increasing the risk of UTI

Factors increasing the risk of UTI
• Infrequent voiding allowing the bacteria to multiply • Incomplete voiding leading to incomplete flushing of urine • Sexual activity causing trauma to urethra, increasing the susceptibility to infection • Use of spermicidal contraception leading to death of normal vaginal flora and colonization by pathogenic organisms • Bacterial virulence factors (surface antigens, adhesins, etc.) conferring enhanced ability to infect anatomically normal urinary tracts can predispose to UTI • Genetic predispositions allowing the vaginal and urethral mucosa to express certain receptors that allow attachment of certain bacteria that later ascend into the bladder. This attachment to receptors prevents flushing effect during micturition • Lack of estrogen seen in post-menopausal women leads to thinning of vaginal tissue and also changes the pH of the vagina allowing colonization of bacteria and increased risk of UTI • Diabetes, an immunosuppressive state leads to increased incidence of UTI. This is more common with uncontrolled blood sugars which act as a good medium for the growth of bacteria • Immunosuppressive state (transplant patients, HIV patients) can cause UTI due to decreasing ability to fight infection

Table 9.3 Common symptoms of UTI

Cystitis
• Frequent small volume urination • Burning micturition • Foul smelling and turbid urine • Hematuria • Lower abdominal pain
Pyelonephritis
• Severe or dull flank or back ache • Fever with chills or rigor • Vomiting
Prostatitis
• Rectal or perineal pain in males • Fever with rigors • Urgency and frequency

Table 9.4 Symptoms of UTI in pediatric patients

- Frequent small volume urine
- Crying while passing urine
- Foul-smelling urine
- Fever without localization
- Vomiting and loose stools
- Poor feeding, unexplained hypothermia and excess bed-wetting in neonates

features of pyelonephritis, which may defervesce very slowly or presents with recurrent symptoms.

Emphysematous pyelonephritis is infection of kidneys, ureter and bladder by gas-forming bacteria. It is seen frequently in diabetics or patients with obstruction. The causative organism is usually *E.coli, Klebsiella pneumoniae* and *Proteus mirabilis*. The patients may present with features of acute pyelonephritis and sometimes with septic shock. Treatment is to initiate appropriate parenteral antibiotic and relieving the obstruction if the patient is stable or else will require nephrectomy.

Genitourinary tuberculosis can present with renal abscess, ureteral obstruction due to stricture, cystitis and epididymitis. Fibrosis of the ureteral orifices can lead to reflux. Urine may show sterile pyuria. Acid-fast bacilli (AFB) stain and culture may be positive.

Fungal infection of the urinary tract can affect the bladder and the kidney. *Candidal* infection in lower urinary tract usually occurs in patients with indwelling urinary catheter or who have persistent bacterial infection on long-term antibiotics or with malignancy. Renal infection is usually due to hematogenous infection and can be of serious consequence. It is most commonly seen in diabetics or immunosuppressed patients or cancer patients on chemotherapy or AIDS patients. These patients may be asymptomatic or have signs of obstruction due to fungal ball in ureter or bladder or may be very sick due to parenchymal involvement.

Acute prostatitis may present with fever, chills, dysuria, urinary frequency and urgency, perineal, back or pelvic pain. There may be symptoms of bladder outlet obstruction. Physical examination may reveal a tender, enlarged and indurated prostate. Chronic prostatitis may be occult or present with recurrent bacteriuria or pelvic pain.

DIAGNOSIS

Diagnosing UTI in neonates and pediatric patients below the communicative age is difficult. One should have an extreme degree of suspicion. Moreover, children with asymptomatic bacteriuria are at a higher risk of developing UTI. Detecting asymptomatic bacteriuria in children is problematic as the question is who should be screened? Screening school-going children may be too late as earlier infection would have caused scarring of the kidneys. Moreover, the implications of cost incurred in screening the entire pediatric population has to be considered. These patients usually have increased morbidity, long-term complications such as renal scarring, hypertension and chronic kidney disease. UTI in pediatric patients and male at any age will require detailed investigations to rule out urinary tract abnormality.

Microscopic Examination

Microscopic examination of clean-catch midstream urine is the first step in the laboratory diagnosis of UTI. The urine may be cloudy, malodorous or bloody. The vast majority of patients have *pyuria* (at least 10 leukocytes/mm^3). The dipstick leukocyte esterase test is a rapid screening test for detecting pyuria. Microscopic or sometimes gross *hematuria* is occasionally seen though it is more commonly indicative of other conditions like ureteric calculi or tumor. *Bacteriuria* is demonstrable on Gram stain of unspun urine in over 90% of patients with significant bacteriuria (colony counts >10^5 bacteria per mL). The presence of white cell casts is indicative of pyelonephritis. Proteinuria is also observed in UTI. Gram stain of the centrifuged urine may show bacteria.

Urine Culture and Sensitivity

Culture of a midstream urine specimen showing at least 10^5 bacteria/mL (significant bacteriuria) is indicative of infection. It is important to remember that one third of young women with symptoms of lower UTI have fewer bacteria in their urine. Hence, recent studies have re-evaluated the definition of significant bacteriuria in symptomatic women to >10^2 bacteria/mL. Women with dysuria and pyuria, who have less than 10^2 bacteria/mL have urethritis caused by chlamydia, *Neisseria gonorrhea, Herpes simplex* or *Trichomonas vaginalis.* Polymicrobial growth is usually indicative of contamination. Moreover, the presence of squamous epithelial cells in a urine specimen is strongly suggestive of contamination. False positive cultures are caused by contamination or incubation of urine prior to processing. False negative cultures may be caused by prior antibiotic therapy, obstruction of the urinary tract below infection, renal tuberculosis and presence of fastidious organisms. The practice of forcing fluids before cultures reduces the yield.

Acute urethral syndrome is the name used to categorize patients, especially women with acute onset of dysuria, frequency or urgency whose urine culture shows insignificant bacteriuria. Once vaginitis and herpes genitalis is excluded, the possibilities include UTI or urethritis due to chlamydia, mycoplasma or gonorrhea.

Imaging Studies

Imaging studies is generally carried out in patients in whom one suspects predisposing cause leading to UTI. In general, imaging is carried out 4–6 weeks after an acute infection. In conditions like obstruction or abscess, imaging is done during the acute stage.

- A plain *X-ray abdomen* is done to look for renal calcification or calculi in the urinary tract. It is not very sensitive. It can detect gas in the perirenal region or pelvis and bladder suggestive of emphysematous pyelonephritis.
- *Ultrasound abdomen* can detect hydronephrosis due to various causes. It is also useful in detecting space occupying lesions in the urinary tract, for evaluation of bladder outlet obstruction including the size of the prostate.
- *Intravenous urography* shows the anatomical details of the pelvicalyceal system and ureter. This imaging technique is usually carried out to rule out obstruction.
- *Computed tomography* is much more sensitive in detecting obstruction and the cause for it. Intravenous contrast is used to detect abscess and tumors in the urinary tract. It is also useful in diagnosing emphysematous pyelonephritis.
- *Micturating urethrogram* is performed in those patients with suspicion of vesicoureteric reflux or posterior urethral valve. Cystogram can reveal thimble bladder suggestive of tuberculosis.

- *Renal scintigraphy* with Di mercaptosuccinic acid (DMSA) scan can detect renal parenchymal infection and renal cortical scars.
- *Cystoscopy* is useful in demonstrating tubercles and or golf-hole appearance of bladder suggestive of tuberculosis.

MANAGEMENT

All symptomatic UTI should be treated. Asymptomatic pregnant women, preschool children with vesicoureteral reflux and patients on whom urethral manipulation is planned also require treatment. Males with UTI need to be evaluated for bladder emptying and obstruction.

Forceful hydration has not been found to be beneficial. Urinary acidification for purported benefits with antibiotics is not warranted. Most antibiotics exhibit adequate antibacterial activity at usual urinary pH. More recently, cranberry juice has been shown to disable the ability of *E. coli* to adhere to the epithelial cells of the urethra. Urinary analgesics like phenazopyridine hydrochloride (pyridium) play a negligible role in the management of symptomatic UTI. It may help in patients with dysuria, without UTI.

Antimicrobial Therapy

Antimicrobial therapy is warranted for all symptomatic UTI. The choice of therapy, dose and duration of therapy depends on the site of infection and the presence of complicating conditions. Even though the species of pathogens causing uncomplicated cystitis in healthy women is highly predictable, rising resistance among these bacteria is posing problems in empiric therapy. In India, a majority of UTI are caused by coliform gram-negative bacteria which produce an extended spectrum beta-lactamase (ESBL) enzyme which render them resistant to all third generation cephalosporins. They also show cross-resistance to fluoroquinolones and cotrimoxazole. Hence, it is strongly recommended that all patients with suspected UTI in India have a urine culture sent-off before initiating empiric therapy. A three days course appears optimal for all cases of uncomplicated cystitis. A seven days course may be pertinent in diabetics or patients with protracted symptoms or recurrent cystitis. For upper UTI, a minimum of 10–14 days of antibiotic is recommended. Prostatitis may require 6–12 weeks of therapy. **Tables 9.5 and 9.6** show oral and parenteral options for treatment of ESBL organism.

Treatment of Recurrent UTI

Simple interventions such as periodic voiding, post-coital voiding and using a contraceptive method other than a diaphragm or spermicide should be advised. Ingestion of cranberry juice helps reduce bacteriuria and pyuria in the elderly and rate of UTI in younger women. This is independent of urinary acidification. One has to rule out anatomical defects and urinary obstruction (organic or functional) before embarking on antimicrobial prophylaxis. Either continuous or post-coital (if infections are temporally related to intercourse) prophylaxis is indicated for frequent recurrences. A single tablet of CTX or nitrofurantoin for 6–12 months is effective.

Table 9.5 Oral regimens for uncomplicated cystitis with ESBL organisms	
Trimethoprim-Sulfamethoxazole (CTX)	160/800 mg BID
Nitrofurantoin	100 mg BID or TID
Oral Fosfomycin	4 g stat

Table 9.6 Parenteral options for ESBL organisms	
Cefoperazone-sulbactum	3 g BID
Piperacillin-tazobactum	4.5 g QID
Ertapenem	1 g OD
Imipenem	500 mg TID/QID
Meropenem	1 g TID

Treatment of Relapsing Infection

The same strain of bacteria causes recurrent episodes of UTI. This is usually due to an obstructed urinary system due to calculi or sloughed off papillae, especially in diabetics. Inadequate (less than 2 weeks of therapy for pyelonephritis) or inappropriate antibiotics (especially with resistant strains) can result in relapses. The presence of deep infection in the form of renal abscess may also necessitate a more prolonged course of antibiotics (3–6 weeks) to eradicate infection. In all such cases, radiologic and urologic evaluation is mandated.

Treatment in Pregnancy

Pregnant women need proactive evaluation to rule out asymptomatic bacteriuria. They require a more prolonged course of therapy (at least 7 days) and a lower threshold for initiation of prophylactic antibiotics, if recurrence of bacteriuria occurs. Antibiotics that are safe in pregnancy have to be used (Nitrofurantoin, Cephalosporins or Carbapenems).

Treatment of UTI in Men

Any episode of UTI in men warrants evaluation of the urinary tract to rule out obstructive uropathy (calculi, prostatic hypertrophy, and structural abnormalities). Foci of infection in the prostate also need to be excluded, as it requires a prolonged course of treatment. In general, all UTI in men require 10–14 days of antibiotics (as in complicated UTI).

Catheter-associated UTI

Catheter-associated UTI (CAUTI) is the most common nosocomial infection. Significant bacteriuria is inevitable in all patients with indwelling Foley's catheter. The presence of bacteriuria in a patient with an indwelling catheter does not automatically warrant therapy. Treatment of CAUTI requires good clinical judgment. If a patient has high fever with chills, loin pain and cloudy urine, pyelonephritis should be suspected and work-up is essential **(Table 9.7)**.

Table 9.7 Prevention of catheter-associated urinary tract infection (CAUTI)

CAUTI bundle
Core measures
• Insert catheters only for appropriate indications • Leave catheters in place only as long as needed • Only properly trained persons insert and maintain catheters • Insert catheters using aseptic technique and sterile equipment • Maintain a closed drainage system • Maintain unobstructed urine flow • Hand hygiene and standard (or appropriate isolation) precautions
Supplemental measures
• Alternatives to indwelling urinary catheterization • Portable ultrasound devices to reduce unnecessary catheterizations • Antimicrobial/antiseptic impregnated catheters

SUMMARY

- UTI is one of the most common infections worldwide. It is associated with significant morbidity and healthcare expenditure.
- Clinical presentation may vary depending upon upper or lower urinary tract involvement.
- Proper collection of urine for routine and microscopic examination and culture is important to guide antimicrobial therapy.
- A good understanding of the local epidemiology and resistance patterns is essential in the approach to treat UTI.
- Ensuring that complicated UTIs are diagnosed and appropriately treated will prevent complications and deterioration of renal function.

Multiple Choice Questions

1. **All the following are considered complicated UTI except:**
   a. UTI in children
   b. Underlying comorbid conditions
   c. Immunocompromised patient
   d. Presence of indwelling Foley's catheter

2. **A 21-year-old pregnant woman who is asymptomatic is found to have the following results: Urine routine shows 4–6 pus cells and urine culture grows *E.coli* >10^5 colonies/mL. You would:**
   a. Repeat a urine culture
   b. Treat with antibiotics
   c. Observe
   d. Put her on cranberry juice twice a day for 10 days

3. **UTI is seen more commonly in males who are:**
   a. Sexually active; due to prostatitis
   b. Diabetics
   c. Elderly
   d. Abstaining from alcohol

4. **95% of all UTI are caused by:**
   a. *S. epidermidis* b. *Candida*
   c. Enterococci d. *E. coli*

5. **Women are more prone to UTI because:**
   a. They void frequently
   b. They lack antibody receptors on the urethral mucosa
   c. Lactobacilli in tha vagina act as inducers
   d. Of a short urethra

6. **A 65-year-old diabetic with a history of recurrent UTI requiring multiple courses of antibiotics in the past one year, presents with dysuria, frequrncy and a low grade fever. You will start her on empirical:**
   a. Nitrofurantoin b. Amoxycillin
   c. Ciprofloxacin d. Cephalexin

7. **A 66-year-old male with a history of prostatic hypertrophy, presents with terminal dysuria, frequency and fever. His creatinine is 3.4. He looks comfortable and hemodynamically stable. The urine culture grows *Klebsiella*, sensitive to nitrofurantoin, meropenem and imipenem. You would treat him with:**
   a. Nitrofurantoin b. Ertapenem
   c. Cranberry extract d. Ampicillin

8. **A 23-year-old asymptomatic female, who is not sexually active, is found to have plenty of pus cells on a routine urine examination. You would:**
   a. Not treat her
   b. Send a urine culture
   c. Start on empiric antibiotics while awaiting treatment
   d. Start her on treatment for chlamydia

9. **You would suspect genitourinary tuberculosis when:**
   a. There is sterile pyuria
   b. Golf-ball appearance of bladder on cystoscopy
   c. Thimble bladder
   d. All of the above

10. **A 41-year-old diabetic male presents with recurrent episodes of fever, chills, loin pain and dysuria. The symptoms respond to antibiotics, based on urine cultures but recur soon after antibiotics are discontinued. Further management includes:**
    a. Cystoscopy to rule out papillary necrosis
    b. Chronic antibiotic prophylaxis
    c. Antifungal therapy along with antibiotics
    d. PSA to rule out prostatitis

Answers

1. a 2. b 3. c 4. d 5. d 6. a 7. b 8. a
9. d 10. d

SUGGESTED READING

1. Eshwarappa M, et al. Clinico-microbiological profile of urinary tract infection in south India. Indian J Nephrol. 2011;21(1):30-6.
2. Fihn SD. Clinical Practice: Acute uncomplicated urinary tract infection in women. N Engl J Med. 2003;349(3):259-66.
3. Komala M, Sampath Kumar KP. Urinary tract infection: Causes, symptoms, diagnosis and its management. Indian Journal of Research and Biotechnology. 2013;1(2):226-33.
4. Najar MS, Saldanha CL, Banday KA. Approach to urinary tract infection. Indian J Nephrol. 2009;19:129-39.
5. Robert W Schrier. Cystitis and Urethritis: Diseases of the Kidney and Urinary Tract, 8th edn; 2012.pp.832-44.
6. Taal M, Chertow G, MassdennP, Skorecki K, Yu A. Brenner and Rector's Urinary Tract Infection. The Kidney, 9th edn; 2011.pp.1356-79.

CHAPTER

10 Contrast-induced Nephropathy

Pranaw Kumar Jha

INTRODUCTION

Contrast-induced nephropathy (CIN) is an important form of acute kidney injury (AKI) in hospital setting and accounts for almost 11% of AKI cases. It has been defined as *more than 25% increase of serum creatinine or absolute increase in serum creatinine of ≥0.5 mg/dL, 48–72 hours after radiographic examination using a contrast administration.* The renal dysfunction in CIN may vary from minimal increase in serum creatinine to oliguria requiring dialysis. It is associated with significant morbidity and mortality and can have significant impact on outcome of basic disease. As more and more investigative procedures are being done requiring IV contrast administration in population at high risk, it is necessary to be vigilant in order to prevent and reduce CIN. This is more important as there is no treatment once CIN sets in.

CONTRAST MEDIA

The contrast media causing contrast-induced nephropathy are chemically modified derivatives of 2-, 4-, 6-triiodinated benzene ring. They are further classified on the basis of:

- Ionization (ionized and non-ionized)
- Osmolality (high, low or iso-osmolal)
- Iodine content.

Although very frequently used in radiology due to its relative harmlessness, it is still toxic for the kidneys and can lead to acute kidney injury. **Table 10.1** shows various contrast media in common use.

The more the number of iodine atoms per molecule (i.e. higher osmolarity), the better is the resolution. Nephrotoxicity can vary depending upon the type of iodinated contrast media used. Ionic contrast media have higher osmolality and usually cause more side effects.

PATHOPHYSIOLOGY

The pathogenesis of CIN involves interplay of multiple factors leading to renal ischemic injury to relatively hypoxic medulla. Most of the information on pathogenesis of contrast-induced nephropathy has come from animal models, as most of the patients developing CIN are not biopsied due to the self-limiting nature of the disease.

Table 10.1 Types of iodinated contrast media

Contrast media	*Osmolality (mOsmols/kg)*
HOCM (5–8 times blood osmolality)	
Ionic	
• Diatrizoate sodium	1550
• Iothalamate meglumine	2100
• Metrizoate	1000
LOCM (2–3 times blood osmolality)	
Ionic	
• Ioxaglate meglumine	
	580
Nonionic	
• Iopamidol	796
• Ioversol	640
• Iohexol	884
IOCM (osmolality equals that of blood)	
Iodixanol	290

Abbreviations: HOCM, high-osmolality contrast media; LOCM, low-osmolality contrast media; IOCM, iso-osmolal contrast media

Postulated mechanisms of CIN include as follows:

- *Medullary hypoxia*: Administration of IV contrast causes short-term vasodilatation followed by long-term vasoconstriction, leading to reduced glomerular filtration rate (GFR). Contrast also leads to an osmotic diuretic effect in ascending loop thereby increasing the oxygen requirement. The overall effect is worsening hypoxia and ischemia of renal medulla. Adenosine and endothelin play important role in this.
- *Direct cytotoxicity*: It has been proposed that direct cytotoxicity of the contrast media on the proximal tubule is a major contributor to the pathogenesis of CIN. It has been seen in in vitro studies that contrast can lead to vacuolization and cytoplasmic injury with rapid loss of important cellular proteins, such as NA^+K^+ ATPase pump and mitochondrial proteins.
- *Role of endothelin 1*: It has been proposed that IV contrast administration leads to endothelin release and tubular necrosis due to worsening of outer medullary ischemia.
- *Reactive oxygen species*: Generation of oxygen-free radical can lead to medullary vasoconstriction and renal ischemia. This is the basis for use of N-acetyl cysteine for prevention of CIN by free radical scavenging.

The pathogenesis of contrast-induced nephropathy is shown in **Figure 10.1**.

RISK FACTORS

There are multiple risk factors for contrast-induced nephropathy. Most important of these are presence of diabetes, pre-existing renal insufficiency and dehydration.

Table 10.2 enlists various modifiable and nonmodifiable risk factors for CIN.

It is important to identify these risk factors in patients undergoing investigations requiring IV contrast administration so as to implement necessary preventive

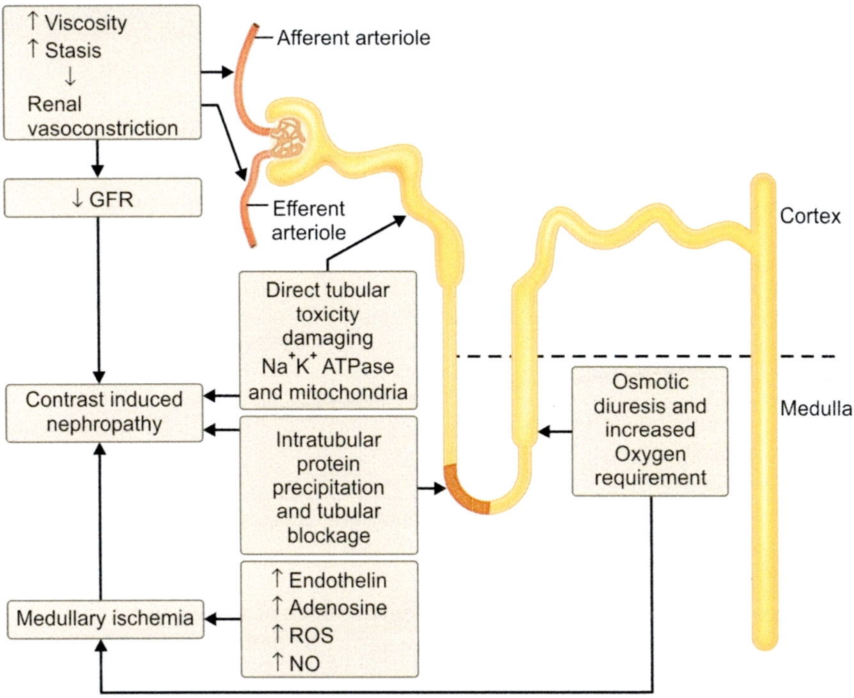

Figure 10.1 Pathogenesis of contrast-induced nephropathy
ROS, reactive oxygen species

Table 10.2 Risk factors for contrast-induced nephropathy
Modifiable risk factors
• Dehydration • Volume of contrast agent used • Type of contrast agent • Presence of other nephrotoxic medications and NSAIDs • Repeated administration of IV contrast within 72 hours • Hypotension • Anemia • Use of intra-aortic balloon pump (IABP)
Nonmodifiable risk factors
• Old age (>75 years) • Underlying renal insufficiency • Diabetes mellitus particularly with renal insufficiency • Left ventricular dysfunction and advanced heart failure • Acute myocardial infarction • Renal transplant recipient

Table 10.3 Mehran contrast-induced nephropathy risk scoring system

Risk factor	*Score*
• Systolic blood pressure <80 mm Hg—5 points • Intra-arterial balloon pump—5 points • Congestive heart failure (Class III–IV or history of pulmonary edema)—5 points • Age >75 years—4 points • Hematocrit level <39% for men and <35% for women—3 points • Diabetes—3 points • Contrast media volume—1 point for each 100 mL • *Renal insufficiency*: – Serum creatinine level >1.5 g/dL—4 points or – eGFR 40–60 mL/min/1.73 m^2—2 points – eGFR 20–40 mL/min/1.73 m^2—4 points – eGFR <20 mL/min/1.73 m^2—6 points	• 5 or less points – Risk of CIN—7.5% – Risk of dialysis—0.04% • 6–10 points – Risk of CIN—14.0% – Risk of dialysis—0.12% • 11–16 points – Risk of CIN—26.1% – Risk of dialysis—1.09% • >16 points – Risk of CIN—57.3% – Risk of dialysis—12.8%

Abbreviations: eGFR, estimated glomerular filtration rate; CIN, contrast-induced nephropathy
Source: Mehran et al. J AM Coll Cardiol. 2004;44(7):1393-9.

measures at the right time. A scoring system has been proposed and validated by Mehran et al. to stratify the risk of CIN in a particular patient **(Table 10.3)**.

CLINICAL FEATURES AND DIAGNOSIS

In CIN, serum creatinine starts increasing within 12–24 hours of IV contrast administration in almost 80% of cases. Recovery starts within 3–5 days but can take up to 2 weeks. Usually, CIN leads to non-oliguric renal failure. Patients with high baseline serum creatinine and low GFR are at high risk of dialysis requirement. Dialysis is required in <10% of the cases.

While diagnosing CIN, one must rule out other causes of renal dysfunction in the patient. Other important differential diagnosis in these cases is atheroembolic renal disease. This is usually associated with embolic lesions at other sites as well, hypocomplementemia and transient eosinophilia. There may be acute kidney injury due to hemodynamic changes or overdiuresis. One must rule out any recent intake of nephrotoxic medication.

As early detection of contrast induced nephropathy is important and serum creatinine increases relatively late after the kidney injury has set in, various other molecules are being tried to diagnose it at an early stage. These include kidney injury molecule-1 (KIM), cystatin-C, serum beta-2 microglobulin, N-terminal fragment of Pro-B natriuretic peptide.

Contrast induced nephropathy has been graded by Harjai et al. into 3 grades:
- *Grade 0*: Serum creatinine increase <25% above baseline and absolute increase <0.5 mg/dL above baseline
- *Grade 1*: Serum creatinine increase ≥25% above baseline and absolute increase <0.5 mg/dL above baseline)
- *Grade 2*: Serum creatinine increase and absolute increase ≥0.5 mg/dL above baseline)

  Prognosis worsens with higher grades.

PREVENTING CONTRAST-INDUCED NEPHROPATHY

Treatment of CIN is mainly supportive. So, it is important to identify risk factors and use preventive measures. General measures include the followings:

- Avoiding procedures requiring IV contrast administration as much as possible. These procedures should be used only when absolutely necessary.
- Trying alternative and safer radiological procedures first.
- Restricting the amount of IV contrast administered.
- Using low or iso-osmolar contrast agent—it has been proposed that low or iso-osmolar contrast agents should be tried instead of the ones with high osmolarity, more so in diabetic patients and in those with pre-existing renal insufficiency. Although NEPHRIC trial showed that incidence of CIN is less with iso-osmolal contrast media (IOCM) than low osmolality contrast media (LOCM), subsequent metaanalysis failed to show similar benefit.
- Avoiding concomitant use of nonsteroidal anti-inflammatory drugs (NSAID) or any other nephrotoxic drugs.
- Withholding angiotensin converting enzyme inhibitors (ACEI) and angiotensin receptor blockers (ARB)—in one of the studies (CAPTAIN trial), a nonsignificant reduction in CIN incidence was seen in patients with moderate renal insufficiency undergoing coronary angiogram (CAG) if ACEI/ARB was withheld before CAG.

Other measures to prevent contrast-induced nephropathy include the following:

Intravenous Hydration with Normal Saline and Bicarbonate

Hydration with normal saline (NS) is one of the most well proven, effective, safe and economical way of preventing CIN. Its efficacy in preventing CIN has been well proven in randomized trials. How it reduces the risk of CIN is not clear, although few mechanisms proposed are as follows:

- Increase intravascular volume
- Promotes diuresis
- Dilution of IV contrast
- Renin angiotensin aldosterone axis suppression
- Antidiuretic hormone (ADH) release suppression.

It has been seen that diabetics, female patients, those receiving large quantity of IV contrast and those requiring emergency procedures benefit most from IV hydration. The trials comparing NS and 0.45% saline found the former to be superior for CIN prevention. There is no fixed duration or amount of hydration, though, continuing for longer duration and administering as much as possible, is better.

It has been proposed that at least 500 mL of IV fluids should be given in three hours preceding procedure while it should be continued for at least 8–10 hours postprocedure. One needs to be careful while hydrating patients with cardiac or renal dysfunction to avoid fluid overload.

Intravenous Hydration with Normal Saline and Forced Diuresis

Role of saline infusion and furosemide-induced diuresis with renal guard system was evaluated in two different studies in patients undergoing CAG. Although the incidence of CIN reduced, volume overload and electrolyte abnormalities remained important concerns.

Sodium Bicarbonate

There has been mixed results about the role of IV sodium bicarbonate. It has additional benefits when compared to IV normal saline, such as alkalinization of the medulla and urine, thereby reducing free radical damage. But the initial enthusiasm for its use is not sustained anymore. To make the solution, add 154 mL of 1 mEq/mL sodium bicarbonate to 846 mL of 5% dextrose. This is approximately three 50 mL ampoules of bicarbonate (8.4%) in 850 mL of water with 5% dextrose. This solution can be given at the rate of 3 mL/kg/hour for 1 hour pre- and 6 hours post-IV contrast administration.

Oral Hydration with Water

A recent meta-analysis and review of PubMed, EMBASE and the Cochrane Central register of controlled trials (CENTRAL) databases searched until April 2015 showed that systematic oral hydration was at least as effective as IV hydration with saline to prevent CIN, although few previous studies did not show beneficial effect of oral hydration.

N-acetyl Cysteine

- N-acetyl cysteine (NAC) is a glutathione precursor. It is derived from amino acid cysteine and replenishes intracellular glutathione. It has poor bioavailability and a large first pass effect but has vasodilatory effects and also reduces oxygen free radical generation. Despite its controversial role in prevention of CIN, it has been used widely due to its low-risk profile and good tolerability. It is administered in dose of 600–1200 mg twice daily orally. Intravenous route has also been tried
- Various trials have shown conflicting results regarding use of NAC to prevent CIN. A recent metanalysis of databases of MEDLINE, EMBASE, and Cochrane library showed that NAC reduced the incidence of CIN among patients with pre-existing renal insufficiency.
- Kidney Disease Improving Global Outcomes (KDIGO) guidelines (2012) suggest administering oral NAC to patients at high risk of CIN.

It has been proposed that NAC may reduce serum creatinine without affecting kidney function.

Prophylactic Hemodialysis or Hemofiltration

Hemodialysis and hemofiltration can remove a large portion of contrast media, but despite this, performing hemodialysis or hemofiltration immediately after IV contrast administration has not been shown to prevent contrast-induced

Flow chart 10.1 An approach to prevention of contrast-induced nephropathy

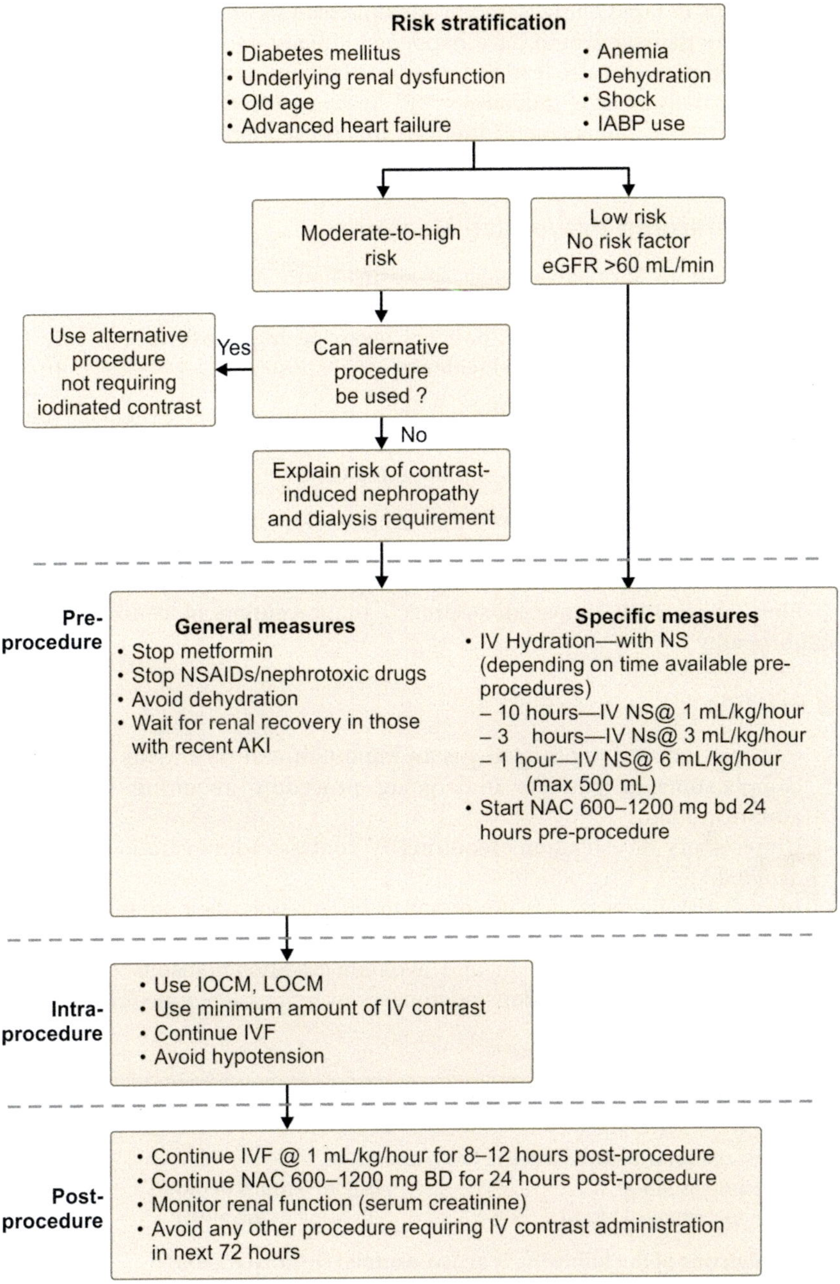

Abbreviations: IABP, intra-aortic balloon pump; NS, normal saline; NSAID, nonsteroidal anti-inflammatory drugs; AKI, acute kidney injury; IOCM, iso-osmolal contrast media, LOCM, low-osmolal contrast media; NAC, n-acetyl cysteine

nephropathy. This may be because of many reasons. Contrast administration usually leads to rapid damage and by the time dialysis or hemofiltration is done much of the damage would have happened already. Moreover, hemodialysis/ hemodiafiltration can also lead to activation of inflammatory pathways.

A meta-analysis of hemodialysis and hemodiafiltration did not show any benefit of renal replacement therapy for prevention of contrast-induced nephropathy, if given prophylactically.

Other Emerging Preventive Measures

Rosuvastatin: In Protective effect of rosuvastatin and Antiplatelet Therapy On contrast-induced acute kidney injury and myocardial damage in patients with ACS (PRATO-ACS) study, patients receiving high dose rosuvastatin had significant relative reduction in incidence of CIN post CAG.

Single bolus erythropoietin: Although there were reports of beneficial role of erythropoietin (EPO) in prevention of CIN, a randomized control trial did not show any such benefit in patients undergoing CAG.

Trimetazidine: One study showed that trimetazidine in combination was more effective than isotonic saline alone in prevention of renal function deterioration in patients with renal dysfunction undergoing CAG.

Flow chart 10.1 shows an approach to prevention of contrast-induced nephropathy.

SUMMARY

- Contrast-induced nephropathy is an important and potentially preventable complication in patients undergoing procedure requiring IV contrast administration.
- Unnecessary investigations requiring IV contrast administration should be avoided.
- In high-risk patients, it is important to inform them beforehand about the probability of renal function deterioration and dialysis requirement.
- Adequate, timely hydration and avoiding additional insults can help in preventing this complication and improve overall patient outcome.

Multiple Choice Questions

1. **High-osmolar contrast media has osmolality:**
   a. Same as blood
   b. 2 to 3 times of blood
   c. 5 to 8 times of blood
   d. None of the above
2. **Which one of the following is an iso-osmolal contrast media?**
   a. Ioversol
   b. Iodixanol
   c. Iohexol
   d. Iothalamate meglumine
3. **Risk factors for contrast-induced nephropathy include:**
   a. Diabetes mellitus
   b. Chronic kidney disease
   c. Hypotension
   d. All of the above

4. Postulated mechanism in pathogenesis of contrast-induced nephropathy include:
   a. Medullary hypoxia
   b. Direct cytotoxic effect on renal tubular cells
   c. Generation of oxygen free radicals
   d. All of the above

5. Single most effective strategy for prevention of contrast-induced nephropathy is:
   a. Dialysis as soon as possible after IV contrast administration
   b. Oral N-acetylcysteine
   c. Hydration with IV normal saline
   d. Oral hydration with water

6. A 58-year-old patient with long-standing history of type 2 diabetes mellitus, hypertension and chronic kidney disease with serum creatinine of 1.5 mg/dL presented with history of stable angina and needs coronary angiogram for evaluation. His investigations revealed serum creatinine of 1.6 mg/dL. What should be done to minimize the risk of contrast-induced nephropathy in this patient:
   a. IV hydration with 0.45% saline
   b. IV hydration with normal saline
   c. Oral N-acetylcysteine 600 mg bid for one day pre- and post-procedure
   d. Both a and c

7. The patient in the above question is on multiple medications. Which medication should be withheld before the procedure?
   a. Metformin
   b. Aspirin
   c. Metoprolol
   d. None of the above

8. The patient in Q.6 was found to have coronary artery disease and now needs revascularization with angioplasty and stenting. His serum creatinine after 24 hours is 1.5 mg/dL. Which one is the most appropriate next step?
   a. Tell the patient that it is too risky and should not be done
   b. Wait for 72 hours after the coronary angiogram before going for revascularization
   c. To do the revascularization immediately
   d. All of the above

9. The patient in Q.6 needs revascularization with angioplasty and stenting for the coronary artery disease. His serum creatinine after 24 hours is 2.5 mg/dL. Which one is the most appropriate next step?
   a. Tell the patient that it is too risky and should not be done at all
   b. Wait for another 72 hours after the coronary angiogram for revascularization
   c. Wait for the serum creatinine to return to the baseline value before proceeding with the revascularization
   d. To do the revascularization immediately

10. After revascularization the above patient's serum creatinine increased to 3.5 mg/dL after 2 days. How will you manage this patient?
   a. Start oral N-acetylcysteine immediately
   b. Start intravenous N-acetylcysteine

c. Start hydrating the patient immediately with IV normal saline to reduce the damage
d. Conservative management appropriate to the signs and symptoms as the damage is already done and the renal recovery will start on its own

Answers

1. c	2. b	3. d	4. d	5 c	6. d	7. a	8. b
9. c	10. d						

SUGGESTED READING

1. Agarwal SK, Mohareb S, Patel A, et al. Systematic oral hydration with water is similar to parenteral hydration for prevention of contrast-induced nephropathy: an updated meta-analysis of randomised clinical data. Open Heart. 2015;5:2(1): e000317. doi: 10.1136/openhrt-2015-000317.
2. Cruz DN, Goh CY, Marenzi G, et al. Renal replacement therapies for prevention of radiocontrast-induced nephropathy: a systematic review. Am J Med. 2012;125:66-78.
3. Gruberg L, Mintz GS, Mehran R, et al. The prognostic implications of further renal function deterioration within 48 h of interventional coronary procedures in patients with pre-existent chronic renal insufficiency. J Am Coll Cardiol. 2000;36:1542-8.
4. Harjai KJ, Raizada A, Shenoy C, et al. A comparison of contemporary definitions of contrast nephropathy in patients undergoing percutaneous coronary intervention and a proposal for a novel nephropathy grading system. Am J Cardiol. 2008;101(6):812-9.
5. Jha PK, Kher V, Radiocontrast agents and contrast induced nephropathy. In: Visweswaran RK. Prescribing Drugs in Renal Diseases, 1st edn. Mumbai: Tree Life Media; 2014. pp.110-8.
6. Kang X, Hu DY, Li CB, et al. N-acetylcysteine for the prevention of contrast-induced nephropathy in patients with pre-existing renal insufficiency or diabetes: a systematic review and meta-analysis. Ren Fail. 2015;13:1-7 (Epub ahead of print).
7. Kunadian V, Zaman A, SpyridopoulosI, et al. Sodium bicarbonate for the prevention of contrast-induced nephropathy: a meta-analysis of published clinical trials. Eur J Radiol. 2011;79(1):48-55.
8. Liu W, Ming Q, Shen J, et al. Trimetazidine prevention of contrast-induced nephropathy in coronary angiography. Am J Med Sci. 2015;350(5):398-402.
9. Mehran R, Aymong ED, Nikolsky E, et al. A simple risk score for prediction of contrast-induced nephropathy after percutaneous coronary intervention: development and initial validation. J Am Coll Cardiol. 2004;44(7):1393-9.
10. Merten GJ, Burgess WP, Gray LV, et al. Prevention of contrast induced nephropathy with sodium bicarbonate: a randomized trial. JAMA. 2004;291: 2328-38.
11. Mueller C, Buerkle G, Buettner HJ, et al. Prevention of contrast media- associated nephropathy: randomized comparison of 2 hydration regimens in 1,620 patients undergoing coronary angioplasty. Arch Intern Med. 2002;162:329-36.
12. Persson PB, Hansell P, Liss P. Pathophysiology of contrast medium-induced nephropathy. Kidney Int. 2005;68:14-22.

13. Shem-Didi L, Kristal B, Eizenberg S, et al. Prevention of contrast-induced nephropathy with single bolus erythropoietin in patients with diabetic kidney disease. A randomized controlled trial. Nephrology. 2015;15. doi: 10.1111/nep.12609. [Epub ahead of print].
14. Topeano F, Leoncini M, Toso A, et al. Impact of Rosuvastatin in contrast-induced acute kidney injury in the elderly: post hoc analysis of the PRATO-ACS trial. J Cardiovasc Pharmacol Ther. 2015; 25. pii: 1074248415599062. [Epub ahead of print].
15. Trivedi H, Nadella R, Szabo A, et al. Hydration with sodium bicarbonate for the prevention of contrast-induced nephropathy: a meta-analysis of randomized controlled trials. Clin Nephrol. 2010;74(4):288-96.
16. Weisberg LS, Kurnik PB, Kurnik BR. Radiocontrast-induced nephropathy in humans: role of renal vasoconstriction. Kidney Int. 1992;41:1408-15.

CHAPTER

11 Urology for Nephrologist

Sohrab Arora, Rajesh Ahlawat

INTRODUCTION

To summarize urology in one chapter is a daunting task. The aim of this chapter was not to present a comprehensive review, but to summarize key topics that are relevant to nephrologists in day-to-day practice. The authors have tried to keep the discourse short, keeping the theory to a minimum and summarizing "key points" and "rules of thumb" that may be helpful to a nephrologist.

TERMS USED FOR LOWER URINARY TRACT SYMPTOMS

The term "prostatism", which was used in the 1990s to describe the symptoms of benign prostatic hyperplasia (BPH), has been replaced by the purely descriptive term "lower urinary tract symptoms" (LUTS). These symptoms are nonspecific to prostate. In fact, these symptoms correlate poorly with prostate size, flow rates or even urodynamic bladder outlet obstruction.

Since this term is nonspecific for prostate, it can also be used for females, patients with urinary tract infections, patients with neurogenic bladder dysfunction or even patients of bladder cancer which can present with "LUTS".

The relationship between LUTS, BPH and bladder outlet obstruction (BOO) is best described by Tag Hald's rings **(Fig. 11.1)**

The classification of LUTS into "obstructive" and "irritative" types has also been replaced by "voiding" and "storage" types which are more descriptive terms and don't pre-suppose the diagnosis as suggested by the corresponding older terms. In addition to storage and voiding LUTS, it is important to know that some patients may have predominantly "post-micturition LUTS" which can be elicited by proper history taking.

COMMON INVESTIGATIONS IN THE EVALUATION OF LUTS

Uroflowmetry

Uroflowmetry is a simple non-invasive test used in the clinic. It is simply the measurement of volume of urine voided per unit time and depends on two factors—the detrusor contractility and the urethral resistance. Therefore a poor flow might indicate, simplistically, an underactive detrusor or an obstruction to flow.

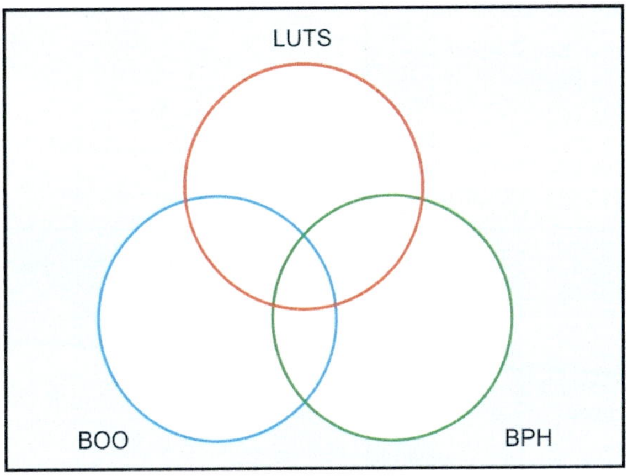

Figure 11.1 Tag Hald's rings
Abbreviations: LUTS, lower urinary tract symptoms; BOO, bladder outlet obstruction; BPH, benign prostatic hyperplasia

Uroflowmetry is best used in conjunction with frequency volume charts, as over-distended and under-distended bladder can both produce erroneous results. The voided volume should be at least 130–150 mL and less than 700 ml to produce accurate curves. Though the "normal" flow depends on age, gender and race, males <40 years usually have a maximum flow (Q_{max}) >25 mL/s, and in females, Q_{max} is 5–10 mL/s more than males at a given bladder volume. Flow <15 mL/s was generally defined as abnormal in literature, but it is now accepted that absolute flow rates correlate poorly with obstruction. About a third of patients with flow between 15–20 mL/s may be obstructed. Similarly, a third of patients with a flow between 11–14 mL/s may be non-obstructed. Therefore, the shape of uroflowmetry graph is as important as the maximum flow rate.

Common uroflowmetry curves are shown in **Figure 11.2**. The normal curve is shaped like a bell with Q_{max} achieved within the initial 1/3rd of voiding time **(Fig. 11.2A)**. Falsely high maximum flow rates may be produced by artifacts **(Fig. 11.2B)**. An intermittent curve **(Fig. 11.2C)** indicates a straining pattern, which further suggest detrusor underactivity. "Constrictive" obstruction, as in stricture urethra produces a flat, box shaped plateau curve **(Fig. 11.2D)**. "Compressive" obstruction, as in BPH leads to curve with Q_{max} achieved early in flow, followed by a prolonged tail **(Fig. 11.2E)**.

This test, despite being non-specific, is still widely used because of the sheer simplicity and ease, and also for follow up after treatment of obstruction.

Post-void Residual Urine

Post-void residual (PVR) urine is defined as volume of urine remaining in the bladder at the end of micturition.

PVR varies considerably from day-to-day and from void-to-void. The circumstances and the environment of the clinic and the pre-void volume may also affect the result. Partially filled or over-filled bladder can both produce

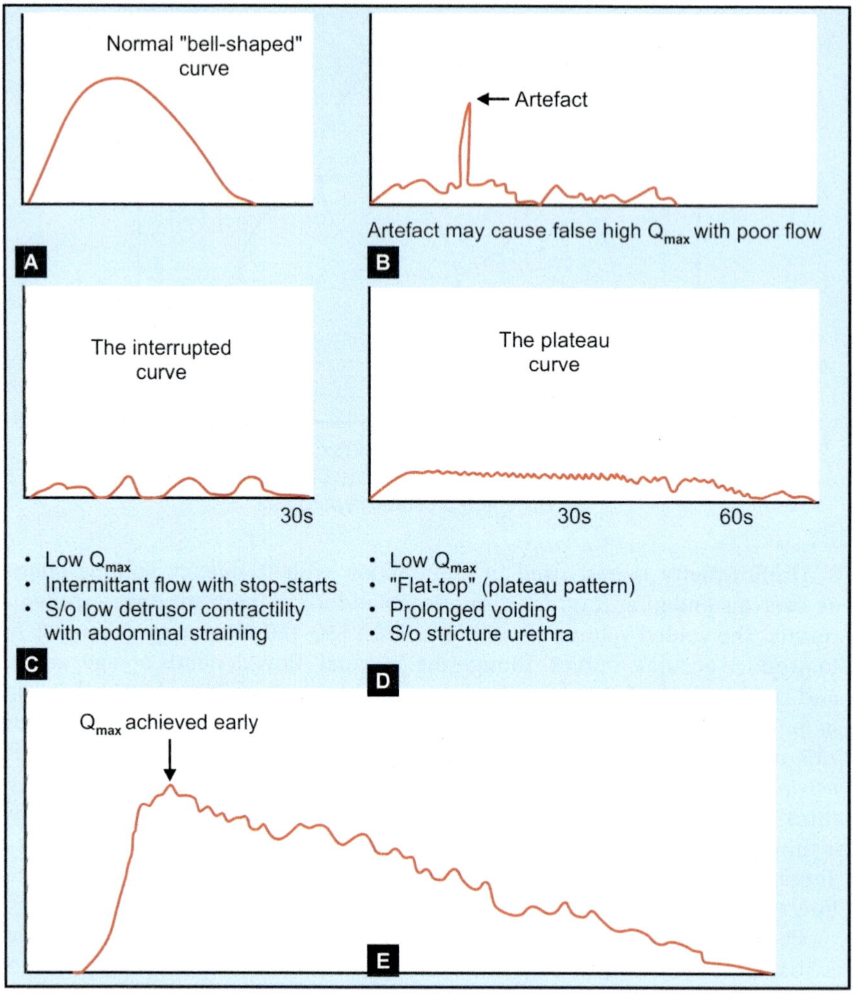

Figures 11.2A to E Common uroflowmetry curves: (A) Normal bell-shaped curve; (B) Artefact; (C) Interrupted curve; (D) Plateau curve; (E) Compressive
Abbreviations: Qmax, maximum flow rate; S/O, suggestive of

erroneous results of PVR. The absolute value of PVR does not correlate with symptoms neither can it predict the outcome of surgery unless at the extremes. It is also important to note that PVR is not specific to bladder outlet obstruction and it could be raised in neurological disease.

Raised PVR is an indication for further testing. For example, very high PVR (>500 mL) may prompt urodynamics which may reveal an under-active detrusor and we can counsel the patient about high chances of failing to void after transurethral resection of prostate (TURP). Similarly, high post-void residual urine associated with renal failure might indicate high-pressure chronic retention (discussed later).

Urodynamics

As noted in the section on uroflowmetry, poor flow may be due to decreased detrusor contractility or due to urethral resistance or obstruction. It is clinically important to distinguish between the two.

In addition, as Whitaker once noted, "Obstruction exists in a fluid-transporting system if the fluid pressure proximal to a relative narrowing must be raised to transmit the usual rate of flow through this area". Simply stated, "normal" flow may be present in an obstructed system, with flow being maintained by high detrusor pressures or abdominal straining.

Urodynamics is a study where the bladder is slowly filled through a catheter and bladder pressures, abdominal pressures and flow rates are measured simultaneously during both the storage and voiding phases. Unfortunately, real life voiding is very different from voiding in an artificial environment with a catheter in place. To make things more complex, the symptoms often don't correlate with flow or even urodynamic obstruction. Therefore, the results of urodynamic testing must be interpreted cautiously, taking the history, physical examination and other investigations into consideration. A working diagnosis should be made *before* the urodynamic study and the study should be designed and customized to answer specific questions. Urodynamics is an invasive investigation and may lead to exacerbation of existing urinary tract infection (UTI). Therefore, it should be deferred in the presence of active UTI.

For the purpose of this chapter, we assume that all artifacts of urodynamics have been eliminated, and only representative diagrammatic graphs are being shown. The phases of urodynamics are being shown in **Figure 11.3**.

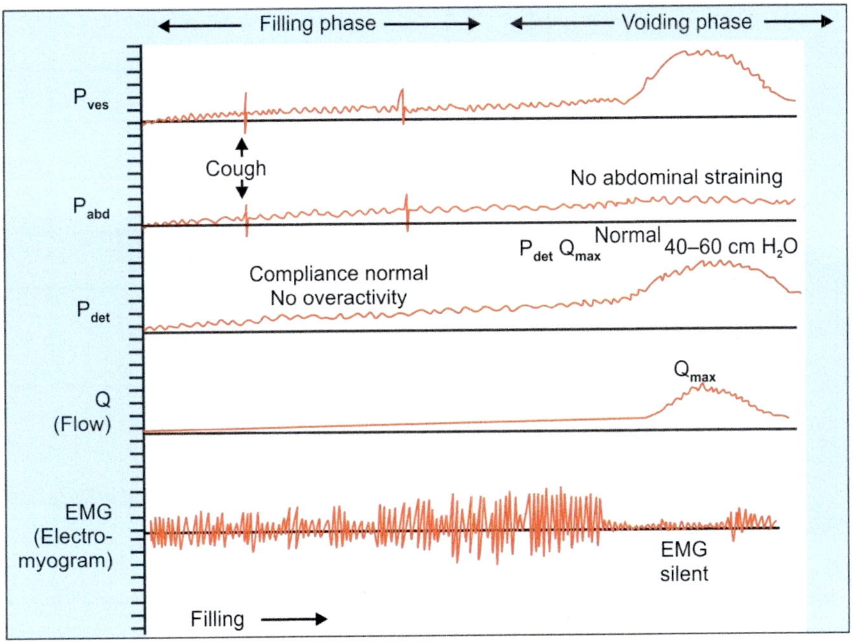

Figure 11.3 Normal cystometrogram (CMG)
Abbreviations: P_{ves}, vesical pressure; P_{abd}, abdominal pressure; P_{det}, detrusor pressure; Q, flow; Q_{max}, maximum flow

Interpretation of the Urodynamics Graph

In a normal urodynamic study, during the filling phase, under physiological filling rates, the bladder should have constant low pressure that does not reach more than 6–10 cm H_2O above the baseline at the end of filling. **Figures 11.4 to 11.6** represent simplified diagrammatic representation of common diagnoses during urodynamics. **Figure 11.3** represents normal urodynamics study. Any transient rise of detrusor pressure above baseline with or without sensation of urgency is defined as detrusor overactivity **(Fig. 11.4)**. The volume at first sensation, normal desire, strong desire, any leak during filling phase and bladder capacity must be noted (**Figure 11.4B** indicates leak associated with detrusor overactivity). A steep rise of detrusor pressure on filling may be due to low compliance of the bladder **(Fig. 11.5)**. Compliance is the relationship between change in bladder volume and change in detrusor pressure. Though "normal" compliance has been variably defined, but generally, a value less than 20 mL/cm of H_2O is considered poor compliance. Absolute pressure during filling phase is more useful than the absolute value of compliance. A storage pressure more than 40 cm of H_2O is associated with adverse effects on the upper tracts.

Normal male patient voids with a detrusor pressure of 40–60 cm H_2O at the maximum flow, and as previously discussed, during the voiding phase, detrusor pressure >100 cm H_2O at maximum flow indicates bladder outlet obstruction even if the flow is normal.

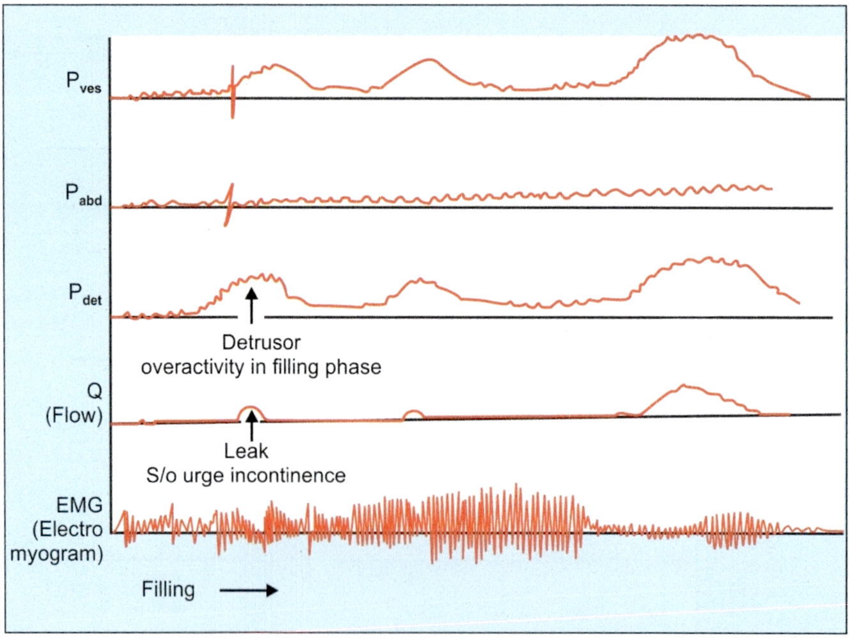

Figure 11.4 Detrusor overactivity with leak

BENIGN PROSTATIC HYPERPLASIA

Incidence of Histological BPH

Benign prostatic hyperplasia (BPH) is a purely histological diagnosis. Over 80% of all men will develop BPH in their lifetime, with an incidence of 50% at the age of 60 years, and 90% at 85 years. Only about 15–30% of these men will develop LUTS and only about 25% of men are symptomatic from BPH at the age of 50.

Static and Dynamic Component of BPH

Rich sympathetic innervation is found in the prostate, prostatic capsule and bladder neck with a predominance of α1-adrenergic receptors. This is the basis of the concept of "dynamic component" of BPH and the basis of α blocker use. α blockers decrease the tone of bladder neck, prostate smooth muscle and capsule, thus relieving the dynamic component.

The static component is provided by the enlarged transition zone producing pressure on the prostatic urethra. The static component can be reduced by reducing the volume of the prostate by using 5α-reductase inhibitors or by surgical management of BPH.

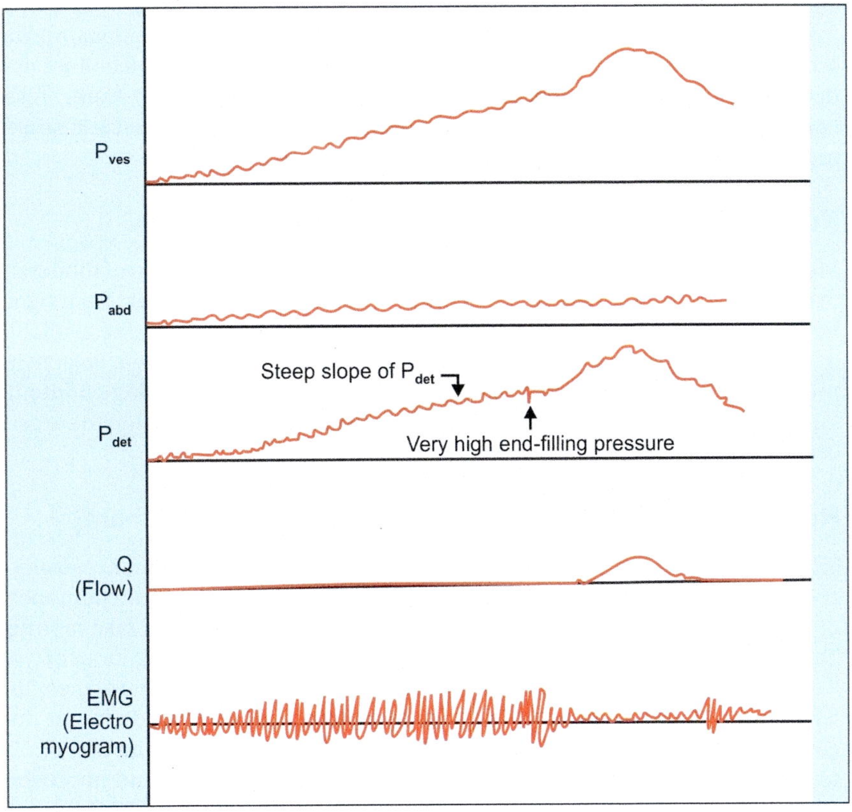

Figure 11.5 Poor compliance with high end filling pressures

The concept of static and dynamic components of BPH is an oversimplification but is a convenient model to understand the pathophysiology of the disease.

Symptoms: The Americal Urological Association Symptom Score (AUASS) and "Bother" International Prostate and Symptom Score (IPSS)

The American Urological Association (AUA) Symptom Score Index is a patient reported score based on a 7-question survey (incomplete emptying, frequency, intermittency, urgency, weak stream, straining, and nocturia), with each question scored from 0 to 5. This score is non-specific to the causes of LUTS but has been validated only for bladder outlet obstruction. The interpretation of the score is as follows:

- Score > 0–7—Mild symptoms
- Score > 8–19—Moderate symptoms
- Score > 20–35—Severe symptoms.

The IPSS adds an additional question on this survey, which qualitatively measures the effect of LUTS on patient's quality of life ("bother"). It is interesting to note that the "bother" does not correlate with the AUA score. A patient may want to defer treatment if the "bother" is low even when the AUA score is high and vice versa.

The AUA score is dynamic and many factors may cause variations on the score. Most common of these factors are drugs. Drugs like anticholinergics, decongestants, and diuretics can cause worsening of AUA score. Also, comorbidities like diabetes, congestive heart failure and neurological diseases may cause increased score.

Role of α Blockers

Medical therapy has been recommended as the first line treatment of moderate to severe symptoms of BPH by the AUA guidelines. The α blocker treatment significantly improves flow rates, quality of life, and symptom scores. The available α blockers (alfuzosin, tamsulosin, silodosin etc.), differ in their selectivity towards α 1a adrenergic receptors but have similar effect on relieving symptoms and improving flow rates. The α blockers do no decrease progression to surgery or the risk of acute urinary retention at 2 years.

Role of 5α Reductase Inhibitors and Combination Therapy

The 5 α reductase inhibitors cause shrinkage of the prostate epithelium causing a reduction in the size of prostate, resulting in a reduction of dynamic component of BPH. This reduction in size is a slow process and the effect may take months. The commonly used drugs are finasteride, which is a competitive inhibitor of type 2 enzyme, and dutasteride which inhibits both type 1 and type 2 isoenzymes. The landmark Medical Therapy of Prostatic Symptoms (MTOPS) study found that combination therapy with an α blocker and a 5 α reductase inhibitor is superior to either α-blocker or 5-ARI therapy in preventing progression and improving symptoms in large prostates. An international multi-centre Combination of

Avodart and Tamsulosin (CombAT) trial showed similar results with combination therapy resulting in significantly greater improvements over α blocker or 5 α reductase inhibitors alone in symptoms at 3 months, BPH related health status at 12 months, peak flow rate at 6 months and decreased progression to retention or surgery. On the other hand, this study found a significant increase in drug related adverse events with combination therapy.

Role of Antimuscarinics

In patients with predominantly storage LUTS and presumed bladder outlet obstruction, if post-void residual is low, anticholinergics may be prescribed safely. Tolterodine is effective in this group of patients and the risk of urinary retention is not increased and there is no exacerbation of LUTS. However, It should be used with caution in high post-void residuals >250–300 mL.

Patient Selection for Surgery

Surgery should be done for patients with complications of BPH, namely refractory retention (at least one failure of trial without catheter), recurrent UTI, bladder calculi, or renal insufficiency. Surgery may also be considered in patients with moderate to severe symptoms scores and high degree of bother who have failed medical management, or patients who choose surgery over medical management. For patients who have failed medical management, pressure-flow studies may be prudent.

ACUTE AND CHRONIC RETENTION

Acute Urinary Retention

Acute urinary retention (AUR) is the sudden, painful inability to void and is usually a dramatic presentation in the emergency room. In majority of cases, no cause can be found (spontaneous AUR) and in some cases, factors like drugs, excessive water or alcohol intake, UTIs, constipation or anesthesia may precipitate AUR (precipitated AUR).

Immediate management of AUR is catheterization. The drained volume is usually less than 1 liter. If the volume drained within the first 10 minutes following catheterization is more than 1 liter, the condition is termed as "acute-on-chronic" retention and is a predictor of failed trial without catheter (TWOC) and are more likely to be offered surgery.

Factors predicting successful TWOC include younger patient, precipitating cause identified, and retained volume <1 liter. The duration of catheterization also affects the chances of successful TWOC. A successful TWOC was achieved in 44% of patients after 1 day of catheterization, 51% of patients after 2 days, and in 62% of patients after 7 days. On the flip side, catheterization more than 3 days is associated with increased morbidity. Alfuzosin has been shown to double the likelihood of a successful TWOC. Therefore, patients should be put on α blocker medication and a TWOC may be tried after 2–3 days. In cases of failed TWOC, surgery should be considered.

Chronic Urinary Retention

Chronic urinary retention has a vague definition in literature. Some authors suggest post-void residual volume >300–500 mL as a definition for chronic retention. The LUTS are usually mild in nature. Indeed, some patients may retain liters of urine without any symptoms! The only symptoms in chronic retention may be dribbling and nocturnal incontinence due to loss of urethral resistance at night.

Chronic retention is usually classified into low-pressure chronic retention (LPCR) and high pressure chronic retention (HPCR).

In HPCR, voiding pressures are high with outlet obstruction and poor flow rates, resulting in upper tract deterioration and renal failure. In LPCR, the bladder is highly compliant and thus, the upper tracts are normal and there is no renal failure. These patients have low detrusor pressures on urodynamics and very large retained volumes.

Catheterization is not an emergency in chronic retention unless renal dysfunction or upper tract deterioration (HPCR) is present. In these cases, catheterization may be followed by post-obstructive diuresis due to osmotic diuresis of retained salt, water and urea, and loss of medullary gradient. Brisk diuresis requires careful fluid replacement which should be around 80% of the output in the first 24 hours. There may be hematuria after catheterization which should not be mistaken for traumatic catheterization and is due to decompression of upper tracts. It usually settles within 48–72 hours. There is no need for gradual decompression and rapid decompression is safe.

URINARY TRACT OBSTRUCTION: OBSTRUCTIVE UROPATHY

Terminology and Impact

It is important to know the various terms often (wrongly) used interchangeably to define obstruction.

Hydronephrosis is a simply a dilation of the renal pelvis or calyces. It may or may not be associated with obstruction of the urinary tract or may be physiological as in pregnancy.

Obstructive uropathy refers to the functional or anatomic obstruction of the urinary tract.

Obstructive nephropathy is when obstructive uropathy causes functional or anatomic damage to the kidneys.

Obstructive uropathy is a common cause of acute and chronic renal failure. Acute obstruction usually presents with severe pain and decreased urine output, but symptoms of chronic obstruction are highly variable, often mild, and require a high index of clinical suspicion. Early diagnosis with appropriate imaging is warranted, and treatment can prevent permanent renal loss.

Obstructive uropathy can be *supravesical* or *infravesical*. We focus our discussion on the supravesical obstructive uropathy in this section.

Diuretic Renal Scan

The diuretic renal scan is a commonly used investigation to evaluate the functional significance of hydronephrosis (to distinguish between obstruction versus non-obstructive dilatation of the pelvicalyceal system).

Principle of Diuretic Renal Scan

A radiotracer filtered by the kidney is injected intravenously and scintigraphic images of the kidney are obtained at serial intervals and are plotted over time. (Tc)99m-diethylene-triamine-penta-acetate (DTPA) which is mainly filtered by the glomerulus and (Tc)99m-mercaptoacetyltriglycine (MAG3) which is mostly secreted by the tubule are the most commonly used radio tracers for the evaluation of obstruction.

An accumulation of radiotracer in the pelvicalyceal system might indicate a hypotonic system (a large extra renal pelvis, for example) or an obstructed system with hydronephrosis. To distinguish between these two, a diuretic is injected after 15–20 minutes (The F+20 protocol), which leads to increased urine flow. If the system is not obstructed, the tracer will wash out and vice versa.

Interpretation of Diuretic Renal Scan

Three distinct phases of renogram are described. The 'uptake' phase corresponds to the speed of injection of the radioisotope and the renal blood flow. An abnormal uptake phase may be due to impaired renal function. The second phase renal 'handling' phase, which corresponds to transfer of isotope across the tubule cell. The 'washout' or drainage phase corresponds to the rate of excretion of tracer in the urine.

The rate of washout can be quantified as T1/2 (the time taken for 50% washout of tracer from the PCS) and also as a visual graph. Conventionally, a half life less than 10 minutes is considered normal, between 10 and 20 minutes is considered equivocal and more than 20 minutes is obstructed. In case of equivocal cases, the F+0 and F-15 protocols may be used when the diuretic is injected along with radio tracer and 15 minutes before radio tracer respectively. A T1/2 more than 10 minutes in the F-15 protocol is considered obstructed. It is important to interpret T1/2 in perspective with the shape of the renogram curve. The types of curves obtained are diagrammatically shown in **Figure 11.6**.

Management of Pain

Pain in renal or ureteric colic is due to collecting system pressure and wall tension. Non-steroidal anti-inflammatory drugs (NSAIDs) are the first line drugs for management. These drugs target the inflammatory pathway of pain and also reduce the pressure in collecting system due to reduction in renal blood flow. These drugs should not be used in renal insufficiency due to the adverse effect on renal function. Narcotic analgesics are also effective and have a rapid onset of action but have the adverse effects of nausea, constipation and urinary retention apart from the physical and psychological addiction and the potential for abuse. Patients of ureteric colic often have anorexia and vomiting associated with pain. Intravenous hydration is advised till the pain is relieved.

Renal Drainage

In ureteral obstruction prompt renal drainage is prudent in the following situations:

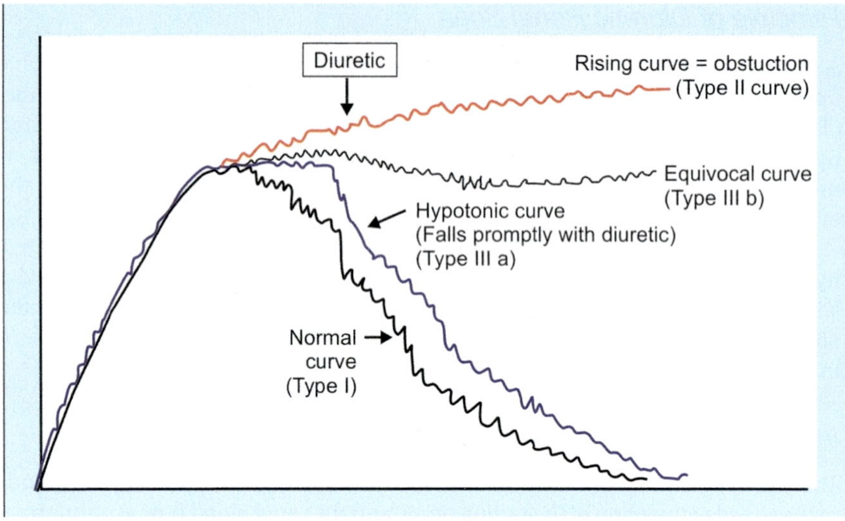

Figure 11.6 Typical curves on a diuretic renogram

- Bilateral obstruction
- Obstruction in a solitary kidney, associated with renal failure
- Patient is highly symptomatic, with high-grade fever or signs of sepsis.

Ureteral stents and percutaneous nephrostomy are options for drainage. Both are equally effective, but have their own advantages and disadvantages summarized in **Tables 11.1 and 11.2**. One of the major complications of ureteral stents is a forgotten DJ stent which is an entirely preventable and potentially fatal complication.

Recovery of Renal Function after Drainage

The recovery of renal function depends on duration of obstruction. Prompt drainage in acute, complete ureteral obstruction leads to full recovery of global glomerular filtration rate (GFR). Tubular function improves in the first 2 weeks of drainage and GFR improves over the next 10 weeks.

Definitive Management of Obstructive Uropathy

Once drainage has been achieved with either a stent or a nephrostomy, definitive management depends on the cause of obstruction. Discussion of individual causes of obstructive uropathy and their management is beyond the scope of this chapter. Renal function deterioration in an obstructed kidney is reversible in cases of acute obstruction and partially reversible in chronic obstruction. Assessment of renal function should be done only 6–8 weeks after adequate drainage. This assessment can be done either using nuclear imaging or by directly measuring creatinine or inulin clearance from the nephrostomy output in case of a percutaneous nephrostomy (PCN) in situ.

The decision of nephrectomy is based on various factors. As a rule of thumb, if the kidney has enough function to prevent dialysis dependence if the other

Table 11.1 Advantages and disadvantages of ureteral stents

- No need of collecting bags
- Associated with stent related symptoms (voiding or storage LUTS)
- Can be used in coagulopathy or platelet dysfunction
- Greater X-ray exposure than PCN insertion (caution in pregnant patients)
- Not effective for extrinsic obstruction
- Can get encrusted, forgotten. Even mortality has been reported with forgotten stents!

Table 11.2 Advantages and disadvantages of percutaneous nephrostomy (PCN)

- Consider if infected/purulent hydronephrosis is suspected
- Ultrasound guided–can be used in pregnant patients
- Allows estimation of differential function of the kidneys by calculating creatinine clearance
- If stent insertion fails, PCN is the only option.

kidney is removed, nephrectomy may be delayed. This corresponds to about 10% contribution to global renal function or about 10 mL/min/1.73 m^2 if the other kidney is normal. The decision of nephrectomy, however should not be based on the above criteria alone. In a patient with severely decreased global renal function, the kidney may be contributing enough function to delay dialysis dependence. In these cases, long-term stenting or PCN or a chance with reconstructive surgery is prudent.

STONE DISEASE

A small overview of two commonly encountered clinical situations is appropriate here.

Small Renal Stones

The incidence of small asymptomatic renal stones is increasing with increasingly better imaging modalities and more people undergoing imaging than before. This comes with a dilemma of treating or managing these stones conservatively.

In a cohort of 347 patients from Korea, majority of these stones did not cause any stone related events at a mean follow up of 31 months and only a quarter of these stones required any intervention. Only 4.6% needed surgical intervention. In a similar study, Benjamin et al. followed 160 stones with an average size of 7 mm and found that most remained asymptomatic through an average follow up of more than 3 years. Less than 30% caused renal colic, less than 20% underwent surgical intervention for pain and 7% spontaneously passed away.

Staghorn Renal Calculi

The term "staghorn" is used to refer to any branched stone occupying more than one portion of the collecting system, i.e., renal pelvis with one or more caliceal extensions. The most common composition is a mixture of magnesium ammonium phosphate (also called struvite) and/or calcium carbonate apatite.

Struvite staghorn calculi have a strong association with UTI by urease producing bacteria like proteus. Indeed, cultures of the stone fragments from both the surface and the inside of the stone demonstrate bacteria, implying that the stone itself is infected. This becomes a chronic focus for recurrent UTIs and may cause life-threatening sepsis if left untreated, and also lead to decrease in kidney function in almost a third of the patients if managed "conservatively".

Patients with staghorn calculi often present with infected hydronephrosis and sepsis. The goal in these patients should be prompt drainage, intravenous antimicrobials followed by complete removal of the stone. Drainage and antimicrobials allow for limiting sepsis following stone fragmentation. Complete removal of the stone should be the goal in all cases as even residual fragments may grow and be a source of recurrent UTI.

Stone free rates are highest for percutaneous nephrolithotomy (PCNL) (78%) and lowest for extracorporeal shock wave lithotripsy (ESWL). Almost all the cases can be managed with a combination of endourological procedures with open surgery being rarely used nowadays. Nephrectomy should be considered when the affected renal unit has negligible function as even in a nonfunctioning kidney, staghorn calculus can be a source of morbidity and when associated with recurrent UTI and chronic obstruction, may lead to development of Xanthogranulomatous pyelonephritis.

SUMMARY

- LUTS replaces all terms previously used for prostate symptoms
- Symptoms poorly correlate with prostate size or flow rates
- Uroflowmetry results are affected by voided volumes and voiding conditions.
- Poor flow is not specific for obstruction. Similarly, "normal" flow does not rule out obstruction
- PVR is not specific to bladder outlet obstruction and does not correlate with symptoms
- Raised PVR in absence of neurological disease does not predispose to UTI
- In a normal urodynamics study, bladder should have a constant low pressure that does not reach more than 6–10 cm H_2O above the baseline at the end of filling. Storage pressures above 40 cm H_2O are associated with deterioration of upper tracts.
- BPH is a histological diagnosis and not all men with "BPH" are symptomatic
- Symptom scores should be interpreted in relation to "bother"
- α blockers significantly improve flow rate and symptoms but do not decrease risk of urinary retention or progression to surgery. 5 α reductase inhibitors decrease the size of the prostate but the effect takes months
- Trial without catheter is best given after 2–3 days of catheterization. α blocker medication doubles the chance of successful trial without catheter
- Upper tract deterioration/renal failure present—suspect high pressure chronic retention—surgery may help
- Normal upper tracts/no renal failure—suspect low pressure chronic retention—long term catheterization of clean intermittent catheterization (CIC) is the solution.

Multiple Choice Questions

1. **70-year-old Mr Kapoor walks into your OPD and states that he is extremely bothered over the last one year with his urinary stream. His wife says that nowadays he takes such a long time in the urinal that she sometimes wonders if he has slept inside the washroom! On the other hand, he barely sleeps at night and has to urinate every hour. He does not have any neurological disease, no diabetes, is not taking any over the counter medications and has never had urinary retention. You examine him and find no bladder lump and no costovertebral angle tenderness. Digital rectal examination reveals a normal anal tone, and a prostate which is 4 cm in breadth, smooth, and non-tender with no nodules. You suspect BPH. At this point, what further evaluation(s) should be performed by you on Mr Kapoor to work-up his likely BPH? (please select all appropriate answers)**
   a. IPSS score
   b. Urinalysis
   c. Urine culture and sensitivity
   d. Serum creatinine/ultrasound
   e. Uroflowmetry/PVR
   f. Urodynamics

2. **Mr Kapoor fills out his IPSS questionnaire which reveals severe symptoms. His urinalysis is normal and PVR is low (20 cc). An ultrasound reveals a 50 gram prostate. Most appropriate next step would be (please select single correct answer)**
   a. Treat him with an alpha blocker medication
   b. Treat him with alpha blocker and 5 alpha reductase inhibitor
   c. Refer to a urologist for a urodynamic study
   d. Refer to a urologist for transurethral resection of prostate

3. **Regarding uroflowmetry/urodynamics, which of the following is correct:**
   a. On uroflowmetry, flow rates > 15 mL/s effectively rule out obstruction
   b. Maximum flow rate <10 mL/s are diagnostic of bladder outlet obstruction
   c. In the filling phase, storage pressured above 40 cm H_2O lead to deterioration of upper tracts
   d. Normal male patient voids with a detrusor pressure of 100 cm H_2O

4. **Regarding post-void residual urine, which of the following is incorrect:**
   a. PVR varies from day-to-day and from void-to-void
   b. PVR has poor correlation with symptoms
   c. High PVR predicts the failure of surgery for BPH
   d. A raised PVR in absence of neurological disease does not predispose to UTI

5. **Regarding medical therapy for LUTS due to BPH, which of the following is true**
   a. Tamsulosin is more effective than older alpha blockers such as alfuzosin and doxazosin.
   b. Alpha blocker medication does not decrease the risk of acute urinary retention in a patient of BPH
   c. Alpha blocker medication decreases progression to surgery
   d. Antimuscarinic drugs are contraindicated in BPH due to the risk of precipitating urinary retention

6. **65-year-old Mr Amarjeet presented to the casualty with painful retention of urine. He is non-diabetic and has no neurological disease. He was catheterized and in the next 10 minutes, 800 mL of urine was drained. His ultrasound reveals**

normal upper tracts and a 34 gram prostate. He wants to know how long will he be kept on catheter. What is the next appropriate step?

a. Refer the patient to a urologist for a transurethral resection of prostate
b. Refer the patient to a urologist for a urodynamic study
c. Start an alpha blocker medication and give a trial without catheter after 3 days
d. Start an alpha blocker medication and give a trial without catheter after 7 days
e. Start an alpha blocker medication and remove catheter next morning

7. **Regarding drainage in obstructive uropathy, which of the following options are correct for drainage of urine in an obstructed system?**
   a. A double J stent is more effective than a percutaneous nephrostomy
   b. A percutaneous nephrostomy is more effective than a double J stent
   c. Stenting is preferred option in case of extrinsic obstruction of ureters (for example, retroperitoneal lymphadenopathy)
   d. Stenting can be done in cases of coagulopathy and platelet dysfunction

8. **70-year-old Mr Khan is having mild LUTS but complains of some bedwetting at night. Besides that, he is largely asymptomatic. During evaluation for a recent febrile illness, his bladder was palpable and serum creatinine was found to be 2.0. An ultrasound showed bilateral moderate hydronephrosis and large post- void residual urine. He was catheterized, and in the following 10 minutes, 1.5 liters of urine was drained. He had post obstructive diuresis which was managed conservatively. Which of the following statements is true for Mr Khan (mark all true statements)**
   a. The diagnosis is most likely low pressure chronic retention
   b. The diagnosis is most likely high pressure chronic retention
   c. The dribbling in his case is due to loss of urethral resistance at night
   d. Urodynamics is likely to reveal underactive detrusor
   e. A transurethral resection is likely to fail in his case

9. **Which of the following statements is incorrect about the definitive management of obstructive uropathy?**
   a. Renal function assessment should be done after 2–3 weeks of drainage via a percutaneous nephrostomy or a stent
   b. Tubular function improves first after drainage of obstruction
   c. NSAIDs are the first line drugs for management of pain of obstructive uropathy
   d. Prompt drainage of acute complete obstruction leads to full recovery of renal function

10. **65-year-old Mr Singh has frequency and bothersome nocturia with an IPSS score of 15. History and physical examination are normal. Urinalysis is negative. The next step is:**
    a. Frequency-volume chart
    b. Serum creatinine
    c. Uroflowmetry
    d. Cystoscopy
    e. Urodynamics

Answers

1. All options except c and f are correct 2. b 3. c 4. c 5. b
6. c 7. d 8. b and c 9. a 10. a

SUGGESTED READING

1. Conway JJ, Maizels M. The "well tempered" diuretic renogram: a standard method to examine the asymptomatic neonate with hydronephrosis or hydroureteronephrosis. A report from combined meetings of The Society for Fetal Urology and members of The Pediatric Nuclear Medicine Council—The Society of Nuclear Medicine. J Nucl Med. 1992;33(11):2047-51.
2. Kaplan SA, et al. Urinary retention and post-void residual urine in men: separating truth from tradition. J Urol. 2008;180(1):47-54.
3. McVary KT, et al. Update on AUA guideline on the management of benign prostatic hyperplasia. J Urol. 2011;185(5):1793-803.
4. Odunayo Kalejaiye, Mark J Speakman. Management of acute and chronic retention in men. European Urology Supplements. 2009;8:523-9.
5. Roehrborn CG, et al. Clinical outcomes after combined therapy with dutasteride plus tamsulosin or either monotherapy in men with benign prostatic hyperplasia (BPH) by baseline characteristics: 4-year results from the randomized, double-blind Combination of Avodart and Tamsulosin (CombAT) trial. BJU Int. 2011; 107(6):946-54.
6. Schafer W, et al. Good urodynamic practices: uroflowmetry, filling cystometry, and pressure-flow studies. Neurourol Urodyn. 2002;21(3):261-74.
7. Wein Alan J. Campbell-Walsh Urology. Philadelphia: Elsevier Saunders, 2012. Print.

CHAPTER

12

Hypertension

Vinay Sakhuja, Indranil Ghosh

INTRODUCTION

Hypertension remains one of the most important preventable contributors to the disease and death. It can lead to the various end-organ damages such as myocardial infarction, stroke, renal failure, and death if not detected early and treated appropriately. The American Society of Hypertension no longer regards hypertension as a single disease entity and recognizes it as the part of a bigger disease conglomerate accompanied by obesity, diabetes, kidney disease or many other co-existing lifestyle problems. Abundant evidence from randomized controlled trials (RCTs) has shown benefit of antihypertensive drug treatment in reducing important health outcomes in persons with hypertension.

The clinicians want guidance on hypertension management using the best scientific evidence; the modalities and cut-offs on treatment of hypertension is a continuously evolving process. The Joint National Committee in their 8th published guidelines in 2014 (JNC 8) has taken into account the rigorous, evidence-based approach to recommend the treatment thresholds, goals, and medications in the management of hypertension in adults. The evidence was drawn from randomized controlled trials, which represent the gold standard for determining efficacy and effectiveness.

DEFINITION

The definition is arbitrary, because blood pressure is not distributed bimodally in the population; an arbitrary level of blood pressure (BP) must be defined as the threshold above which hypertension can be diagnosed. The correlation between the levels of systolic BP (SBP) and diastolic BP (DBP) and cardiovascular risk has long been recognized. Increasing BP clearly has an adverse effect over the entire range of recorded pressures, even those generally considered to be in the normal range. The goal of identifying and treating high BP is to reduce the risk of cardiovascular disease and associated morbidity and mortality.

The seventh report of the Joint National Committee (JNC) on Prevention, Detection, Evaluation, and Treatment of High Blood Pressure (JNC 7) had established criteria for the diagnosis and classification of BP in adult patients **(Table 12.1)**. The *optimal* BP in an individual who is not acutely ill is lower than 120/80 mm Hg. Individuals with an SBP of 120 to 139 mm Hg or a DBP of 80 to 89 mm Hg were defined as *prehypertensive*. These patients are at twice the risk of developing hypertension as those with lower values. These prehypertensive

Table 12.1 Stages of hypertension

BP classification	*Systolic BP (mm Hg)*		*Diastolic BP (mm Hg)*
Normal	<120	and	<80
Prehypertension	120–139	or	80–89
Stage 1 hypertension	140–159	or	90–99
Stage 2 hypertension	≥160	or	≥100

a. Adults aged 18 years and older.
b. Classification should be based on the mean or two or more properly measured seated blood pressure readings obtained on each of two or more office visits.
c. When systolic and diastolic BP fall into different categories, classify based on the higher category.

The seventh report of the Joint National Committee on Prevention, Detection, Evaluation and Treatment of High Blood Pressure. The JNC 7 Report. JAMA. 2003;289: 2560-72.

patients need to be monitored to exclude the development of hypertension. *Hypertension* is arbitrarily defined as an SBP of 140 mmHg or greater or a DBP of 90 mmHg or greater, or by virtue of the patient taking antihypertensive medications. The stage of hypertension (stage 1 or 2) is determined by the levels of both SBP and DBP **(Table 12.1)**. This classification should be based on the average of two or more BP readings at each of two or more visits after the initial BP screening. When SBP and DBP fall into different categories, the higher category should be selected to classify the individual's BP.

The JNC 8 guideline which has come out in 2014 were an evidence-based hypertension guideline focusing on three important questions:

1. Whether starting anithypertensive drug at above a particular BP threshold will improve the health outcomes?
2. Whether treating with antihypertensive drugs to achieve a specific BP goal improves health outcomes?
3. Is there any specific advantage or disadvantage of using a particular class of drug?

EPIDEMIOLOGY

Hypertension is the biggest contributor to the global burden of disease and to global mortality, according to 2010 data from the Institute for Health Metrics and Evaluation. Hypertension is estimated to contribute to 9·4 million deaths each year and prevalence estimates are as much as 1 billion individuals worldwide. The World Health Organization reports that suboptimal BP (115 mm Hg SBP) is responsible for 62% of cerebrovascular disease and 49% of ischemic heart disease, with little variation by sex. In addition, suboptimal blood pressure is the number one attributable risk for death throughout the world.

Data from the National Health and Nutrition Examination Survey (NHANES) indicate that approximately 28% of the adult population in the United States are hypertensive and the prevalence increases sharply with age. The increasing burden of hypertension is due to increasing population along with increased prevalence of obesity and the overall aging of the population. Overall, the prevalence of hypertension in obese adults is 41.4% for men and 37.8% for women; compared with 14.9% for men and 15.2% for women with body mass index (BMI) ≤ 25 kg/m^2. Further proof of the significant relationship between body weight and BP is found in the observation that BP falls with even modest weight reduction. Black men and women have a two-fold higher prevalence of hypertension (30%) than white men and women (15%) in a sampling of almost 18,000 American adults aged 48–75 years in the NHANES data. Prevalence appears to be equal in men and women in most of the surveys. Data from the Framingham Heart Study indicate that even individuals who are normotensive at 55 years have a 90% lifetime risk of developing hypertension. Many hypertensive patients have a positive family history of parental hypertension.

The mode of inheritance is polygenic in most instances. The intake of dietary salt (sodium chloride) has significant effect on BP, especially in patients with other factor predisposing to the development of hypertension, such as advancing age, obesity, adult-onset diabetes, positive family history of hypertension, black race, or underlying renal disease. Animal experiments, epidemiologic studies, and clinical trials have provided compelling evidence for a detrimental association of sodium intake and the blood pressure levels of individuals across the population. Northern Japanese fishermen who ingest 450 mEq of sodium daily have a 40% prevalence of hypertension. In the 1950s, there was a large decline in blood pressure across the Japanese population potentially due to a broad reduction in sodium consumption. There has been significant reduction in SBPs, DBPs and mean blood pressures (MBPs) ever since. In contrast, indigenous Alaskan populations and the Yanamamo Indians in Brazil and Venezuela, who have dietary intake of 1 mEq of sodium daily, do not develop hypertension at any age. In Bangladesh, recent studies have determined the daily intake of sodium to be 21 g which radically supersedes all recommended levels. Intersalt, an international epidemiologic study, examined the relation between dietary sodium intake (based on 2–4 hours urinary sodium excretion) and BP in more than 10,000 individuals with ages from 20 to 59 years from 52 countries around the world. The results demonstrated a significant correlation between median SBP and DBP and dietary sodium intake. In Nepal and Nigeria, the important contributors for their rise in hypertension are increased sodium intake along with rising levels of obesity. In Nigeria approximately 30.5% had elevated SBP and 38.7% had elevated DBP out of which, the overall prevalence of hypertension was 42.2%. With respect to Nepal, the prevalence has increased from 18% in 1981 to 33.8% in 2006.

The continued high prevalence of hypertension and hypertension-related complications such as stroke, cardiovascular complications, heart failure and end stage renal disease (ESRD) represents a major public health challenge.

Indian Scenario

In India, 6–15% of the adults in different survey have been reported to be suffering from hypertension. In an Indian study done at West Bengal, the overall prevalence of hypertension was found to be 61% (30% prehypertensive and 31% hypertensive) for boys and 33% (19% prehypertensive and 14% hypertensive) for girls. 76% overweight and obese males and 49% overweight and obese females were hypertensive, whereas it was 58% and 29% respectively for healthy males and females. Significant association was noted between hypertension and BMI as well as hypertension and male sex.

Table 12.2 Recent studies (2004–2012) on prevalence of hypertension in urban and rural Indian population

First Author	*Year*	*Place*	*Age (yrs)*	*Sample Size*	*Prevalence (%)*
Urban population					
Gupta PC	2004	Mumbai	≥ 35	88,635	47.9
Reddy KS	2006	National	20–69	19,973	27.24
Mohan V	2007	Chennai	≥ 20	2,350	20.0
Yadav S	2008	Lucknow	≥ 30	1,746	32.2
Momin MH	2012	Gujarat	≥ 20	1,493	30.4
Rural population					
Hazarika	2004	Assam	> 30	3,180	33.3
Thankappan	2006	Kerala	> 30	2,159	36
Krishnan A	2008	Haryana	15–64	2,828	9.3
Yuvaraj BY	2010	Davangere	≥ 18	1,900	18.3
Rajasekar VD	2012	Tamil Nadu	≥ 30	1,905	19.1

The studies conducted in 2012 in Puducherry, India, have indicated that out of 79 persons taking in sodium-rich food, 53 developed hypertension. A study from India emphasizes the need for government intervention to impose control measures and to improve awareness about sodium-rich food **(Table 12.2)**.

PATHOGENESIS

A large body of experimental data has demonstrated the importance of the kidney in the pathogenesis of hypertension. To date, each of the genetic causes of hypertension that have been elucidated, has been shown to relate to an abnormality of renal sodium handling. For example, Liddle's syndrome results from enhanced distal tubular sodium reabsorption due to an abnormality in sodium channels in the distal nephron. Cross-transplant experiments in hypertensive and normotensive rat strains validate the importance of the kidney in the pathogenesis of hypertension, because the presence or absence of hypertension depends on the donor source of the kidney.

Guyton's hypothesis states that the most important and fundamental mechanism in determining the long-term control of BP is the renal fluid-volume feedback mechanism. In simple terms, through this basic mechanism, the kidneys regulate arterial pressure by altering renal excretion of sodium and water, thereby controlling circulatory volume and cardiac output. Changes in BP, in turn, directly influence the renal excretion of sodium and water, thereby providing a negative feedback mechanism for the control of extracellular fluid (ECF) volume, cardiac output, and BP. For instance, an increase in systemic BP will lead to an increase in sodium excretion, a process known as *pressure natriuresis*. The hypothesis is that derangements in this renal fluid-volume pressure control mechanism are the fundamental cause of virtually all hypertensive states **(Fig. 12.1)**. In every hypertensive state, an underlying abnormality exists in the intrinsic

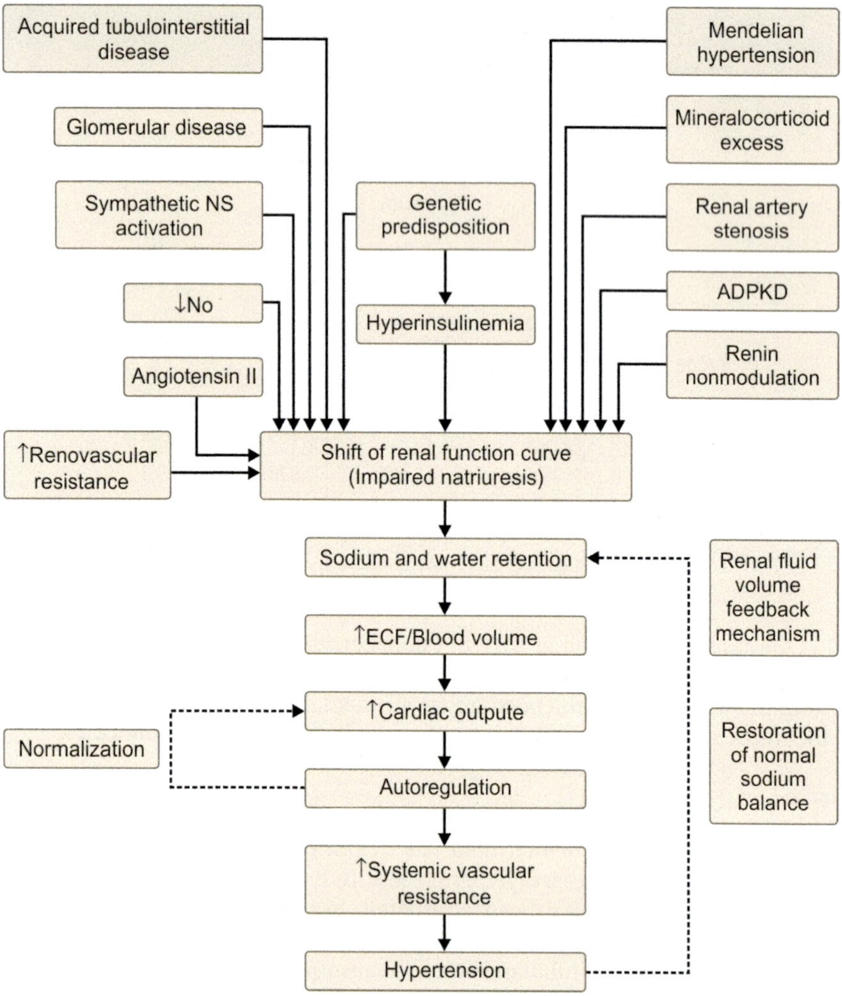

Figure 12.1 Abnormal renal sodium handling in the pathogenesis of hypertension (Guyton's hypothesis). In the setting of essential hypertension, primary renal disease, mineralocorticoid excess, or insulin resistance with hyperinsulinemia, a defect in the intrinsic natriuretic capacity of the kidney is present that prevents sodium balance from being maintained at a normal level of BP. Initially, this impairment in natriuresis leads to increases in extracellular fluid (ECF) volume and cardiac output. Circulatory autoregulation occurs to maintain normal perfusion of the tissues, resulting in an increase in the systemic vascular resistance (SVR). The increase in SVR leads to systemic hypertension. With pressure-induced natriuresis, the renal fluid-volume feedback mechanism returns sodium balance, EVF volume, and cardiac output to normal. (ADPKD, autosomal dominant polycystic kidney disease; NS, nervous system: AII, angiotensin II.) (Adapted from Nolan CR, Schrier RW. The kidney in hypertension. In: Schrier RW (Ed). Renal and electrolyte disorders, 6th edn. Philadelphia, PA: Lippincott Williams & Wilkins, 2003).

natriuretic capacity of the kidney, so that the daily salt intake cannot be excreted at a normal BP, and the development of hypertension is necessary to induce a pressure natriuresis that allows the kidney to excrete the daily salt intake. Normal sodium balance and ECF volume are maintained, but at the expense of systemic hypertension.

In patients with obesity and insulin resistance (metabolic syndrome), hyperinsulinemia increases proximal tubular sodium reabsorption. Increased *angiotensin II levels* and *sympathetic nervous system* activity also enhance sodium reabsorption. Mineralocorticoids enhance distal tubular sodium reabsorption. Renal parenchymal disease causes nephron loss, resulting in an impaired natriuretic defect. Abnormalities in renal endothelin or nitric oxide levels may also impair natriuresis. Guyton's hypothesis states that this decreased natriuretic capacity of the kidney initially leads to renal salt and water retention. ECF volume expansion, and increased cardiac output with hypertension. This phase of volume expansion and high cardiac output is short lived. In the setting of high cardiac output, autoregulatory vasoconstriction of each vascular bed matches the blood flow to the metabolic requirements of the tissues. This phenomenon of circulatory autoregulation leads to an increase in systemic vascular resistance (SVR). Therefore, hypertension that was initially caused by high cardiac output becomes high SVR hypertension.

The development of hypertension represents a protective mechanism, because it induces the kidney to undergo a pressure natriuresis and diuresis, thereby resorting normal salt balance and returning ECF volume to normal. This mechanism explains why an underlying problem with sodium excretion, as in salt-sensitive hypertension, is manifest as high-SVR hypertension without evidence of overt fluid overload. In the absence of pressure natriuresis, patients with a primary disorder in sodium retention would progressively develop overt fluid overload and consequences such as pulmonary edema. To substantiate the role of direct pressure-induced natriuresis in the regulation of sodium balance in mineralocorticoid hypertension, Hall et al. compared the systemic BP and natriuretic effect of aldosterone infusion in a dog model in which the renal perfusion pressure was either allowed to increase or mechanically servo-controlled to maintain renal artery pressure at normal levels. In the intact animal, continuous aldosterone infusion caused a transient period of sodium and water retention with a mild increase in BP. This sodium retention lasted only a few days however, and was followed by an *escape* from the sodium retaining effects of aldosterone and a restoration of normal sodium balance. In contrast, when the renal perfusion pressure was servo-controlled to maintain normal renal perfusion pressure during aldosterone infusion, no aldosterone escape occurred, and a relentless increase in sodium and water retention occurred, accompanied by severe hypertension, edema, ascites and pulmonary edema. When the servo-control device was removed and the renal perfusion pressure was allowed to rise to the systemic level, a prompt natriuresis and diuresis ensued, with the restoration of sodium balance and a fall in BP. Moreover, the observation that abnormal renal sodium handling is central in the pathogenesis of all forms of hypertension, provides a sound pathophysiologic rationale for the JNC 7 recommendation regarding thiazide-type diuretics as first-line antihypertensive therapy in most patients.

Endothelial dysfunction: An important reason for hypertension in patients with vascular disease is endothelial dysfunction which leads to an imbalance between vasodilatory factors (such as nitric oxide and prostaglandin E1) and vasoconstrictors (such as angiotensin II and endothelin). Endothelial injury leads to loss of vasodilatation. It also leads to the release of chemotactic cytokines and adhesion molecules on injured endothelial surface thereby participating in inflammation and atherosclersis. Medial smooth muscle cells proliferate and migrate subintimally. Decreased vasodilatory factors lead to increased arterial stiffness and isolated systolic hypertension.

Salt in kidney disease: Salt intake promotes progression of chronic kidney disease and hypertension. It can lead to increased extracellular volume and glomerular hyperfiltration leading to progressive renal injury. There is an increase in pro-inflammatory cytokines [e.g. transforming growth factor (TGF) beta] which promotes renal and cardiac fibrosis. Also, there is increased oxidative stress as documented in normal rats receiving high salt diet.

Various new mechanisms implicated in pathogenesis of high-salt induced hypertension have been proposed. How exactly high intake of salt leads to hypertension is largely unclear. It has been proposed that high sodium intake can lead to vascular dysfunction. A newly discovered hormone, endogenous ouabain (EO), which is secreted by adrenal glands and hypothalamus, has also been proposed to contribute to increased vascular resistance and thereby hypertension.

DIAGNOSTIC EVALUATION OF HYPERTENSION

Detection of hypertension begins with proper measurement of BP at each health-care encounter. Repeated BP measurements are used to determine whether initial elevations persist and require prompt attention or have returned to normal values and require only periodic surveillance. Blood pressure measurement should be standardized **(Table 12.3)**.

Table 12.3 Guidelines for measuring blood pressure
Posture • After at least 5 minutes of rest, the patient should be seated in a chair with the back supported and one arm bared and supported at heart level.
Circumstances: • The patient should refrain from smoking or ingesting caffeine for 30 minutes before the examination.
Equipment: • For an appropriately sized cuff, the bladder should encircle at least 80% of the arm. Many patients require a large adult cuff. • Measurements should ideally be taken with a mercury sphygmomanometer. Alternatively, a recently calibrated aneroid manometer or a validated electronic device can be used.
Technique: • The first appearance of sound (phase 1) is used to define SBP. The disappearance of sound (phase 5) is used to define DBP. • The BP should be confirmed in the contralateral arm.

Measurement of BP outside of the physician's office may provide some valuable information with regard to the diagnosis and treatment of hypertension. **Self-measurement** is useful in distinguishing sustained hypertension from *"white-coat hypertension"*, a condition in which the patient's pressure is consistently elevated in the clinician's office but normal at other times. Self-measurement may also be used to assess the response to antihypertensive medications and as a tool to improve patient adherence to treatment. **Ambulatory monitoring** is useful for the evaluation of:

- Suspected white-coat hypertension
- Patients with apparent drug resistance
- Hypotensive symptoms with antihypertensive medications
- Episodic hypertension

In elderly patients, the possibility of **pseudohypertension** should always be considered. Pseudohypertension is a condition in which the indirect measurement of arterial pressure using a cuff sphygmomanometer is artificially high in comparison to direct intra-arterial pressure measurement. Pseudohypertension can result from Monckeberg's medial calcification (a clinically benign form of arterial calcification) or advanced atherosclerosis with widespread calcification of intimal plaques. Here stiffening of the arterial wall prevents its collapse to externally applied pressure, resulting in artificially high indirect BP readings. The presence of a *positive Osler's maneuver*, in which the radial or brachial artery remains palpable despite being made pulseless by proximal inflation of a cuff above systolic pressure, is an important physical examination finding that should suggest the diagnosis. Roentgenograms of the extremities frequently reveal calcified vessels. The diagnosis can only be confirmed by a direct measurement of intra-arterial pressure. Patients with pseudohypertension are often elderly and therefore, may have a critical limitation of blood flow to the brain or heart, such that inappropriate BP treatment may precipitate life-threatening ischemic events.

History and physical examination of patients with hypertension should assess lifestyle, identify other cardiovascular risk factors, and identify the presence of target organ damage **(Table 12.4)** that may affect prognosis and impact treatment decisions. Although the vast majority of hypertensive patients have essential (primary) hypertension without a clearly definable etiology, the initial evaluation

Table 12.4 Target organ damage in hypertension
Heart • Left ventricular hypertrophy • Angina or prior myocardial infarction • Prior coronary revascularization • Heart failure
Brain Prior stroke or transient ischemic attack
Chronic kidney disease
Peripheral arterial disease
Retinopathy (see **Table 12.6**)

Table 12.5 Secondary causes and symptomatology of hypertension

• Metabolic syndrome – Obesity – Insulin resistance – Impaired glucose tolerance – Dyslipidemia
• Obstructive sleep apnea – Day time somnolence – Morbid obesity – Headache – Snoring or fitful sleep
• Drug-induced hypertension
• Chronic Kidney Disease – Fatigue – Loss of appetite – Swelling feet
• Primary hyperaldosteronism – Muscle weakness
• Renovascular disease – Flash pulmonary edema – Labile BP
• Chronic steroid use/Cushing's syndrome
• Pheochromocytoma – Episodic anxiety – Headache – Diaphoresis – Palpitations
• Coarctation of the aorta – Claudication of limbs
• Thyroid or parathyroid disease – Weight gain

Adapted and modified from the seventh report of the Joint National Committee on Prevention, Detection, Evaluation and Treatment of High Blood Pressure. The JNC 7 Report. JAMA. 2003;289:2560-72.

is also designed to screen for identifiable causes of secondary hypertension **(Table 12.5)**.

Medical history should include information about prior BP measurements, to assess the duration of hypertension and details about adverse effects from any prior antihypertensive therapy. History or symptoms of coronary heart disease, chronic heart failure (CHF), cerebrovascular disease, peripheral vascular disease, or renal disease should be carefully evaluated. Symptoms suggesting unusual secondary causes of hypertension should be queried for **(Table 12.5)**. Information regarding other risk factors, such as diabetes, tobacco use, hyperlipidemia, physical activity, and any recent weight gain, should be obtained. Dietary assessment regarding the intake of salt, alcohol and saturated fat is also important. Detailed information should be sought regarding all the prescription

Table 12.6 Classification of hypertensive retinopathy

Retinal arteriosclerosis and arteriosclerotic retinopathy (Characteristic of benign hypertension)
Arteriolar narrowing (focal or diffuse) Arteriovenous crossing changes Broadening of the arteriolar light reflex Copper or silver wiring changes Perivasculitis Solitary round retinal hemorrhages Hard exudates Central or branch venous occlusion
Hypertensive neuroretinopathy (Sine qua non of malignant hypertension)
Generalized arteriolar narrowing Striate (flame-shaped) hemorrhages Cotton wool spots (soft exudates) Bilateral papilledema Star figure at the macula

These features distinguish retinal arteriosclerosis (benign hypertension) from hypertensive neuroretinopathy (malignant hypertension). Adapted with permission from Nolan CR. Malignant hypertension and other hypertensive crises. In: Schrier RW (Ed). Diseases of the kidney and urinary tract, 8th edn. Boston MA: Lippincott Williams & Wilkins; 2007. pp. 1370-436.

and over-the-counter medication use, including herbal remedies and illicit drugs, some of which may raise BP or interfere with the effectiveness of antihypertensive therapy. For example, nonsteroidal anti-inflammatory drugs impair the response to virtually all antihypertensive agents and increase the risk of hyperkalemia or renal insufficiency with angiotensin-converting enzyme (ACE) inhibitor therapy. Stimulus such as cocaine, ephedra, amphetamines, and anabolic steroids can raise BP. A family history of hypertension, diabetes, premature cardiovascular disease, or renal disease should be sought.

Physical examination should include the anthropometric data, fundoscopy to identify characteristic findings of hypertensive neuroretinopathy (HNR) **(Table 12.6)**, which are indicative of the presence of malignant hypertension. Examination for carotid bruit, distended neck veins, and thyromegaly is important. Cardiac examination should include investigation for abnormalities of rate or rhythm, murmurs and third or fourth heart sounds. The lungs should be examined for rales and evidence of bronchospasm. Abdominal examination should include auscultation for bruits (an epigastric bruit present in both systole and diastole suggests renal artery stenosis), abdominal or flank masses (polycystic kidney disease), or increased aortic pulsation (abdominal aortic aneurysm). Peripheral pulses should be examined for quality and bruit. The lower extremities should be examined for edema. A neurologic screening examination is used to identify prior cerebrovascular events. Routine laboratory tests are recommended before the initiation of antihypertensive therapy to identify other risk factors and screen for the presence of target organ damage.

Most patients with hypertension have *primary (essential) hypertension* in which no clearly definable underlying etiology is apparent. In contrast, a wide variety of uncommon conditions can lead to so-called *secondary hypertension*, some of which are potentially amenable to surgical correction **(Table 12.5)**. Secondary causes of hypertension amenable to surgical intervention are so uncommon that extensive diagnostic testing is not warranted. Secondary hypertension should be considered when:

- The patient has onset of hypertension at an early age (younger than 30 years) or late age (older than 55 years)
- Inadequate BP control in a complaint patient on a three-drug regimen which includes a diuretic (resistant hypertension)
- Previously well-controlled hypertension becomes uncontrolled in a compliant patient
- Hematuria or proteinuria (underlying renal disease) or elevated serum creatinine (renal disease or ischemic nephropathy due to bilateral renal artery stenosis)

The initial history, physical examination, and routine laboratory tests **(Table 12.7)** are usually all that is required to evaluate for the possibility of secondary hypertension. Few common causes are:

- *Renal parenchymal disease:* A normal estimated creatinine clearance and urinalysis are usually sufficient to exclude underlying renal disease as a secondary cause of hypertension. Detection of abdominal or flank masses may indicate polycystic kidney disease, a diagnosis that can be confirmed with ultrasound.
- *Primary hyperaldosteronism (PHA):* Because most of these patients have unprovoked hypokalemia while not on diuretic therapy, a measurement of serum potassium is a suitable screening test, and routine measurement of aldosterone levels or plasma aldosterone/renin ratio is not necessary.

Table 12.7 Basic investigations for evaluation of hypertension

- Serum Biochemistry
  - Electrolytes: sodium, potassium
  - Renal function test: Blood urea, serum creatinine
  - Fasting glucose
  - Lipid profile [total cholesterol, low-density lipoprotein and high-density lipoprotein (HDL) cholesterol]
- Complete blood cells-count
- Urinalysis that would suggest the presence of underlying primary renal disease
  - Proteinuria
  - Hematuria
- A 12-lead electrocardiogram
  - Left arterial enlargement, left ventricular hypertrophy (LVH) or prior myocardial infarction (MI)
- Optional tests, depending on the clinical situation
  - 24-hour creatinine clearance
  - 24-hour urine protein or a spot urine protein to creatinine ratio
  - Serum uric acid
  - Glycosylated hemoglobin
  - Thyroid function tests
  - Echocardiogram to identify the presence of LVH

Creatinine clearance should be estimated using either the Cockcroft-Gault or the Modification of Diet in Renal Disease (MDRD) formulae.

However, some patients with PHA are normokalemic (when not receiving diuretic therapy). Although routine screening of all patients with hypertension for PHA is not warranted, in a patient with drug resistant hypertension or significant hypokalemia induced by low dose diuretic therapy, the possibility of PHA should be considered. In this regard, patients with resistant hypertension due to PHA often have a dramatic BP response following the initiation of a mineralocorticoid antagonist (spironolactone or eplerenone).

- *Vascular:* Assessment for any delay or diminution of pulses in the lower extremities, or a discrepancy between arm and leg BP can be used to screen for coarctation of the aorta.
- *Pheochromocytoma:* A careful assessment of a history of episodic hypertension, associated with headache, palpitations, diaphoresis and pallor, is all that is usually required to screen for pheochromocytoma. The routine measurement of serum or urine catecholamines is not warranted.
- *Cushing's syndrome:* Evaluation for truncal obesity and abdominal purple striae is all that is usually required to screen for Cushing's syndrome, therefore, routine measurement of serum cortisol or cortisol suppression testing is unnecessary.
- *Obstructive sleep apnea (OSA)* is an important treatable cause of hypertension. The diagnosis can be confirmed with a sleep study to document apneic episodes. Appropriate treatment with a continuous positive airway pressure device may result in a significant reduction in BP.

Several tests are notably absent from the recommended list of routine screening tests for secondary hypertension. Intravenous pyelography, renal scanning, captopril renography, and arterial digital subtraction angiography all lack sufficient specificity to be of any value as routine screening tests for renovascular hypertension. In this regard, the prevalence of renovascular hypertension in the general hypertensive population is so low that the predictive value of a positive test from any of these procedures is abysmal when used as a general screening test.

TREATMENT

Goals of Treatment

The goal of treating hypertension is the reduction of cardiovascular and renal morbidity and mortality. The BP target is < 150/90 mm Hg for patients > 60 years of age in the JNC 8 guidelines. The goal of treatment is an SBP less than 140 mmHg and a DBP less than 90 mmHg in younger patients and for patients with Diabetes or CKD. This is in contrary to the previous JNC 7 guidelines wherein hypertensive patients with diabetes or underlying CKD, a BP goal of less than 130/80 mm Hg was recommended. Control of BP leads to an approximate 50% reduction in heart failure, 40% reduction in stroke and 20–25% reduction in myocardial infarction (MI).

Nonpharmacologic Treatment

Lifestyle modification helps in prevention of hypertension and also in reaching target blood pressure. However, this is not sufficient in at least 50% of patients

Table 12.8 Lifestyle modifications to manage hypertension

Modification	*Recommendation*	*Appropriate SBP reduction*
Weight Loss	Maintain normal weight (BMI 18.5–24.9)	5–20 mm Hg/10 kg
Dietary sodium restriction	Limit dietary sodium intake to <100 mEq/d (2.4 g sodium or 6 g sodium chloride)	2–8 mm Hg
Adopt DASH diet	Consume diet rich in fruits, vegetables, and low-fat dairy products with a reduced content of saturated and total fat	8–14 mm Hg
Increase physical activity	Engage in regular aerobic physical activity such as brisk walking (at least 30 mins, most days of the week)	4–9 mm Hg
Moderate alcohol consumption	Limit consumption to no more than two drinks per day (1 oz or 30 mL ethanol per d; e.g. 24 oz beer, 10 oz wine, 3 oz 80-proof whiskey) in most men, and no more than one drink per day in women and lighter weight men	2–4 mm Hg

Abbreviations: BMI, body mass index; DASH, dietary approaches to stop hypertension; SBP, systolic blood pressure.

Adapted from the seventh report of the Joint National Committee on Prevention, Detection, Evaluation and Treatment of High Blood Pressure. The JNC 7 report. JAMA. 2003;289:2560-72.

with hypertension who are insulin resistant and have a metabolic profile known to increase risk of cardiovascular disease. All patients should be encouraged to adopt the lifestyle modifications outlined in **Table 12.8**, especially if they have additional cardiovascular risk factors such as hyperlipidemia or diabetes. Modest weight reduction of as little as 4 kg (10 lb) significantly reduces BP. In addition to the positive effects on overall health, regular aerobic exercise is associated with a significant reduction in BP.

Dietary changes: Changes in diet can have significant effects on BP.

- Dietary sodium intake in the form of table salt has a strong epidemiologic link to hypertension. The restriction of sodium intake has been shown to reduce the need for antihypertensive medication, reduce diuretic-induced renal potassium wasting, lead to regression of left ventricular hypertropy (LVH), and prevent renal stones through a reduction in renal calcium excretion. The recommended daily value for sodium intake as per the Canadian Journal of Cardiology is approximately 2000 mg (5 g of salt or 87 mmol of sodium) per day. Same has also been endorsed by the report of a joint World Health Organization-Food and Agriculture Organization Expert Consultation Committee. The therapeutic implications of these observations include dietary sodium restriction as part of nonpharmacologic therapy and the recommendation of thiazide diuretics as a first-time drug therapy for the treatment of hypertension in most patients. Various guidelines have recommended reducing salt intake in general population to less than 100 mmol/day (i.e. <2.3 g/day). In hypertensives, CKD patients, African Americans and those above 50 years of age, it has been further reduced to 65 mmol/day (1.5 g/day).

- The Dietary Approaches to Stop Hypertension (DASH) study group compared a diet rich in fruits and vegetables to a control diet in patients with mild diastolic hypertension (DBP > 95 mm Hg). The DASH diet lowered both SBP and DBP significantly in this population. A follow-up study, the DASH sodium study, randomized patients with stage 1 hypertension to the DASH diet or a control diet. Within each group, patients were randomized to three levels of sodium intake. Sodium reduction decreased BP and the DASH diet decreased BP at all levels of sodium intake.

Ethanol intake: Excessive intake of ethanol is an important risk factor for high BP, and it can lead to resistant hypertension. Ethanol intake should be limited to not more than 30 mL (1 oz) per day in men and 15 mL (0.5 oz) per day in women and lighter -weight men. This type of moderate ethanol intake may be associated with a reduction in the risk of coronary heart disease.

Others: Smoking cessation and reductions in dietary fat and cholesterol are also recommended to reduce the overall cardiovascular risk. Although caffeine may acutely raise BP, tolerance to this effect develops quickly. Most epidemiologic studies have found no direct relationship between caffeine intake and BP.

The Association of Socioeconomic Status (SES) with nutrients intakes attracts public attention worldwide. The Socioeconomic Status is Significantly Associated with Dietary Salt Intakes and Blood Pressure in Japanese Workers (J-HOPE Study) concluded that SES is an independent determinant of salt intake and blood pressure, in order to lower the risk of hypertension, the efforts to narrow the social status gaps should be considered by the health policy-makers.

Pharmacologic Treatment

The decision to treat hypertension with medications after the failure of lifestyle modifications to adequately control BP, or initially as an adjunct to lifestyle modifications, is based on an assessment of the risk of cardiovascular morbidity, given the presence of other cardiovascular risk factors and pre-existing target organ damage or cardiovascular disease **(Table 12.4)**. Reducing BP with drugs clearly decreases cardiovascular morbidity and mortality regardless of age, gender, race, stage of hypertension, or socioeconomic status. Benefit has been demonstrated for stroke, coronary events, heart failure, progression of primary renal disease, prevention of progression to malignant hypertension, and all-cause mortality. Numerous clinical trials have demonstrated that lowering BP with several classes of drugs, including thiazide-type diuretics, angiotensin-converting enzyme (ACE) inhibitors, angiotensin receptor blockers (ARBs), B-blockers and calcium channel blockers (CCBs), reduces all the complications of hypertension.

Nine recommendations were made in JNC 8 based on the systematic evidence review **(Table 12.9)**.

In the *general population aged 60 years or older*, initiate pharmacologic treatment to lower BP at systolic blood pressure (SBP) of 150 mm Hg or higher or diastolic blood pressure (DBP) of 90 mm Hg or higher and treat to a goal SBP lower than 150 mm Hg and goal DBP lower than 90 mm Hg [**Recommendation 1**]. This was a Grade A strong recommendation based on available evidence. Corollary to that based on expert opinion (Grade E) if pharmacologic treatment for high BP resulted in lower achieved SBP (for example, <140 mm Hg) and treatment is not associated with adverse effects on health or quality of life, treatment does not need to be adjusted.

In the *general population younger than 60 years,* initiate pharmacologic treatment to lower BP at DBP of 90 mm Hg or higher and treat to a goal DBP of lower than 90 mm Hg [**Recommendation 2**]. It was a Grade A recommendation For ages 30 through 59 years, and was a Grade E recommendation based on expert opinion for ages 18 through 29 years. This recommendation is based on high-quality evidence from 5 DBP trials (HDFP, Hypertension-Stroke Cooperative, MRC, ANBP, and VA Cooperative) that demonstrated improvements in health outcomes among adults aged 30 through 59 years with elevated BP. Initiation of antihypertensive treatment at a DBP threshold of 90 mm Hg or higher and treatment to a DBP goal of lower than 90 mm Hg reduces cerebrovascular events, heart failure, and overall mortality. In the general population younger than 60 years, the guidelines were to initiate pharmacologic treatment to lower BP at SBP of 140 mm Hg or higher and treat to a goal SBP of lower than 140 mm Hg [**Recommendation 3**]. This was based on expert opinion (Grade E).

In the population *aged 18 years or older with CKD* [**Recommendation 4**], *Diabetes* [**Recommendation 5**] , initiate pharmacologic treatment to lower BP at SBP of 140 mm Hg or higher or DBP of 90 mm Hg or higher and treat to goal SBP of lower than 140 mm Hg and goal DBP lower than 90 mm Hg.

There is an evidence of moderate quality demonstrating no benefit in slowing the progression of kidney disease from treatment with antihypertensive drug therapy to a lower BP goal (for example, < 130/80 mm Hg) compared with a goal of lower than 140/90 mm Hg. Three important trials looking at the effect of antihypertensive treatment on GFR change were AASK, MDRD and REIN-2. None of these showed any significant benefit of further lowering BP to <130/80 mm Hg on CKD progression. SHEP, UKPDS trials showed that there are cardiovascular and cerebrovascular health outocmes in diabetic and hypertensive patients if SBP is lowered to less than 150 mm Hg. This recommendation is also supported by the ACCORD-BP trial, in which the control group used this goal and had similar outcomes compared with a lower goal. The usual recommendation of SBP goal was < 130 mmHg (JNC 7); however, this lower SBP goal is not supported by any RCT. In the HOT trial, which is frequently cited to support a lower DBP goal, investigators compared a DBP goal of 90 mmHg or lower vs a goal of 80 mmHg or lower. The lower goal was associated with a reduction in a composite CVD outcome, but the evidence was graded low quality. In UKPDS trial as well, a significant benefit was found in cardiovascular outcomes in patients where BP control was more intensive (<150/85 mm Hg).

It has been recommended that *in nonblack population including ones with diabetes mellitus* calcium channel blockers, thiazide diuretics, ACEI or ARBs should be used as initial drugs for hypertension management [**Recommendation 6**]. Any of these 4 classes would be good choices as add-on agents as well [**Recommendation 9**]. Medications should be dosed adequately. β-blockers, α-blockers, dual α1- + β-blocking agents (e.g. carvedilol), vasodilating β-blockers (e.g. nebivolol), central α_2-adrenergic agonists (e.g. clonidine),

Table 12.9 Joint National Committee (JNC) 8 recommendations for management of hypertension

Recommendation 1

In the general population aged ≥60 years, initiate pharmacologic treatment to lower blood pressure (BP) at systolic blood pressure (SBP) ≥150 mm Hg or diastolic blood pressure (DBP) ≥90 mm Hg and treat to a goal SBP <150 mm Hg and goal DBP <90 mm Hg. (Strong Recommendation – Grade A)

Corollary Recommendation

In the general population aged ≥60 years, if pharmacologic treatment for high BP results in lower achieved SBP (e.g. < 140 mm Hg) and treatment is well-tolerated and without adverse effects on health or quality of life, treatment does not need to be adjusted.
(Expert Opinion – Grade E)

Recommendation 2

In the general population <60 years, initiate pharmacologic treatment to lower BP at DBP ≥90 mm Hg and treat to a goal DBP <90 mm Hg. (For ages 30–59 years, strong Recommendation – Grade A; For ages 18–29 years, Expert Opinion – Grade E)

Recommendation 3

In the general population <60 years, initiate pharmacologic treatment to lower BP at SBP ≥140 mmHg and treat to a goal SBP <140 mm Hg. (Expert Opinion – Grade E)

Recommendation 4

In the population aged ≥18 years with chronic kidney disease (CKD), initiate pharmacologic treatment to lower BP at SBP ≥140 mm Hg or DBP ≥90 mm Hg and treat to goal SBP <140 mmHg and goal DBP <90 mm Hg.
(Expert Opinion – Grade E)

Recommendation 5

In the population aged ≥18 years with diabetes, initiate pharmacologic treatment to lower BP at SBP ≥140 mm Hg or DBP ≥90 mm Hg and treat to a goal SBP <140 mm Hg and goal DBP <90 mm Hg.
(Expert Opinion – Grade E)

Recommendation 6

In the general nonblack population, including those with diabetes, initial antihypertensive treatment should include a thiazide-type diuretic, calcium channel blocker (CCB), angiotensin-converting enzyme inhibitor (ACEI), or angiotensin receptor blocker (ARB). (Moderate Recommendation – Grade B)

Recommendation 7

In the general black population, including those with diabetes, initial antihypertensive treatment should include a thiazide-type diuretic or CCB.

Recommendation 8

In the population aged ≥18 years with CKD, initial (or add-on) antihypertensive treatment should include an ACEI or ARB to improve kidney outcomes. This applies to all CKD patients with hypertension regardless of race or diabetes status.
(Moderate Recommendation – Grade B)

Recommendation 9

The main objective of hypertension treatment is to attain and maintain goal BP. If goal BP is not reached within a month of treatment, increase the dose of the initial drug or add a second drug from one of the classes in recommendation 6 (thiazide-type diuretic, CCB, ACEI, or ARB). The clinician should continue to assess BP and adjust the treatment regimen until goal BP is reached. If goal BP cannot be reached with 2 drugs, add and titrate a third drug from the list provided. **Do not use an ACEI and an ARB together in the same patient.** If goal BP cannot be reached using only the drugs in recommendation 6 because of a contraindication or the need to use more than 3 drugs to reach goal BP, antihypertensive drugs from other classes can be used. Referral to a hypertension specialist may be indicated for patients in whom goal BP cannot be attained using the above strategy or for the management of complicated patients for whom additional clinical consultation is needed. (Expert Opinion – Grade E)

direct vasodilators (e.g. hydralazine), aldosterone receptor antagonists (e.g. spironolactone), adrenergic neuronal depleting agents (reserpine), and loop diuretics (e.g. furosemide) have not been recommended for the initial treatment of hypertension because there are no RCTs of good or fair quality comparing the four recommended classes of drugs. β-blockers have been shown to increase composite outcome of myocardial infarction, cardiovascular death and stroke when compared with ARB in one of the studies although other studies have not shown this equivocally. Similarly, α-blockers have been shown to lead to worse cardiovascular outcomes when compared to diuretics.

In *patients with CKD and hypertension,* initial (or add-on) antihypertensive treatment should include an ACEI or ARB to improve kidney outcomes [**Recommendation 8**]. This applies to all CKD patients with hypertension regardless of race or diabetes status. This had a moderate Grade B Recommendation.

The Kidney Disease Improving Global Outcomes (KDIGO) recommend treating patients to a goal BP < 140/90 mm Hg in nondiabetic kidney disease patients with nonproteinuric kidney disease (<300 mg/day). The evidence for this BP goal comes from long-term follow up of patients in the African-American Study of Kidney Disease and Hypertension (AASK) trial. For one component of the study, AASK study randomized patients with hypertension and CKD to two goal BPs-mean arterial pressure (MAP) ≤92 or 102–107 mm Hg. During the trial, the low BP group had a mean BP of 130/78 mm Hg and the other group had a BP of 141/86 mm Hg. After 9 years of follow-up, there was no difference in outcomes in patients with little proteinuria. The modification of diet in renal disease (MDRD) study, however, did show a benefit with lower BP goals. The MDRD study also randomized non-diabetics with CKD to two different BP goals. In the low BP goal group, the achieved BP was 126/77 mm Hg; and in the other group, the BP was 134/81 mm Hg. The patients in the low BP group were less likely to reach the primary endpoint of renal failure or mortality; however, the patients in the low BP group were more likely to receive ACE inhibitors. In the Ramipril Efficacy in Nephropathy (REIN) trial, patients with nondiabetic renal disease were randomized to ramipril or placebo plus other antihypertensive therapy as needed to achieve DBP below 90 mm Hg. The trial was terminated prematurely among patients excreting more than 3 g protein per day because of a significant benefit with ACE inhibitor treatment with regard to ameliorating the rate of decline of renal function.

Tighter control has some cardiovascular benefits but has some potential harm. In proteinuric diabetic nephropathy, KDIGO recommends a goal BP of 130/80 mmHg and treatment with an ACE inhibitors or ARB. If goal BP is not achieved then a diuretic is to be added with the premise of improving natriuresis taking care of the pathogenesis of hypertension in CKD. Thiazides may be effective in the early stages of CKD but a loop diuretics may be necessary in advance stages or in the setting of secondary nephrotic syndrome.

Effects of treatment of hypertension on CAD: A significant benefit in CVD risk reduction has been achieved with effective antihypertensive therapy and this has been shown in many randomized trials. A specific class effect for ACEI on CVD outcomes has been seen in Heart Outcomes Prevention Evaluation [HOPE], Survival and Ventricular Enlargement [SAVE], and European Trial on Reduction of Cardiac Events with Perindopril in Stable Coronary Artery Disease [EUROPA] trials.

Lower BP goals and diabetes mellitus: In the International Verapamil-Trandolapril Study (INVEST) trial, patients in diabetic cohort of subjects with hypertension and CAD, did not have improved cardiovascular outcomes if SBP control was tight (<130 mm Hg vs 130–139 mm Hg). However in Appropriate Blood Pressure Control in Diabetes (ABCD) trial, a beneficial effect was seen in all cause mortality in a group with tighter BP control.

In the elderly a J curve association has been seen between DBP control and all cause mortality, non-fatal MI and stroke [INVEST study and Hypertension in the Very Elderly Trial (HYVET) study]. This may be due to these patients have higher likelihood of CAD and low coronary reserve.

Strategies to Dose Antihypertensive Drugs

How should clinicians titrate and combine the drugs? The strategy should be adjusted based on the individual circumstances, clinician and patient preferences, and drug tolerability. Patient's BP should be assessed regularly and lifestyle interventions must be promoted. Fixed-dose combinations, it is hoped, will improve adherence in patients needing more than one drug and might be better for control and avoidance of adverse events than higher-dose monotherapy. The recommendations from the European Society of Hypertension and European Society of Cardiology, issued in 2013 differ from those of the joint guideline by the American Society of Hypertension and the International Society of Hypertension, and from those of the JNC 8.

SUMMARY

- Hypertension is an important cause of morbidity and mortality worldwide.
- Although primary hypertension is commonest, one must rule out a secondary cause as it is treatable.
- Lifestyle interventions should be tried first for BP control and, if not achieved, pharmacological treatment is required.
- Adequate BP control requires combination of the various antihypertensive drugs.

Multiple Choice Questions

1. **As per the JNC, prehypertensive is defined as**
   a. SBP 120–139 & DBP 80–89
   b. SBP 140–159 & DBP 90–99
   c. SBP 110–139 & DBP 70–89
   d. SBP 110–129 & DBP 70–79

2. **Secondary hypertension should be suspected if**
   a. Hypertension onset is in < 30 years and > 55 years
   b. If BP is inadequately controlled despite being on a three-drug regimen including a diuretic
   c. Hypertension which was well-controlled initially becomes poorly controlled in a compliant patient
   d. All of the above

3. **Hperaldosteronism is characterized by**
   a. Unprovoked hypokalemia
   b. Poor BP control on conventional antihypertensive
   c. Good response to aldosterone
   d. All of the above

4. **BP target as per the JNC 8 guidelines for a patient > 60 years of age, is**
   a. SBP/DBP < 130/80 mm Hg
   b. SBP/DBP < 150/90 mm Hg
   c. SBP/DBP < 140/90 mm Hg
   d. SBP/DBP < 120/80 mm Hg

5. **49-year-old Mr RM is a known diabetic for the past 8 yrs. He also has hypertension, diabetic retinopathy and chronic kidney disease. He is not on any anithypertensives. His BP during OPD visit is 170/90 mm Hg. His blood test showed blood urea 54 mg/dL, serum creatinine of 1.7 mg/dL, serum sodium 143 mmol/L and serum potassium 4.9 mmol/L. Which class of antihypertensive should be started for him?**
   a. Beta-blockers
   b. Calcium channel blockers
   c. ACE inhibitors or ARBs
   d. Alpha-blockers

6. **Above patient (Q. 5) was started on Tab Telmisartan 40 mg once daily. During further OPD visit after 2 weeks his BP is 146/86 mm Hg and lab tests revealed serum creatinine of 1.9 mg/dL and serum potassium 5.5 mmol/L. What should be the next line of management?**
   a. Stop Telmisartan and evaluate for renal artery stenosis
   b. Add calcium channel blockers
   c. Add thiazide diuretic
   d. Add alpha blocker

7. **A 37-year-old gentleman, Mr XL, who is an African-American, presents in a clinic for routine evaluation. He has been recently diagnosed to have hypertension and has tried lifestyle modification but his blood pressure continues to be high and during his OPD visit, it is found to be 150/94 mm Hg. He does not have any other comorbidities. His renal functions and serum electrolytes are normal and other causes of secondary hypertension have been ruled out. Which is the best first-line drug for the management of hypertension in this case?**
   a. Beta-blockers
   b. Calcium channel blockers
   c. ACE inhibitors or ARBs
   d. Alpha-blockers

8. **As per the JNC guidelines, which of the following is not recommended as a first-line antihypertensive agent for essential hypertension?**
   a. Calcium channel blockers
   b. Thiazide diuretic
   c. ACE inhibitors
   d. Alpha blockers

9. **Hyponatremia is a common complication of treatment with**
   a. Thiazide diuretics
   b. Calcium channel blockers
   c. ACE inibitors
   d. None of these

10. **Which of the following is not a side effect of amlodipine?**
   a. Pedal edema
   b. Tachycardia
   c. Dizziness
   d. Hyperkalemia

Answers

1. a	2. d	3. d	4. b	5. c	6. c	7. b	8. d
9. a	10. d						

SUGGESTED READING

1. Prevention of stroke by antihypertensive drug treatment in older persons with isolated systolic hypertension. Final results of the systolic hypertension in the elderly program (SHEP). SHEP Cooperative Research Group. JAMA: The Journal of the American Medical Association. 1991;265(24):3255-64.
2. Beckett NS, Peters R, Fletcher AE, et al. Treatment of hypertension in patients 80 years of age or older. New England Journal of Medicine. 2008/05 2008;358(18):1887-98.
3. Staessen JA, Fagard R, Thijs L, et al. Randomised double-blind comparison of placebo and active treatment for older patients with isolated systolic hypertension. The Lancet. 1997;350(9080):757-64.
4. Conlin PR. Eat your fruits and vegetables but hold the salt. Circulation. 2007;116(14):1530-1.
5. Cutler JA, Follmann D, Allender PS. Randomized trials of sodium reduction: an overview. Am J Clin Nutr. 1997;65(2 Suppl):643S-651S.
6. Elliott P. Observational studies of salt and blood pressure. Hypertension. 1991;17(1 Suppl):I3-I8.
7. Elliott P, Walker LL, Little MP, et al. Change in salt intake affects blood pressure of chimpanzees: Implications for human populations. Circulation. 2007;116(14):1563-8.
8. Graudal NA, Galløe AM, Garred P. Effects of sodium restriction on blood pressure, renin, aldosterone, catecholamines, cholesterols, and triglyceride. JAMA. 1998;279(17):1383.
9. Midgley JP. Effect of reduced dietary sodium on blood pressure. JAMA. 1996;275(20):1590.
10. Miura K. Epidemiology and prevention of hypertension in Japanese: how could Japan get longevity? The EPMA Journal. 2011;2(1):59-64.
11. Islam AK, Majumder AA. Hypertension in Bangladesh: A review. Indian heart journal. 2012;64(3):319-23.
12. Bi Z, Liang X, Xu A, et al. Hypertension prevalence, awareness, treatment, and control and sodium intake in Shandong Province, China: baseline results from Shandong-Ministry of Health Action on Salt Reduction and Hypertension (SMASH), 2011. Preventing Chronic Disease. 2014;11:E88.
13. Addo J, Agyemang C, Smeeth L, de-Graft Aikins A, Edusei AK, Ogedegbe O. A review of population-based studies on hypertension in Ghana. Ghana Medical Journal. 2012;46(2 Suppl):4-11.
14. Dalai N, Cui H, Yan M, Rile G, Li S, Su X. Risk factors for the development of essential hypertension in a Mongolian population of China: a case-control study. Genetics and molecular research: GMR. 2014;13(2):3283-91.
15. Ulasi, II, Ijoma CK, Onwubere BJ, Arodiwe E, Onodugo O, Okafor C. High prevalence and low awareness of hypertension in a market population in Enugu, Nigeria. International Journal of Hypertension. 2011;2011:Article ID 869675.
16. Vaidya A, Pathak RP, Pandey MR. Prevalence of hypertension in Nepalese community triples in 25 years: a repeat cross-sectional study in rural Kathmandu. Indian Heart Journal. 2012;64(2):128-31.
17. Changing concept in medical practice. Delhi: Institute of Health and Nutrition. 1994; 1994.
18. Ganesh Kumar S, Deivanai Sundaram N. Prevalence and risk factors of hypertension among bank employees in urban Puducherry, India. The

International Journal of Occupational and Environmental Medicine. 2014;5(2):94-100.
19. Bhadoria AS, Kasar PK, Toppo NA, Bhadoria P, Pradhan S, Kabirpanthi V. Prevalence of hypertension and associated cardiovascular risk factors in Central India. Journal of Family & Community Medicine. 2014;21(1):29-38.
20. Linde CI, Karashima E, Raina H, et al. Increased arterial smooth muscle Ca^{2+} signaling, vasoconstriction, and myogenic reactivity in Milan hypertensive rats. American Journal of Physiology. Heart and Circulatory Physiology. 2012;302(3):H611-20.
21. Padilha AS, Salaices M, Vassallo DV, Batista PR, Siman FD. Hypertensive effects of the iv administration of picomoles of ouabain. Brazilian Journal of Medical and biological research = Revista brasileira de pesquisas medicas e biologicas/ Sociedade Brasileira de Biofisica ... [et al.]. 2011;44(9):933-8.
22. Pulina MV, Zulian A, Berra-Romani R, et al. Upregulation of Na^{+} and Ca^{2+} transporters in arterial smooth muscle from ouabain-induced hypertensive rats. American Journal of Physiology. Heart and Circulatory Physiology. 2010;298(1):H263-74.
23. Takahashi H, Yoshika M, Komiyama Y, Nishimura M. The central mechanism underlying hypertension: a review of the roles of sodium ions, epithelial sodium channels, the renin-angiotensin-aldosterone system, oxidative stress and endogenous digitalis in the brain. Hypertension research: official journal of the Japanese Society of Hypertension. 2011;34(11):1147-60.
24. Wenceslau CF, Davel AP, Xavier FE, Rossoni LV. Long-term ouabain treatment impairs vascular function in resistance arteries. Journal of Vascular Research. 2011;48(4):316-26.
25. Hamlyn JM, Manunta P. Endogenous ouabain: a link between sodium intake and hypertension. Current Hypertension Reports. 2011;13(1):14-20.
26. Blaustein MP, Leenen FH, Chen L, et al. How NaCl raises blood pressure: a new paradigm for the pathogenesis of salt-dependent hypertension. American Journal of Physiology. Heart and circulatory physiology. 2012;302(5):H1031-49.
27. Wallace SML, Yasmin, McEniery CM, et al. Isolated Systolic Hypertension is Characterized by Increased Aortic Stiffness and Endothelial Dysfunction. Hypertension. 2007;50(1):228-33.
28. Celermajer DS, Sorensen KE, Bull C, Robinson J, Deanfield JE. Endothelium-dependent dilation in the systemic arteries of asymptomatic subjects relates to coronary risk factors and their interaction. Journal of the American College of Cardiology. 1994;24(6):1468-74.
29. Stewart KJ, Sung J, Silber HA, et al. Exaggerated exercise blood pressure is related to impaired endothelial vasodilator function. American Journal of Hypertension. 2004;17(4):314-20.
30. Krikken JA, Laverman GD, Navis G. Benefits of dietary sodium restriction in the management of chronic kidney disease. Current opinion in nephrology and hypertension. 2009;18(6):531-8.
31. Hovater MB, Sanders PW. Effect of dietary salt on regulation of TGF-beta in the kidney. Seminars in nephrology. 2012;32(3):269-76.
32. Weir MR, Fink JC. Salt intake and progression of chronic kidney disease: an overlooked modifiable exposure? A commentary. American Journal of Kidney Diseases: the official journal of the National Kidney Foundation. 2005;45(1): 176-88.

33. Chobanian AV, Bakris GL, Black HR, et al. Seventh report of the Joint National Committee on Prevention, Detection, Evaluation, and Treatment of High Blood Pressure. Hypertension. 2003;42(6):1206-52.
34. McGuire S. US. Department of Agriculture and US. Department of Health and Human Services, Dietary Guidelines for Americans, 2010. 7th Edition, Washington, DC: US Government Printing Office, January 2011. Advances in nutrition (Bethesda). 2011;2(3):293-4.
35. Hypertension. http://www.nice.org.uk/guidance/cg127. October 2013;CG127
36. American Diabetes A. Standards of medical care in diabetes--2013. Diabetes care. 2013;36(Suppl 1):S11-66.
37. Flack JM, Sica DA, Bakris G, et al. Management of high blood pressure in Blacks: an update of the International Society on Hypertension in Blacks consensus statement. Hypertension. 2010;56(5):780-800.
38. Mancia G, Fagard R, Narkiewicz K, et al. 2013 ESH/ESC guidelines for the management of arterial hypertension: the Task Force for the Management of Arterial Hypertension of the European Society of Hypertension (ESH) and of the European Society of Cardiology (ESC). European Heart Journal. 2013;34(28):2159-219.
39. Outcomes KDIG, Group KBP. KDIGO clinical practice guideline for the management of blood pressure in chronic kidney disease. Kidney Int. 2012;2(5): 78.
40. Stern RH. The new hypertension guidelines. Journal of Clinical Hypertension (Greenwich, Conn.). 2013;15(10):748-51.
41. Effects of treatment on morbidity in hypertension. II. Results in patients with diastolic blood pressure averaging 90 through 114 mm Hg. JAMA. 1970; 213(7):1143-52.
42. Effect of antihypertensive treatment on stroke recurrence. Hypertension-Stroke Cooperative Study Group. JAMA. 1974;229(4):409-18.
43. Five-year findings of the hypertension detection and follow-up program. I. Reduction in mortality of persons with high blood pressure, including mild hypertension. Hypertension Detection and Follow-up Program Cooperative Group. JAMA. 1979;242(23):2562-71.
44. The Australian therapeutic trial in mild hypertension. Report by the Management Committee. Lancet (London, England). 1980;1(8181):1261-7.
45. Five-year findings of the hypertension detection and follow-up program. III. Reduction in stroke incidence among persons with high blood pressure. Hypertension Detection and Follow-up Program Cooperative Group. JAMA. 1982;247(5):633-8.
46. MRC trial of treatment of mild hypertension: principal results. Medical Research Council Working Party. British Medical Journal (Clinical research ed.). 1985;291(6488):97-104.
47. Klahr S, Levey AS, Beck GJ, et al. The effects of dietary protein restriction and blood-pressure control on the progression of chronic renal disease. Modification of Diet in Renal Disease Study Group. The New England Journal of Medicine. 1994;330(13):877-84.
48. Ruggenenti P, Perna A, Loriga G, et al. Blood-pressure control for renoprotection in patients with non-diabetic chronic renal disease (REIN-2): multicentre, randomised controlled trial. Lancet (London, England). 2005;365(9463):939-46.
49. Wright JT Jr, Bakris G, Greene T, et al. Effect of blood pressure lowering and antihypertensive drug class on progression of hypertensive kidney disease: results from the AASK trial. JAMA. 2002;288(19):2421-31.

50. Tight blood pressure control and risk of macrovascular and microvascular complications in type 2 diabetes: UKPDS 38. UK Prospective Diabetes Study Group. BMJ. 1998;317(7160):703-13.
51. Curb JD, Pressel SL, Cutler JA, et al. Effect of diuretic-based antihypertensive treatment on cardiovascular disease risk in older diabetic patients with isolated systolic hypertension. Systolic Hypertension in the Elderly Program Cooperative Research Group. JAMA. 1996;276(23):1886-92.
52. Tuomilehto J, Rastenyte D, Birkenhager WH, et al. Effects of calcium-channel blockade in older patients with diabetes and systolic hypertension. Systolic Hypertension in Europe Trial Investigators. The New England Journal of medicine. 1999;340(9):677-84.
53. Group AS, Cushman WC, Evans GW, et al. Effects of intensive blood-pressure control in type 2 diabetes mellitus. The New England Journal of Medicine. 2010;362(17):1575-85.
54. Hansson L, Zanchetti A, Carruthers SG, et al. Effects of intensive blood-pressure lowering and low-dose aspirin in patients with hypertension: principal results of the Hypertension Optimal Treatment (HOT) randomised trial. HOT Study Group. Lancet (London, England). 1998;351(9118):1755-62.
55. Dahlof B, Devereux RB, Kjeldsen SE, et al. Cardiovascular morbidity and mortality in the losartan intervention for endpoint reduction in hypertension study (LIFE): a randomised trial against atenolol. Lancet (London, England). 2002;359(9311):995-1003.
56. Antihypertensive, Lipid-Lowering Treatment to Prevent Heart Attack Trial Collaborative Research G. Diuretic versus alpha-blocker as first-step antihypertensive therapy: final results from the Antihypertensive and Lipid-Lowering Treatment to Prevent Heart Attack Trial (ALLHAT). Hypertension. 2003;42(3):239-46.
57. Neal B, MacMahon S, Chapman N. Blood Pressure Lowering Treatment Trialists C. Effects of ACE inhibitors, calcium antagonists, and other blood-pressure-lowering drugs: results of prospectively designed overviews of randomised trials. Blood Pressure Lowering Treatment Trialists' Collaboration. Lancet (London, England). 2000;356(9246):1955-64.
58. Lewington S, Clarke R, Qizilbash N, Peto R, Collins R, Prospective Studies C. Age-specific relevance of usual blood pressure to vascular mortality: a meta-analysis of individual data for one million adults in 61 prospective studies. Lancet (London, England). 2002;360(9349):1903-13.
59. Yusuf S, Sleight P, Pogue J, Bosch J, Davies R, Dagenais G. Effects of an angiotensin-converting-enzyme inhibitor, ramipril, on cardiovascular events in high-risk patients. The Heart Outcomes Prevention Evaluation Study Investigators. The New England Journal of Medicine. 2000;342(3):145-53.
60. Pfeffer MA, Braunwald E, Moye LA, et al. Effect of captopril on mortality and morbidity in patients with left ventricular dysfunction after myocardial infarction. Results of the survival and ventricular enlargement trial. The SAVE Investigators. The New England Journal of Medicine. 1992;327(10):669-77.
61. Fox KM. Investigators EURopean trial on reduction of cardiac events with perindopril in stable coronary artery disease investigators. Efficacy of perindopril in reduction of cardiovascular events among patients with stable coronary artery disease: randomised, double-blind, placebo-controlled, multicentre trial (the EUROPA study). Lancet (London, England). 2003;362(9386):782-8.
62. Pepine CJ, Handberg EM, Cooper-DeHoff RM, et al. A calcium antagonist vs a non-calcium antagonist hypertension treatment strategy for patients with

coronary artery disease. The International Verapamil-Trandolapril Study (INVEST): a randomized controlled trial. JAMA. 2003;290(21):2805-16.

63. Estacio RO, Jeffers BW, Gifford N, Schrier RW. Effect of blood pressure control on diabetic microvascular complications in patients with hypertension and type 2 diabetes. Diabetes Care. 2000;23 Suppl 2:B54-64.
64. Denardo SJ, Gong Y, Nichols WW, et al. Blood pressure and outcomes in very old hypertensive coronary artery disease patients: an INVEST substudy. The American Journal of Medicine. 2010;123(8):719-26.
65. Beckett NS, Peters R, Fletcher AE, et al. Treatment of hypertension in patients 80 years of age or older. The New England Journal of Medicine. 2008;358(18):1887-98.
66. Aronow WS, Fleg JL, Pepine CJ, et al. ACCF/AHA 2011 expert consensus document on hypertension in the elderly: a report of the American College of Cardiology Foundation Task Force on Clinical Expert Consensus Documents. Circulation. 2011;123(21):2434-506.

CHAPTER

13 Nutrition in Renal Diseases

Anita Saxena, Amit Gupta

INTRODUCTION

Nutritional care of patients with renal disease is complex. The patient has to frequently learn different diets as his medical condition and treatment approach changes with transition of chronic kidney disease (CKD) staging from milder to advanced renal failure. Patients with kidney disease require constant assessment and monitoring of nutritional status and dietary counseling. Protein energy wasting (PEW) is common in CKD and is associated with adverse outcomes anorexia, loss of taste, nausea, vomiting, gastroparesis and edema are frequent complaints. Hence, the patients need quality nutritional care and coaxing to eat. This chapter will discuss issues related to nutrition in renal disease and approach to dietary counseling in CKD.

PROTEIN ENERGY WASTING

The term "protein-energy-wasting" has been proposed to describe conditions such as protein-energy-malnutrition, malnutrition-inflammation complex syndrome, malnutrition-inflammation atherosclerosis syndrome, kidney wasting disease and uremic cachexia which are associated with inadequate nutrient intake, decreased body protein and/or reduced energy reserves. PEW defines loss of somatic and circulating body protein mass and energy reserves. Malnutrition *per se* is defined as an imbalance between nutrient intake and nutrient requirement, which results in altered metabolism. Malnutrition is of two types **(Table 13.1)**. Malnutrition associated with uremia is reversible with dialysis and nutritional repletion. However, malnutrition associated with malnutrition inflammation atherosclerosis (MIA) syndrome is not reversible because of inflammation.

Causes of PEW: Malnutrition and inflammation are two major causes of PEW **(Table 13.2)**

Association between malnutrition and anorexia is given in **Figure 13.1**.

The International society of renal nutrition and metabolism (ISRNM 2013) has issued consensus statement on etiology of PEW syndrome in CKD. During PEW, hunger response is blunted by increased half-life of leptin and ghrelin and by increased inflammation and dialysis. Resting energy expenditure (REE) increases from 12% to 20% because of protein catabolism and inflammation. Loss of protein occurs from muscle because of metabolic acidosis, glucocorticoids, and inflammation leading to increased insulin resistance. Dialysis results in

Table 13.1 Types of malnutrition in kidney disease

Factors	*Type 1*	*Type 2*
	Associated with uremic syndrome	*Associated with MIA syndrome*
Serum albumin	Normal/low	Low
Co-morbidity	Uncommon	Common
Presence of inflammation	No	Yes
Food intake	Decreased	Low/Normal
Resting energy expenditure	Normal	Elevated
Oxidative stress	Increased	Markedly increased
Protein catabolism	Decreased	Increased
Reversed by dialysis and nutritional support	Yes	No

Table 13.2 Causes of protein energy wasting (PEW)

Inflammation
- Associated with infected vascular access sites, systemic infectious illness including tuberculosis, diabetes mellitus, myocardial infarction, stroke, peripheral vascular ischemia, and vasculitis
- Unassociated with clinically apparent disease such as, inflammatory reaction to vascular access catheters, grafts, peritoneal dialysis catheters, dialysis tubing, impure dialysate, old nonfunctioning transplant kidney, kidney failure *per se*

Decreased food intake
- Anorexia caused by uremic toxicity, medication, inflammatory disorders
- Loss of taste, unpalatable prescribed diets, intercurrent illness, emotional stress, impaired ability to procure, prepare or mechanically ingest foods, unpalatable prescribed diets
- Non-anorexic causes (financial constraints), medical or surgical illness, particularly of gastrointestinal tract, impaired cognitive function, other mental disability, physical disability, loss of dentures

Dialysate nutrient losses
- Losses of amino acids, peptides and protein into dialysate
- Losses of water soluble vitamins and minerals during dialysis

Metabolic acidemia

Anemia and loss of blood due to
- Gastrointestinal bleed
- Frequent blood sampling

Hormonal disorders
- Resistance to anabolic hormones such as insulin, growth hormone, insulin-like growth factor-1
- Increased levels of counter regulatory hormones such as glucagon, parathyroid hormone

Increased fecal excretion of nitrogen

Decreased level of antioxidants: Vitamin E, C, selenium, reduced glutathione (GSH)

Physical conditioning

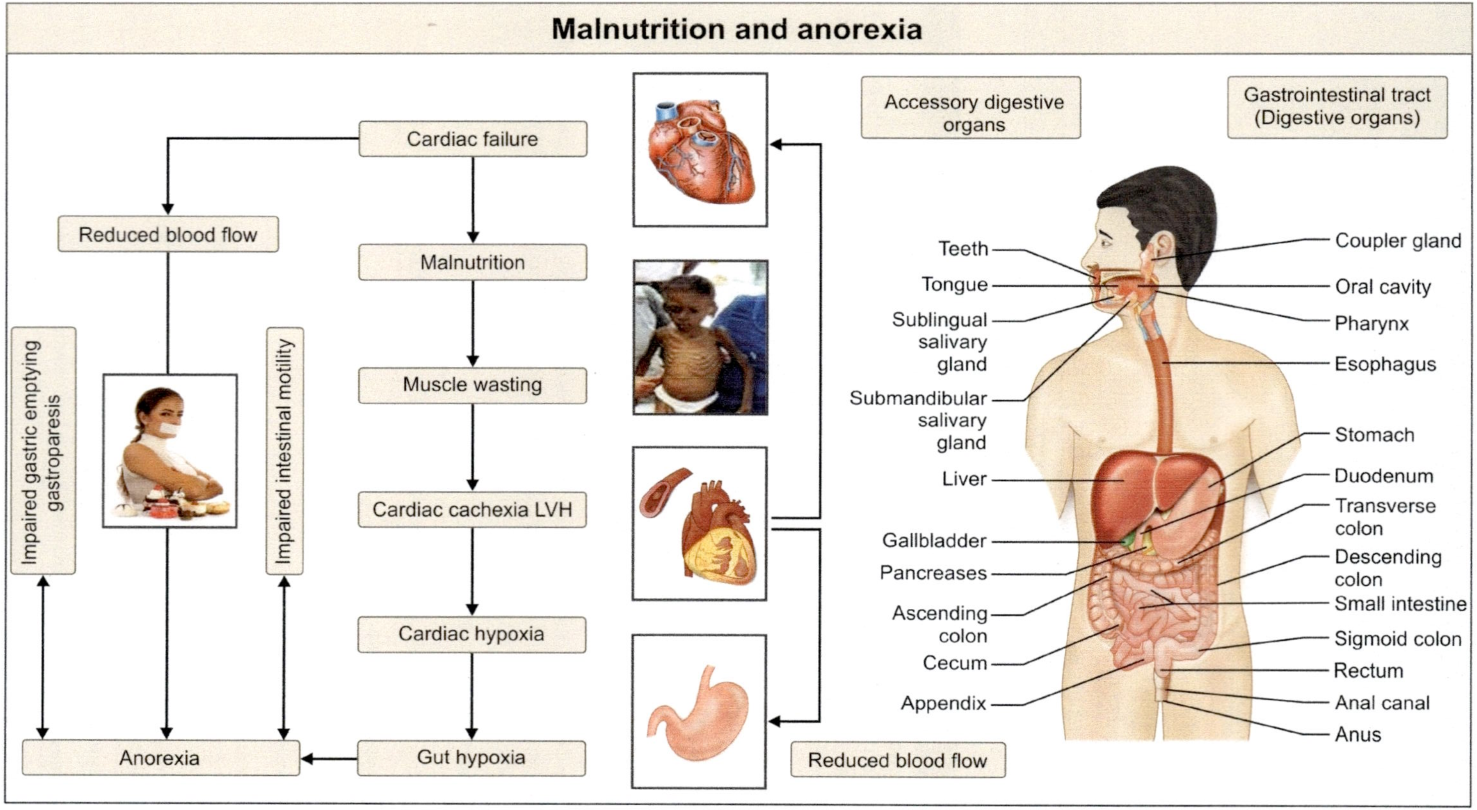

Figure 13.1 Malnutrition causes muscle-wasting leading to cardiac cachexia and left ventricular hypertrophy which causes cardiac hypoxia, reduced blood flow, gut hypoxia and anorexia, impaired gastric emptying, gastroparesis and impaired intestinal motility

loss of amino acids stimulating muscle breakdown. Liver, under the influence of metabolic acidosis (MA) and inflammation makes glutamine for deamination in kidney, increases acute phase reactant proteins and reduces serum albumin. Kidneys increase glucose production from glutamine due to MA.

MANAGEMENT OF NUTRITIONAL STATUS

This involves several aspects like assessment, striking balance between nutrient requirement and nutrient intake despite poor appetite (anorexia), hyperglycemia, hyperinsulinemia, insulin resistance and gastroparesis.

Assessment of Nutritional Status

Renal disease is marked by lean body mass (LBM) wasting. The fat mass is not lost as rapidly as the LBM is. To evaluate protein energy nutritional status combination of valid complementary measures is a must because no single measure provides a comprehensive indication of nutritional status. Measures of intake, visceral and somatic protein stores, body composition, and functional status identify different aspects of nutrition status. Evaluation of protein energy nutritional status assessment includes:

- Medical history and assessment of dietary intake (subjective global assessment and malnutrition inflammation score) which may be through diet history questionnaires, food weighing, or observation
- Physical examination and anthropometry
- Biochemical tests
- Body composition techniques like, DEXA, bioimpedance (BIA), near infrared reactance (NIR) nuclear magnetic resonance spectroscopy, muscle biopsy (for estimation of extracellular water ECW, intracellular water ICW, fat free solids electrolytes proteins, and amino acids).

Diagnosis of Protein Energy Wasting

Timely diagnosis of PEW is important for early initiation of intervention and treatment. Criteria for diagnosing PEW are given in **Table 13.3**.

Goals of Nutritional Therapy

Adequate nutritional support can maintain protein stores and correct pre-existing or disease-related deficits in lean body mass. Over-nutrition, on the other hand, is associated with altered renal hemodynamics, particularly if there is excess of high protein or amino acid intake. Glomerular protein trafficking induces hypermetabolism (hyperfiltration) and oxidative stress, and a low protein diet (LPT), is associated with reduced oxygen consumption and monoaldehyde production. Nutritional intervention is directed towards overall patient outcome and comorbid conditions such as anemia, bone disease, and cardiovascular disease (CVD). As glomerular filtration rate (GFR) declines, the stages of kidney disease change, and consequently nutritional requirements also change.

Table 13.3 Criteria for diagnosing protein-energy-wasting (PEW)

Criteria	
BMI	<22 kg m^2 if age >65 years <23 kg m^2 (age <65 years)
Unintentional weight loss	5% in 3 months or 10% in 6 months
Total body fat	<10%
Muscle wasting (reduced muscle mass)	5% in 3 months or 10% in 6 months
Reduced mid upper arm muscle circumference (MUAC) area	>10% reduction in relation to 50th percentile of reference population
Unintentional low dietary protein intake and Unintentional low dietary energy intake	<0.8 g/kg/day for at least 2 months for maintenance dialysis patients <25 kcal/kg/day for least 2 months
Net protein creatinine appearance (nPCR)	<1.0
For predicting outcome	***Effect***
Low serum albumin levels <3.5g/dL	Poor nutritional status, infection, inflammation, overhydration
Prealbumin <30 mg/dL	Poor nutritional status, infection, inflammation
Decreased edema free/fat-free mass	Muscle breakdown, protein catabolism
Low serum creatinine	Presence of inflammation and hence muscle wasting and protein catabolism
Residual renal function	Better clearance of middle molecules, better nutritional intake
nPCR <1.0 (Decreased total body nitrogen content)	Low protein intake
Serum cholesterol <100 mg/dL	Chronic malnutrition
SGA score: 1–7 normal 7–14 mild malnutrition 15–21 moderate malnutrition 22–35 severe malnutrition *Original rating*: 1–3 severely malnourished 4–5 mild-moderately malnourished 6–7 well nourished	Overall protein and energy nutritional status

Therefore, the primary objective of nutritional intervention for patients with renal-disease is to:

- Prevent appearance of uremic symptoms
- Control progression of disease and to maintain adequate nutritional status
- Delay initiation of renal replacement therapy (RRT)
- Improve outcomes in CKD patients
- Improve nutrition
- Build up body stores for good transplant outcome (if planned)
- Improve quality of life.

Nutrient Requirement

While planning diet of a patient with compromised renal function, the most important constituents of diet, which need to be monitored and controlled, are:

- Energy (kilocalories)
- Protein of high biological value (HBV)
- Sodium
- Potassium
- Phosphorus and calcium for maintaining bone health (bone metabolism) and to prevent hyperparathyroidism
- Fluid management
- Saturated fat and cholesterol
- Vitamins and minerals for proper functioning of enzymes, taste and for preventing anemia.

Primary goal of nutritional therapy in renal patients is to control intake of nitrogen in order to prevent uremic symptoms and muscle catabolism (breakdown) and maintain serum protein levels to prevent edema **(Fig. 13.2)**.

About 20–70% patients on maintenance dialysis show signs of protein energy wasting (PEW). The MDRD study has shown that there is association between dietary intake, serum albumin and GFR. As GFR decreases to below 60 mL/min/1.73 m^2 dietary protein and energy intake decreases and so does serum albumin. Patients with CKD have a decreased ratio of essential to nonessential aminoacids, a pattern that is observed in protein-calorie malnutrition.

The plasma levels of branched chain aminoacids (BCAA) valine, leucine and isoleucine and of their respective ketoacids are decreased, with valine being

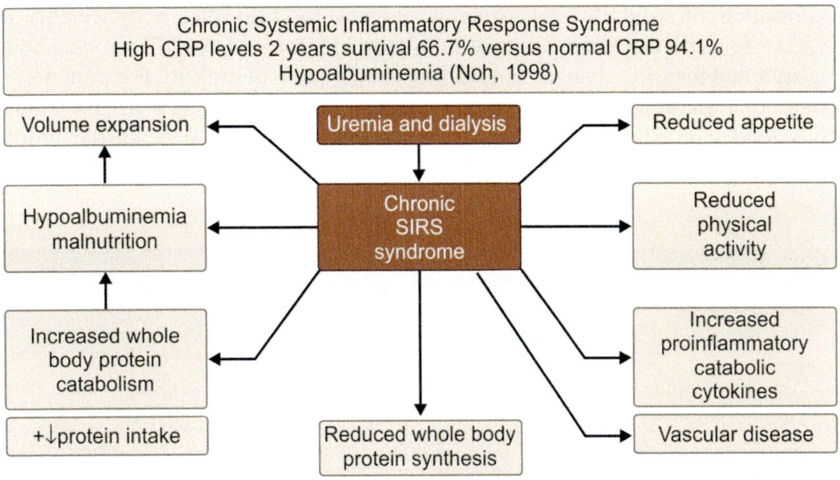

Figure 13.2 *Chronic systemic inflammatory response syndrome*: Uremia and dialysis induce chronic Systemic Inflammatory Response Syndrome (SIRS) which cause reduced appetite, reduced physical activity and increased levels of catabolic cytokines. This causes reduced protein synthesis, increased protein catabolism, hypoalbuminemia and malnutrition and volume expansion

reduced to a greater extent than others. The potential mechanism responsible for this decrease in BCAA might be related to oxidation of such amino acids in skeletal muscle as a consequence of metabolic acidosis.

Nutritional Management in Predialysis Stage: Conservative Management

Indian patients have low energy intake. A study conducted on CKD stage 2 and 3 patients **(Table 13.4)** has shown that energy intake of patients based on body mass index (BMI) is 17 kcal/kg/day compared to recommended intake of 30-35 kcal/kg/day. They also have reduced serum protein level (serum albumin was 2.9 ± 0.9 g/dL and serum protein of 5.7 ± 1.40 g/dL). As appetite worsens, energy intake decreases **(Table 13.4)** (Effect of appetite and body mass index on energy and protein intake in chronic kidney disease Stage 3 and 4 patients unpublished data Saxena A and Gupta A).

In predialysis stages protein intake is restricted. Low protein diet (LPD) is a conservative treatment in patients with CKD to improve uremic symptoms and slow progression of renal dysfunction. LPD, i.e. protein intake 0.6–0.8 g/kg/day (*Stage 1* CKD GFR >90 mL/min. - 0.8 g/kg/day; CKD *Stage 2–5* GFR 15–89 mL/min. - 0.6 g/kg/day) and energy intake of 30–35 kcal/kg/day is recommended for predialysis CKD patients.

Children frequently have poor appetite and require modification of dietary nutrient intake to maintain optimal nutrition, growth, and development. Nutritional counseling should be individualized according to nutritional assessment, child's age, development, food preferences, cultural beliefs, and psychosocial status. Frequent re-evaluation and modification of the nutrition plan should be done with changes in child's condition and nutritional status. Protein and energy requirements for children are according to recommended allowance for children for chronological age (based on ideal body weight). In CKD stage 3 dietary protein intake should be 100–140% of the DRI for ideal body weight and for CKD stages 4–5 it should be 100–120% of the DRI. For patients on hemodialysis, additional increment on anticipated losses of 0.4 g/kg/day should be added to intake and for patients on peritoneal dialysis, 0.8–0.9 g/kg/day should be added to recommended intake. However, if the patient is not gaining weight

Table 13.4 Energy and protein intake based on body mass index and appetite

Based on BMI	*Normal*	*Underweight*	*Severely underweight*
N%	52.8%	15%	5.71%
Energy intake kcal/kg	17.2 ± 9.0	17.0 ± 10.0	15.91 ± 11.1
Protein intake g/kg/day	0.6 ± 0.34	0.5 ± 0.4	0.56 ± 0.44
	Based on appetite		
Appetite	*Normal*	*Average*	*Poor*
Energy intake kcal/kg/day	21.5 ± 4.6	16.4 ± 0.4	13.5 ± 5.8
Protein intake g/kg/day	0.8 ± 0.3	0.6 ± 0.2	0.52 ± 0.2

then height age should be taken as reference for additional energy and protein intake.

In order to maintain basic metabolic rate and to support physical activities while patient is awake, the patient must take sufficient calories. Energy requirement for these patients is 30–35 kcal/kg/day. Patients are usually given simple carbohydrates and mono and polyunsaturated fats. The best combination of fat is two tea-spoons (10 g) of refined or mustard oil and one teaspoon (5 g) of either salt-free butter or clarified butter (ghee) or olive oil. This provides sufficient amount of omega-6 fatty acids and essential fatty acid. Saturated fat in invisible form is consumed in milk, milk products and meat.

Metabolic acidosis (MA) increases breakdown of muscle protein, therefore, correction of MA with sodabicarbonate (0.9 g TID) or with dialysis is must in order to maintain serum bicarbonate level ≥22 mmol/L.

MDRD study has shown that very low protein diet (VLPD) 0.3 g/kg/day supplemented with keto-analogue 5 mg/kg/day (one tablet contains 50 mg essential amino acids) reduces uremic symptoms, preserves residual renal function, slows down rate of progression of the disease, delays onset of dialysis and improves metabolic complications due to renal insufficiency (like proteinuria, disturbances in calcium-phosphate, carbohydrate and lipid metabolism) and preserves nutritional status *provided* it is supplemented with high energy intake. Dietary recommendations for CKD and AKI patients are given in **Table 13.5**.

Sodium intake of patients with renal failure must be restricted to (a) control hypertension (b) prevent water retention and hence edema. Renal hypertension is salt sensitive. High sodium intake worsens hypertension and proteinuria. However, sodium intake below 120 mEq/day can result in atherosclerosis because sodium acts on RAAS (renin-angiotensin-aldosterone system) and renin is profibrotic and causes insulin resistance. Sodium and intravascular volume balance are usually well maintained until the GFR falls below 15 mL/min/1.73 m^2. Sodium chloride less than 6 g/day (or 2 g/day of sodium) is recommended. Patients with a GFR below 20 mL/min/1.73 m^2 in whom, despite sodium restriction, edema appears, respond to loop diuretics. In the absence of edema in predialysis stage, free water intake should be approximately equal to urine output plus an additional 1 L/day to account for insensible losses (depending upon CKD Stage).

Nutritional Management in Chronic Kidney Disease Stage 5 Patients on Maintenance Dialysis

Protein Energy Management

NKF/KDOQI GPG (Guidelines 3–4) recommend maintaining serum albumin at ≥4 g/dL and prealbumin at ≥30 mg/dL. In order to maintain serum albumin level ≥4 g/dL, protein intake for clinically stable maintenance hemodialysis (MHD) patients should be 1.2 g/kg/day necessary to ensure neutral or positive nitrogen balance. Unless a patient on peritoneal dialysis has demonstrated an adequate nutritional status on 1.2 g/kg/day protein diet, prescribe 1.3 g/kg/day to replenish protein loss during peritoneal dialysis. Prevalence of PEW is 18–56% in peritoneal dialysis (PD) patients.

Table 13.5 Dietary recommendations for chronic kidney disease and acute kidney injury patients

(A) CKD patients

(i) Predialysis CKD stage 1–5:

- Low protein diet 0.6–0.8 g/kg/day and energy 30–35 kcal/kg/day
- Very low protein diet (VLPD) 0.3–0.4 g/kg/day plus keto-analogue 5 mg/kg/day (with VLPD energy intake should be high)

Diabetic nephropathy:

- Low protein diet 0.8 g/kg/day
- As GFR declines reduce protein 0.6 g/kg/day
- Energy 30 kcal/kg/day

Pregnancy, diabetes and CKD:

- Protein 1.0–1.2 g/kg preconception body weight/day
- HbA1C as close to normal as possible (<1% above upper limit of normal)
- Appropriate energy intake to prevent hyperglycemia

(ii) Patients on dialysis (i.e. CKD stage 5D)

- Hemodialysis: Protein 1.2 g/kg/day and energy 30–35 kcal/kg/day
- *CAPD*: Protein 1.3 g/kg/day and energy 30–35 kcal/kg/day
- *During PD peritonitis*: Protein 1.5 g/kg/day and energy 25–35 kcal/kg/day
- Energy 30 kcal/kg/day if age ≥60 years; 35 kcal/kg/day if age <60 years

(B) Patients with acute kidney injury:

- Requiring renal replacement therapy—Protein 1.5 g/kg/day and energy 25–35 kcal/kg/day
- Relatively noncatabolic AKI patients with milder nonoliguric forms, not needing RRT and likely to regain renal function in a few days—Protein 0.8 g/kg/day and energy 25–30 kcal/kg/day (excess urea appearance <5%)
- Moderate catabolism and extracorporeal therapy protein 1.0–1.5 g/kg/day (excess urea appearance 5–10%) energy 25–30 kcal/kg/day
- Severe hypercatabolism requiring CRRT or SLED up to 1.7 g/kg/day (excess urea appearance >10%) energy 30–35 kcal/kg/day

Other nutrients:

- *Fat*: 15–20 g/day (3–4 tsps refined oil/day)
- *Sodium*: <2.4 g/day or 1 level tsp
- *Potassium*: 1 mEq/kg/day
- *Calcium*: 1200–1500 mg/day but not more than 2000 mg/day
- *Phosphorus*: 800–1000 mg/day
- Vitamin B complex (B_1, B_6, B_{12})—1 capsule OD
- *Folic acid*: 5 mg/day
- *Zinc*: 15–20 mg/day
- *Vitamin D*: To supplement if deficiency is established
- *Vitamin C*: Supplement 60 mg/day for HD patients. Patients on CRRT require higher intake of vitamin C (up to 150–200 mg)

For parenteral nutrition:

- Glucose (carbohydrate g/kg/day) mild to severe catabolism 3.0–5.0
- *Fat (g/kg/day)*: Moderate catabolism 0.5–1.0; severe catabolism 0.8–1.2
- *Amino acids/protein (g/kg/day)*: Mild catabolism 0.6–1.0; moderate catabolism 0.8–1.2; severe catabolism 1.0–1.5 (g/kg/day)

Measures to correct inadequate food intake because of uremia (nausea, vomiting):

- Prescribe antiemetics half an hour before meals
- Correct uremic intoxication
- Discontinue use of phosphate binders for short period
- Establish adequate urine production, and
- Provide nutritional support (oral nutritional supplement and/or IDPN) until renal function is returned.

Contd...

Contd...

Fruits permitted: One fruit in a day (approx 50 mEq) if serum potassium is <5.0 mgdL, Apple, banana (diabetic to avoid banana), orange, pineapple, rose apple (*jamun*), guava, papaya, pear.
If serum potassium is >5.0 stop fruits

Vegetable permitted: Potato, *turai* (ridge gourd), *lauki* (bottle gourd), *bhindi* (ladies finger), *tinda* (giloda), *parwal* (snake gaurd), *methi saag* (fenugreek leaves), *kaddu* (pumpkin), cabbage, simla mirch (green pepper), green peas.

Dal (pulses) permitted: *Dhuli moong* (green gram), *arhar* (tur dal), *urad dhuli* (black gram), *dhuli masoor* (lentil), kidney beans, chick-peas (choley once a month).
Process for cooking dal: Boil dal. Discard water. Cook dal in fresh water.

Other foods permitted: Bread slice, *chappati* (*roti*), daliya (porridge), *sabut dana* (sorgum), *upma, khichri, poha, suji halwa, idli, dosa* (made on nonstick tawa with negligible oil), *besan cheela* (pancake).
Process for reducing potassium intake (Leaching process)
Leach/remove potassium from vegetables by soaking chopped vegetables in luke warm water for half an hour. Cook in fresh water.

Food items not permitted: Green leafy vegetables like spinach, mustard leaves, bathua, *chaulai, kathal* (jackfruit) *karela* (bitter gourd), shalgam (turnip), *chukandar* (beetroot), *sahjan, kamal kakri* (lotus stem), *gohar phalli* (cluster beans), french beans, *sem* (broad) beans, tomato, cauliflower, sweet lime, lemon, *gajar* (carrots), *mooli* (raddish), raw salad, mango, *awala* (indian gooseberry), mushroom, *singhara* (water chestnut), dry fruits (almond, cashew, coconut, groundnut, pistachio, walnut, etc.), fruit juice, vegetable soup, coconut water, melon, water melon and bhel fruit, bajra . Bakery products like cake, pastry patties, biscuits, chocolate, coffee, baking soda, ajinomotto, eno salt, salted butter, gur (jaggery), pickel, chutney, namkeen mixture, papad, processed cheese, canned foods, deep fried food, popcorns
Use refined flour (sieve flour/*atta* before cooking)
Use tamarind pulp instead of tomatoes to enhance taste
Use garlic, *heeng, methi dana,* and turmeric in cooking. Turmeric is anti-inflammatory
Use coriander powder (*dhania*), cumin seeds (*zeera*) and red chilli powder in small quantity.

High protein food for dialysis patients:

- Curd with high protein powder
- High protein chappati—Add 1 tbsp of soybean flour to wheat flour (*atta*) or mix protein powder to wheat flour (*atta*)
- Others such as *sandesh* (diabetic patients can use sugar-free powder to make sandesh), *chenney ka rasgulla* (not for diabetics), rice pudding/*kheer* (diabetics can use sugar free powder), *paneer ki kheer* (diabetics can use sugar free powder), *moong dal kebabs*, egg white, soyabean and other products (Tofu, nuggets and milk).

CANUSA study has shown that 1 g/L lower serum albumin concentration is associated with 6% increase in relative risk of death and every 1 unit lower SGA score is associated with 25% increased relative risk of death. In dialysis dependent patients, protein requirements are influenced by treatment modality selected by the patient. Fifty percent of protein should be of HBV. At least 0.35–0.45 g/kg body weight protein of HBV should come from low fat milk (preferably skimmed milk), cottage cheese, soya milk and egg white. Other sources of protein are pulses and legumes and high protein preparations or supplements in powder or biscuit form. Peptide based supplements are the preferred choice for sick patients. Wheat flour and rice contain protein, which are not of high biological value. Soy protein diet is safe to maintain the nutritional state (weight, BMI and body composition) of patients on short-term acute peritoneal dialysis (APD). Animal protein foods are usually high in fat and cholesterol; hence their intake should be controlled. Vegetarian sources of protein (incomplete proteins) should be combined with milk products to get complete protein). Energy intake should be 35 kcal/kg/day for those less than 60 years and 30 kcal/day for those above 60 years. American heart association recommends including 1 serving of cold-water fish in the diet 3 times per week. It is possible that 3 servings of cold-water fish, such as salmon, mackerel, herring, and albacore tuna, would provide EPA and DHA in excess of the 10% of adequate intake amounts for men and women. In the opinion of the working group, these recommendations may be considered for the diabetics and CKD population.

Studies have shown that if patients consumed renal specific oral nutritional supplements (ONS) product (16.6 g of protein and 475 calories per 240-mL serving) thrice weekly with each hemodialysis session, their serum albumin values showed a significant benefit after 3 months, compared to controls who did not take ONS. It takes at least 3 months for ONS to show its effect. If ONS is discontinued, calories and protein intake reduces.

Intradialytic Parenteral Nutrition

Intradialytic parenteral nutrition (IDPN) should be considered in patients who are malnourished and unable to eat. IDPN results in substantial increase in whole body protein and forearm muscle protein synthesis in association with a decrease in whole body protein catabolism. Monitor side effects include:

- *Nausea and vomiting (incidence 15–25%)*: In such cases decrease infusion rate and reduce total IDPN by half for 1–2 weeks
- Intradialytic cramping can occur in rare cases of low plasma osmolality if sodium profiling is not used. If this happens, 1 g NaCl/hour of infusion should be added to IDPN
- Adjust insulin dose if hyperglycemia (>300 mg/dL) occurs. Administer short acting insulin 2–6 units to prevent hyperglycemia. Along with IDPN encourage patients to take oral supplements.

Peritoneal Dialysis

Patients on peritoneal dialysis although are better off when it comes to potassium intake compared to those on hemodialysis, it is still important to restrict potassium if patient is on ACEi or ARBs. One gram of protein contains 1 mEq of potassium. Therefore fruits and vegetables given in **Table 13.4** should be preferred to avoid hyperkalemia. If serum potassium is <3.5 mmol/L allow liberal intake of fruits, but if serum potassium is <3 mmol/L, treat hypokalemia with oral/IV potassium chloride.

Intraperitoneal amino acid (IPAA) solutions: One daily exchange of IPAA has been shown to improve nutritional parameters. Results of a randomized study on 22 CAPD patients with serum albumin levels < 3.5 g/dL showed that use of 1.1% AA solution had anabolic response with increase in IGF and lower phosphorous and potassium levels and the nutritional status improved. IPAA should be administered during postprandial state, i.e. start after breakfast, immediately before or after lunch, or after supper, especially if patient eats an evening snack. If two AA dialysate exchanges are used, they should be given immediately after breakfast and supper. In order to gain maximum benefit of IPAA it is important to optimize oral intake of all other essential nutrients, especially energy and vitamins.

Icodextrin-based PD solution: Studies have shown that these solutions effectively clear small solutes, increase ultrafiltration rates, improve blood pressure control, improve cardiovascular parameters, improve lipid profile and better blood sugar, lowers insulin level and improve insulin sensitivity. With icodextrin-based PD solutions lower levels of advanced glycation end products (AGEs) are formed and peritoneal membrane is better preserved. Long dwell can help some anuric patients to be maintained on PD because of better fluid balance.

Phosphorus Management

Renal patients have impaired phosphate excretion. Protein has linear relation with phosphate. One gram protein brings 13–15 mg phosphate, of which 30–70% is absorbed. One regular hemodialysis session clears 500–600 mg phosphate and 1-day peritoneal dialysis clears ~300 mg (2–3 grams per week) phosphate. Phosphorus availability from animal products is greater than 70%, whereas availability from plant products (50%) and mixed meals (50–70%) is lower. To optimally manage elevated phosphate levels, it is important to first assess the presence or absence of other mineral abnormalities, vascular calcifications, and note the administration of concurrent therapies. Among dialysis patients, aim is to maintain serum phosphate levels between 3.5 mg/dL and 5.5 mg/dL. Initial step should be to restrict dietary phosphate to 800–1000 mg/day. Among dialysis patients with elevated phosphate levels that are refractory to maintenance dialysis therapy and diet, administration of phosphate-binding agents is a must. Some patients do not achieve the recommended serum phosphate goals due in part to the use of various agents to help control PTH levels. Vitamin D analogs may contribute, raising both phosphate and calcium concentrations. A possible alternative is the use of cinacalcet, which acts by a different mechanism and produces significant reductions in PTH, calcium, and phosphate levels. More frequent and more intensive dialysis can also lower phosphate levels.

Fluid Management

It is important to prevent intradialytic weight gain. More than 1–1.5 kg of intradialytic weight gain for twice weekly dialysis regimen and more than 750 g–1.0 kg for thrice weekly dialysis regimen is not advisable as the nutritional status is compromised because of associated complications (symptoms of volume overload such as not able to sleep in supine position, dyspnea on exertion, generalized edema). Fluid intake includes liquid like water, tea, curd, milk, lentil (*dal*) of thin consistency. Patients who are unable to control thirst should be counseled to rinse their mouth when they feel thirsty or they can suck ice cubes made with 5 mL of flavored or plain water, or chew gum or cardamom (*green elaichi*) cinnamon (*dalchinni*).

Water-soluble Vitamins

These are dialysed; therefore, vitamin B should be prescribed post dialysis. Vitamin B complex prevents hyperhomocystenemia (folic acid, B_6, B_{12}), and anemia. Patients who are not prone to intradialytic hypotension should be advised to take protein rich supplement or snacks any time after half an hour of starting dialysis. This will prevent muscle and protein catabolism and preserve nutritional status. Intradialytic oral nutritional supplements improve quality of life.

Role of Residual Renal Function

Residual renal function (RRF) may affect nutritional status and protein intake through the continuous characteristic of residual renal solute elimination. The kidneys provide more continuous solute elimination compared with renal replacement therapies such as HD and CAPD. Studies have shown that anorexia is more common in patients who have lost RRF and has significant independent effect on dietary protein intake. Patients with RRF have higher mean dietary protein intake (DPI) and nPNA than patients without RRF (1.08 ± 0.31 vs 0.89 0.31 g/kg/day and 62.1 ± 12.4 vs 54.9 ± 15.3 g/day). Every 1 mL/min/1.73 m^2 increase in GFR is associated with 0.041-fold increase in DPI and 0.838-fold increase in dietary calorie intake (DCI). Studies have shown that PD solutions may also affect RRF. Many current PD solutions are bioincompatible, with low pH.

Preservation of intrinsic renal function also maintains synthesis of erythropoietin and conversion of vitamin D to its active form. Inhibiting the elevation of PTH may have a favorable anabolic effect by reducing amino acid release from muscle tissue. All these factors have a beneficial effect on the quality of life, oral food intake, including energy intake, and protein metabolism in patients with RRF who receive chronic HD.

Reverse Epidemiology

Maintenance dialysis patients often suffer from protein energy malnutrition. This is an important risk factor for increase mortality and morbidity. This is in contrast to the general population and known as reverse epidemiology. Various cardiovascular risk factors (such as body mass, blood pressure, serum cholesterol, etc.) are related to dialysis patient's outcome in a reverse way.

Cachexia in Slow Motion or Malnutrition Inflammation Complex Syndrome

In dialysis population LBM depletes faster compared to fat mass. In overweight patients increased adipose tissue serves as a reserve and the patient will develop frank PEM more slowly compared to patients who are depleted of reserves.

Many studies report a strong association between hypoalbuminemia and CVD in maintenance dialysis patients. Cardiac diseases such as heart failure or other comorbid conditions may engender anorexia and, may induce protein and muscle wasting, which is also known as cardiac cachexia. CVD and PEM in dialysis patients may be caused by cytokine activation due to renal failure or other proinflammatory comorbid condition. This increased activation of inflammatory cytokines (interleukin 6 or TNF-α) suppresses appetite and causes muscle proteolysis and hypoalbuminemia and contributes to atherosclerosis. Condition arising out of combination of PEM and inflammation can be summed up as "malnutrition-inflammation complex syndrome" (MICS). Unique wasting syndrome that develops with increasing number of years on dialysis in these patients has been referred to as "cachexia in slow motion."

Obesity

It potentially attenuates the magnitude of PEM or inflammation in dialysis and CHF patients because patients on dialysis are in a state of undernutrition, which may predispose to infection or other inflammatory processes. Also, when patients are malnourished, they are more susceptible to the ravages of inflammatory diseases.

It has also been seen that in all PD patients—obese or nonobese—use of 1.5–4.25% of dextrose (higher calorie intake) in their peritoneal dialysate (often around the clock), which is estimated to be absorbed at 45%, have survival advantage in contrast to HD patients who are exposed to 1% of dextrose in their dialysate during the 4-hours, thrice-weekly dialysis. Higher biochemical markers of improved nutrition in patients with higher BMI may offset part of the toxic effects of uremia in uremic patients and have positive influence on survival.

Postrenal Transplant

Issues which need attention after renal transplant are: protein catabolism due to surgical trauma and high dose of steroids, hypertension, obesity and diabetes. The daily protein intake recommendation in the immediate post transplant phase is 1.3–1.5 g/kg/day. Protein intake should be controlled in the presence of acute tubular necrosis with associated uremic symptoms. After 4 weeks if the patients has recovered well, then protein intake should be brought down to 1 g/kg/day and should continue till three months post-transplant. At three months protein intake should be brought down to 0.8 g/kg/day. Patient should prefer taking boiled water and avoid eating at roadside joints. They should avoid eating at places where food is being cooked on large scale and hygiene may be compromised. Vegetables should be washed thoroughly to avoid getting infections (gastrointestinal infections). Water intake should be thirst driven but it should not be less than 2 L/day.

The post-transplant nutritional care of diabetic patients is considerably complicated by insulin resistance induced by steroid therapy. Some patients develop clinical diabetes (new onset diabetes after transplantation: NODAT) as a result of immunosuppressive therapy with glucocorticoids and calcineurin inhibitor tacrolimus. Even recipients of renal transplants with overtly normal glucose tolerance have evidence of insulin resistance when studied by the insulin clamp technique. The diabetogenic effect of tacrolimus is dose dependent so that with downward dose adjustment, the long-term prevalence of diabetes decreases and may eventually be similar to the rate observed in cyclosporine treated patients. Insulin therapy is recommended to keep blood sugar under control.

Chronic allograft nephropathy (CAN or chronic renal allograft injury CRAI) is a state, which is similar to predialysis stage wherein renal function is impaired but the patient may or may not require dialysis as he is having good urine output and is able to eat well. If a patient has CAN, he should be put on low protein diet, i.e. 0.6–0.75/kg/day of protein as in case of CKD stage 2–5 patients not on dialysis. If creatinine is above 2 mg/dL, sodium bicarbonate should be supplemented to prevent metabolic acidosis and consequently protein catabolism. To prevent hyperphosphatemia phosphate binders should be prescribed with meals. Water intake will have to be monitored. If patient has edema, water intake should be reduced.

Acute Kidney Injury

It is a common complication affecting approximately 5% of hospitalized patients and 10–30% of patients managed in intensive care units. Acute kidney injury (AKI) induces protein catabolism, impairs glucose and fat metabolism. Biochemical alterations in hypercatabolic AKI include

- Release of endotoxins, TNF, IL-I by underlying catabolic illness,
- Increased concentration of counter-regulatory hormones, e.g. epinephrine, cortisone, and glucagon
- Acidemia promoting catabolism of proteins and amino-acids
- Increased protein catabolism if energy intake is inadequate and
- Nutritional loss during dialysis.

Therefore, issues, which need to be addressed in AKI, are volume overload due to impaired excretory function, metabolic acidosis, hyperkalemia, hypocalcemia, anorexia, poor nutritional intake, hyperglycemia, hypoalbuminemia and infection. RRT should be initiated when life-threatening changes in fluid, electrolyte, and acid-base balance exist. Quantification of extracellular and intracellular volume expansion using bioimpedance technique can be useful in achieving dry weight. Correct interstitial edema by correcting plasma colloid osmotic pressure in order to prevent hypotension during HD. For initial management for expansion of intravascular volume (deficit), use isotonic crystalloids rather than colloids (albumin or starches) in the absence of hemorrhagic shock. However, for patients requiring additional fluid use colloids (albumin). SAFE study has shown that patients treated with albumin received 27% less fluid compared to the saline arm (2247 vs 3096 mL) and were approximately 1 liter less positive in overall fluid balance. Judicious use of loop diuretics for removal of excessive fluid is warranted as overuse can cause electrolyte imbalance such as hypokalemia, hypernatremia and lead to worsening of renal functions and altered sensorium.

When to Initiate Nutritional Support

Renal failure can impair gastrointestinal motility. If a patient has had little or no nutritional intake for 2 weeks, malnutrition is impending. Initiate nutritional support if patient is undernourished for one week or less. Evidence that a patient is malnourished includes poor nutritional intake accompanied by unintentional weight loss or low body weight. Patients with renal injury frequently require volume restriction. If oral feeding is not possible, then enteral feeding (tube feeding) should be initiated within 24 hours.

Enteral Feeding

It may be more difficult in patients with AKI because of impaired gastrointestinal motility and decreased absorption of nutrients secondary to bowel edema. Avoid hyperosmolar enteral nutrition as it predisposes patients to diarrhea or symptoms similar to dumping syndrome if it is infused rapidly. Overnight supplement can improve in nutritional status and overall well-being. Initiate bolus feeding with 50–100 mL and then increase to 300–400 mL per feeding. Continuous feeding should be started with 20–50 mL/hour, followed by 20 mL increase every 2–8 hours. until desired requirement is achieved. Check patient's gastric residual volume prior to increasing the infusion rate. Discontinue infusion if gastric residual volume exceeds 150–250 mL.

Parenteral Nutrition

If gastrointestinal tract cannot be used, or when enteral nutrition appears inadequate to reach nutrient intake goals parenteral nutrition should be initiated. Glucose should be used as the main energy substrate. Glucose intake must be restricted to 3–5 g/kg/day. Neutralize with insulin if required. Parenteral solutions containing both essential amino acids and nonessential amino acids should be used. Provide a portion of the energy by lipid emulsions to reduce risk of developing hyperglycemia. Usually, 1 g fat/kg/day will not increase plasma triglycerides substantially. Total parenteral nutrition (TPN) is associated with increased infectious complications and is significantly more expensive than enteral feedings. Use products with antioxidants and omega-3 fatty acids in a feeding product may have an anti-inflammatory effect.

Gastroparesis characterized by delayed gastric emptying and upper gastrointestinal symptoms can be present in both diabetic and nondiabetic patients. Management of diabetic gastroparesis (DG) should be focused on maintaining good control of blood sugar, hydration, and nutrition, controlling symptoms of delayed gastric emptying. Fullness and bloating are suggestive of delayed emptying and hence DG. In diabetic patients, maintain glucose levels below 180 mg/dL. Advise small meals at frequent intervals that consist of low-fat and complex carbohydrates. Medium-chain triglycerides do not delay gastric emptying to the same extent as common fat does therefore meals containing fat should be avoided. Advise high-calorie liquid supplements if patient is not in fluid overload. Parenteral nutrition may be needed to supply dietary requirements temporarily in severe cases. Use prokinetic drugs, antiemetic agent is advocated to control symptoms of gastroparesis.

Control Hyperglycemia, Insulin Resistance and Hyperinsulinemia

Patients with renal insufficiency have a certain degree of glucose intolerance. Although most patients are euglycemic when fasting, glucose intolerance occurs after oral or intravascular glucose loads. The abnormal glucose metabolism of patients with renal insufficiency is characterized by fasting euglycemia, abnormal glucose intolerance, a delayed decrease in blood glucose in response to insulin, hyperinsulinemia and hyperglucagonemia. A deficiency of calcitriol can contribute to the resistance of peripheral tissues to insulin. Leptin plays an important role in regulating food intake and energy expenditure; its main target is the hypothalamus. Levels of free leptins are generally increased when correlated with body mass in patients with CKD and also correlate with low EPO levels and insulin resistance. The amount and type of carbohydrate (CHO) in food influence blood glucose levels. There are two approaches to manage CHO intake: keep amount of CHO constant and CHO counting. A fixed CHO meal plan is useful for patients who use only diet to control their blood sugar or who are on fixed doses of insulin or other hypoglycemics. In this approach amount of CHO intake is kept constant and the timing of food intake is fixed. Patients, who follow CHO counting method, adjust insulin according to intake. This approach requires good understanding of CHO amount in food item.

SUMMARY

- PEW is a major challenge in CKD patients. A holistic approach to treatment of underlying causes like inflammation, infection, dialysis adequacy and dietary intake is the key to preventing deterioration of renal function.
- To replenish losses of protein in the dialysate ONS are indispensable. They have major role to play in maintenance of amino acid pool and improve nutritional status.
- Identify nutritional deficiencies before they become clinically evident. Assess appetite using tools like appetite and diet assessment tool (ADAT), subjective global assessment (SGA) or kidney disease quality of life-short form
- Prevent MA with bicarbonate supplementation.
- Counsel patient on every visit on dietary intake. Dedicated dietician should stay in touch with the patients through telephonic conversations once in a fortnight in order to motivate the patient to eat well.

Multiple Choice Questions

True or False

1. **A 40-year-old male with chronic kidney disease, diabetes and hypertension, serum creatinine 3.6 mg/dL, serum albumin 2.9 g/dL and 4+ proteinuria presents with anorexia, and generalized edema. Nutritional management will include:**
   a. Protein intake less than 0.6 g/kg/day
   b. Protein intake to 1.2 g/kg/day
   c. Advise protein intake 0.6 g/kg/day plus 1 g of protein lost in urine
   d. Advise oral supplement if dietary intake is <20 kcal/kg/day
   e. Give loop diuretic furosemide 40 mg twice a day

2. **A 6-year-old child presents with edema, 4 g proteinuria, total cholesterol 300 mg/dL and blood pressure 130/90 mm Hg. Management will include:**
   a. A liberal fluid intake
   b. Protein intake to recommended dietary allowance for chronological age
   c. Restrict salt to <2 g/day
   d. Advise dietary cholesterol 300 mg/day
   e. Restrict protein intake

3. **An 8-year-old child presents with facial puffiness, pedal edema, short stature and blood pressure 128/95 mm Hg and 4+ proteinuria. Management will include:**
   a. No antihypertensive medication as blood pressure is normal for age
   b. Advise 4.0 g salt/day
   c. Advise fat intake more than 60 g/day to improve calorie intake
   d. Restrict salt intake and fluid intake
   e. Advise protein intake according to recommended dietary allowance for chronological age

4. **An 8-year-old postrenal transplant patient on triple immunosuppression (prednisolone, tacrolimus and MMF) has serum creatinine of 0.8 mg/dL, blood pressure 110/70 mm Hg, hemoglobin of 12.5 g/dL, serum albumin 3.5 g/dL, serum calcium 6 mg/dL and pedal edema. Management will include:**
   a. Protein intake 0.8 g/kg/day
   b. Restrict dietary calcium intake
   c. Increase fluid intake
   d. Advise grape fruit juice
   e. Restrict fluid intake

5. **A 32-year-old male presents with bilateral small sized kidney, with facial puffiness, generalized weakness, pedal edema, decreased urine output, blood pressure 140/95 mm Hg, serum creatinine 4.3 mg/dL, serum calcium 6.4 mg/dL, serum phosphate 5.8 mg/dL and 4+ proteinuria. Management will include:**
   a. Fluid restriction according to 24 hours urine output
   b. Advise intake of 6 g of sodium
   c. Protein intake should be 0.6 g/kg/day
   d. Correct serum calcium with calcium supplement taken with meals
   e. Advise calcium supplements between two meals or on empty stomach and non calcium based phosphate binder with meals

6. **A 20-year-old female presents with postpartum acute kidney injury. She is edematous, oliguric with serum creatinine of 7.9 mg/dL, blood pressure 135/90 mm Hg, hemoglobin of 6.5 g/dL, serum albumin 3.2 g/dL and serum calcium 6.6 mg/dL. Management will include:**
   a. Liberal fluid intake
   b. Increase protein intake to 1.3–1.5 g/kg/day
   c. Restrict protein intake to 0.6 g/kg/day
   d. Give blood transfusion to correct anemia
   e. Recommend oral protein supplement and intradialytic parenteral nutrition

7. **A 47-year-old postrenal transplant patient presents with severe pain abdomen, diarrhea, high grade fever, raised serum amylase and lipase, rise in serum creatinine from 1.6 mg/dL to 2.5 mg/dL, hemoglobin 13.5/dL, and serum sodium 129 mmol/L, serum potassium 2.9 mmol/L. Urine output is 3000 mL. Management will include:**
   a. Oral protein supplements
   b. Stop oral feeds
   c. Administer intravenous fluids
   d. Provide parenteral nutrition
   e. Supplement potassium chloride and sodium

8. A 46-year-old postrenal transplant patient with chronic allograft nephropathy on triple immunosuppressive medication has serum creatinine of 3.6 mg/dL, blood pressure 140/90 mm Hg, and hemoglobin 11 g/dL, serum albumin 3.5 g/dL and serum potassium 5 mmol/L. Management will be:
   a. Restrict protein intake to 0.6 g/kg/day
   b. Increase protein intake to 1.2 g/kg/day
   c. Restrict fluid intake according to thirst
   d. Restrict fruits, fruit juices and vegetable soups
   e. Target blood pressure below 120/80 mm Hg

9. A 50-year-old male with end stage kidney disease on continuous ambulatory peritoneal dialysis (CAPD) with two 2.5% and one 1.5% exchanges, presents with body weight 55 kg, generalized edema, mild abdominal pain, high grade fever, loose stools, loss of appetite, blood pressure 110/70 mm Hg, rise in creatinine from 7.2 mg/dL to 12.9 mg/dL, hemoglobin of 10.5 g/dL and serum albumin 2.8 g/dL and serum calcium 7 mg/dL. Management will include:
   a. High protein diet 1.3–1.5 g/kg/day
   b. Advise 0.8 g/kg/day protein intake
   c. Advise oral nutritional supplements
   d. Advise liberal intake of fluid
   e. Consider giving few hemodialysis sessions to bring down serum creatinine and to provide intradialytic parenteral nutrition to improve nutritional status

10. Young children suffering from end-stage-renal disease on maintenance dialysis
   a. Should be advised protein according recommended dietary allowances for age plus extra protein for losses due to dialysis
   b. Protein loss is inversely proportional to body size
   c. Salt intake should not be restricted
   d. Recombinant human growth hormone therapy should be considered if growth is stunted
   e. Supplement zinc, selenium and water soluble vitamins if dietary intake is below recommended allowance

Answers

1. FFTTT 2. FTTFF 3. FFFTT 4. FFFFT 5. TFTFT 6. FTFTT 7. FFTTT
8. TFTTT 9. TFTFT 10. TTFTT

SUGGESTED READING

1. Acchiardo S, Riley M. Five Years Experience with Oral Nutritional Supplements (ONS) In Hemodialysis (HD) Patients (Pts). Are They Useful? J Am Soc Nephrol. 2002;13:415A.
2. Adewale B Ajumobi, Ronald A. Griffin Diabetic Gastroparesis: Evaluation and Management Hospital Physician. 2008. pp. 27-35.
3. Anita Saxena. Approach to Nutritional Management of Chronic Kidney Disease (Protocol 28). Journal of Renal Nutrition and Metabolism. Special issue on Society of Renal Nutrition and Metabolism Protocols for Kidney Diseases, 2015;(2).
4. Anita Saxena. Nutritional Approach to Acute Kidney Injury (Protocol 26). Journal of Renal Nutrition and Metabolism. Special issue on Society of Renal Nutrition and Metabolism Protocols for Kidney Diseases, 2015;(2).

5. Anita Saxena. Nutritional Approach to Nephrotic Syndrome (Protocol 13). Journal of Renal Nutrition and Metabolism. Special issue on Society of Renal Nutrition and Metabolism Protocols for Kidney Diseases, 2015;(2).
6. Anita Saxena. Nutritional Approach to Post Renal Transplant Management (Protocol 35). Journal of Renal Nutrition and Metabolism. Special issue on Society of Renal Nutrition and Metabolism Protocols for Kidney Diseases, 2015;(2).
7. Anita Saxena. Nutritional Approach to Primary Hypertension (Protocol 9). Journal of Renal Nutrition and Metabolism. Special issue on Society of Renal Nutrition and Metabolism Protocols for Kidney Diseases, 2015;(2).
8. Anita Saxena. Nutritional Management of Diabetic nephropathy (Protocol 20). Journal of Renal Nutrition and Metabolism. Special issue on Society of Renal Nutrition and Metabolism Protocols for Kidney Diseases, 2015;(2).
9. Cano N. Clinical Nutrition. ESPEN Guidelines on Enteral Nutrition: Adult Renal Failure. 2006;25:295-310.
10. Caravaca F, Arrobas M, Dominguez C. Influence of residual renal function on dietary protein and caloric intake in patients on incremental peritoneal dialysis. Perit Dial Int. 1999;19:350-6.
11. Carrero JJ, Stenvinkel P, Cuppari L, Ikizler TA. Etiology of the protein-energy wasting syndrome in chronic kidney disease: a consensus statement from the International Society of Renal Nutrition and Metabolism (ISRNM). J Ren Nutr. 2013;23(2):77-90.
12. Chaudhary K, Khanna R. Biocompatible peritoneal dialysis solutions: do we have one? Clinical Journal of the American Society of Nephrology. 2010;5(4):723-32.
13. Christian Faul, Ansel P. Amaral, Behzad Oskouei, Ming-Chang Hu. FGF23 induces left ventricular hypertrophy J Clin Invest. 2011;121(11):4393-408.
14. Eustace JA, Coresh J, Kutchey C, et al. Randomized double-blind trial of oral essential amino acids for dialysis-associated hypoalbuminemia. Kidney Int. 2000;57:2527.
15. Finfer SR, Bellomo R, Boyce NW, French J, Myburgh J, Norton RN. SAFE Study Investigators: Comparison of Albumin and Saline for Fluid Resuscitation in the Intensive Care Unit. N Engl J Med. 2004;350:2247-56.
16. Fouque D, Kalantar-Zadeh K, Kopple J, Cano N, Chauveau P, Cuppari L, et al. A proposed nomenclature and diagnostic criteria for protein-energy wasting in acute and chronic kidney disease. Kidney Int. 2008;73:391-8.
17. Han SH, Han DH. Nutrition in patients on peritoneal dialysis. Nature Reviews Nephrology. 2012;8:163-75.
18. Implications of the Canada–USA (CANUSA) study of the adequacy of dialysis on peritoneal dialysis schedule NDT. 1998;13(Suppl 6):158-63.
19. Joel D Kopple, Tom Greene W Cameroon Chumlea. Modification of Diet in Renal Disease Study Group. Relationship between nutritional status and the glomerular filtration rate: Results from the MDRD Study Kidney International. 2000;57:1688-703.
20. Kalantar-Zadeh K. Recent advances in understanding the malnutrition-inflammation-cachexia syndrome in chronic kidney disease patients: What is next? Semin Dial. 2005;18(5):365-9.
21. KDOQI. Clinical Practice Guideline for Nutrition in Children with CKD: 2008 update. Executive summary. Am J Kidney Dis. 2009;53(3 Suppl 2):S11-104.
22. KDOQI. Clinical Practice Guidelines for Nutrition in Chronic Kidney Disease. AJKD, 2000;35(6)Suppl 2.

23. Kim SG, Kim S, Hwang YH, Kim K, Oh JE, Chung W, et al. Korean Balnet Study Group. Could solutions low in glucose degradation products preserve residual renal function in incident peritoneal dialysis patients? A 1-year multicenter prospective randomized controlled trial (Balnet Study). Perit Dial Int. 2008;28(Suppl 3):S117-22.
24. Kris-Etherton PM, Harris WS, Appel LJ. Fish consumption, fish oil, omega-3 fatty acids and cardiovascular disease. Circulation. 2002;106:2747-57.
25. Li FK, Chan LY, Woo JC, Ho SK, Lo WK, Lai KN, et al. A 3-year, prospective, randomized, controlled study on amino acid dialysate in patients on CAPD. Am J Kidney Dis. 2003;42(1):173-83.
26. Macias WL, Alaka KJ, Murphy MH, et al. Impact of nutritional regimen on protein catabolism and nitrogen balance in patients with acute renal failure. J Parenter Enteral Nutr. 1996;20:56-62.
27. Mitch WE, Clark AS. Specificity of the effects of leucine and its metabolism on protein degradation in skeletal muscle, 1984.
28. Mitch WE, Walser M, Steinman TL, Hill S, Zeger S, Tungsanga K. The effect of a keto amino acid supplement to a restricted diet on the progression of chronic renal failure. N Engl J Med. 1984;311:623-9.
29. Myles Wolf. Update on Fibroblast Growth Factor 23. In Chronic Kidney Disease Kidney Int. 2012;82(7):737-47.
30. Saxena Anita, Sharma RK, Gupta Amit. Association of water compartments with hypertension in non-edematous renal transplant recipients. Indian Journal of Transplantation. 2012;6(2);39-45.
31. Scheinkestel CD, Adams F, Mahony L, et al. Impact of increasing parenteral protein loads on amino acid balance in critically ill anuric patients on continuous renal replacement therapy. Nutrition. 2003;19:733-40.
32. Sheard NF, Calrk NG, Brand-Miller JC, et al. Dietary carbohydrate (amount and type) in the prevention and management of diabetes: a statement of American Diabetes Association. Diabetes Care. 2004;27:2226-71.
33. Stenvinkel P[1], Heimbürger O, Lindholm B, Kaysen GA, Bergström J. Are there two types of malnutrition in chronic renal failure? Evidence for relationships between malnutrition, inflammation and atherosclerosis (MIA syndrome). Nephrol Dial Transplant. 2000;15(7):953-60.
34. Taylor GS, Patel V, Spencer S, Fluck RJ, McIntyre CW. Long-term use of 1.1% amino acid dialysis solution in hypoalbuminemic continuous ambulatory peritoneal dialysis patients. Clin Nephrol. 2002;58(6):445-50.
35. The SAFE Study Investigators. Saline or albumin for fluid resuscitation in patients with traumatic brain injury. N Engl J Med. 2007;357(9):874-84.
36. Wang AY. Energy intake and energy expenditure profiles in peritoneal dialysis patients. J Ren Nutr. 2011;21(1):31-4.
37. Wang AY, Sanderson J, Sea MM, et al. Important factors other than dialysis adequacy associated with inadequate dietary protein and energy intakes in patients receiving maintenance peritoneal dialysis. Am J Clin Nutr. 2003;77:834-41.
38. Wilfred Druml. Nutritional management of acute renal failure. J of Renal Nutr. 2005;15(1):63-70.
39. Yashpal P Jadeja, Vijay Kher. Protein energy wasting in chronic kidney disease: An update with focus on nutritional interventions to improve outcomes. Indian J Endocrinol Metab. 2012;16(2):246-51.
40. Zoccali C. The obesity epidemics in ESRD: from wasting to waist? Nephrol Dial Transplant. 2009;24:376-80.

CHAPTER

14

Drug Dosing in Renal Diseases

R Kasi Viswesaran

INTRODUCTION

All substances irrespective of whether they are obtained from nature, plant products or synthesized in a facility are chemical compounds. When these chemical substances are administered, they exert their actions on the body. Drugs are the chemicals used for treatment and should reach the target for its specific action to exert the desired effects with no complications. Since it is not possible to target all drugs to their specific site of action, they may cause harm to normal cells and side effects. This is particularly true of anticancer drugs, most of which cause damage to normal cells as well. The drugs are mainly eliminated by the kidneys although the gastrointestinal, skin or respiratory systems are also involved in drug elimination to some extent.

A clinician should have basic understanding of how much of the oral drug is reaching the bloodstream (*bioavailability*), how much is bound to plasma proteins (protein binding), how much is distributed in the body fluids (*volume of distribution*), how the body handles the drug (*pharmacokinetics and metabolism*), what the drugs do to the body (*pharmacodynamics*), and method of elimination of the drug. In the case of drugs given orally, the absorbed drugs pass through the liver first before reaching the systemic circulation. Some drug may be metabolized in the liver before reaching the systemic circulation. This is called '*first pass metabolism*'. If there is significant first pass metabolism, the bio availability will be lower. Intravenously administered drugs have 100% bioavailability. The half-life of a drug is the time taken for the blood level to reduce by 50%. The half-life of each substance is variable. Those with short half life will have a short duration of action and if it is long, obviously, the duration of action will be longer and only less frequent dosing will be necessary. Short acting barbiturates used for induction of anesthesia have a very short half-life and the action ceases shortly after the injection is stopped. Long acting barbiturates on the other hand act for many hours and have long half-life. It is possible to modify the half-life of drugs to suit the requirement at the manufacturing level. The typical example is addition of substances to the crystalline insulin to prolong the duration of action, e.g. protamine zinc insulin, lente insulin, neutral protamine Hagedorn (NPH) insulin, insulin degludec, insulin glargine, and insulin detemir.

Therapeutic window represents the area between minimum therapeutic and minimum toxic blood level of the drug **(Fig. 14.1)**. If the drug level is below, its effectiveness is diminished and if it is above the minimum toxic level, the side effects are higher **(Figs 14.2A and B)**.

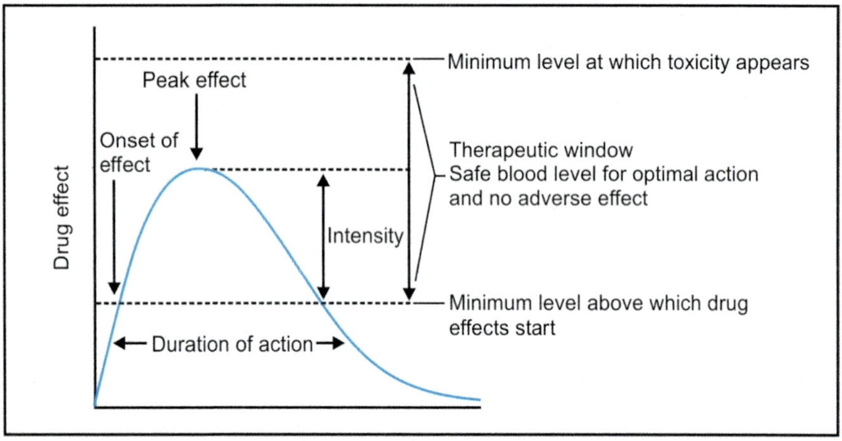

Figure 14.1 Time Therapeutic window (safe blood level between the minimum therapeutic level and minimum toxic level)

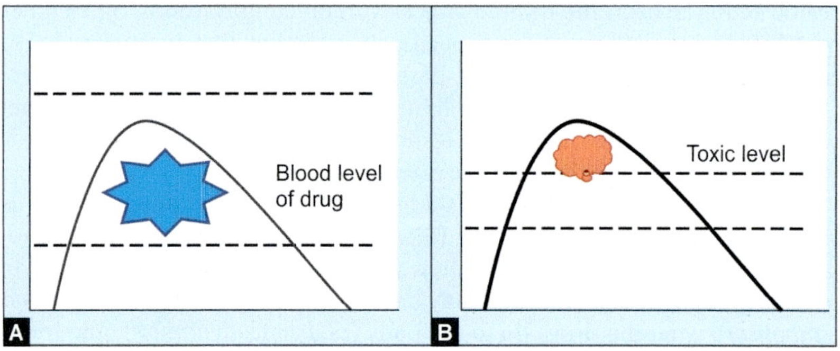

Figures 14.2A and B Wide and narrow therapeutic window: (A) Wide therapeutic range; (B) Narrow therapeutic range

VULNERABILITY OF KIDNEYS

The kidneys are important organs for metabolizing drugs and eliminating them from the body. They are highly vulnerable organs to ischemic and toxic insults because of several unique features and events that occur in them. They include:

- Unique features
  - *Blood flow per gram of renal tissue:* Among the organs, kidneys receive the maximum amount of blood per gram of tissue every minute (weight approximately 300 g and blood flow rate about 1200 mL/min = 4 mL/gram renal tissue/minute). In comparison, the brain and the liver get only about 1 mL/gram/minute (1500 g weight and 1500 mL/min). Thus more of the drug reaches the kidney.
  - *Endothelial surface area:* The renal circulation is peculiar because there are 2 sets of capillary systems between the arteriole and venule, the glomerular capillary and peritubular capillaries. The glomerular capillary endothelium enables formation of 180 L of filtrate and the peritubular capillary is involved in reabsorption of nearly 179 L of the filtrate. Since the filtrate contains

various molecules which have to be reabsorbed or eliminated, the large endothelial surface area is subjected to stress due to transport of molecules across.

- *Metabolic activity and oxygen requirement of tubular cells:* The renal tubular cells are one of the most metabolically active cells in the body. The cells in the proximal tubule and the thick ascending limb of the loop of Henle are metabolically very active and have high oxygen demand.
- *Medullary circulation:* Inside the kidney, the cortex receives 90% of the blood. The blood perfusing the renal medulla is derived from the efferent arterioles of mainly the juxtamedullary glomeruli.
- *Medullary osmolality:* The countercurrent mechanisms maintain the high medullary interstitial osmolality which is essential for the formation of concentrated urine. Therefore, the solute (drug/toxin/urea) concentration achieved in the medullary region is high.
- *Role of vasoactive compounds:* Vasoactive compounds regulate the renal blood flow, maintain autoregulation and glomerular filtration rate (GFR). Extraneously administered compounds or drugs which suppress endogenous production of vasoactive hormones can cause renal damage. Prostaglandin F2alpha, which is produced in the renal medulla in response to diminished GFR, causes afferent arteriolar vasodilatation thereby helping to maintain GFR.

- The events occurring inside the kidney contributing its vulnerability to damage are:
  - *Glomerular filtration:* As the blood travels along the glomeruli, filtration occurs @ 120 mL/min. If the drug is filtered, it reaches the tubule in higher concentration than blood. If it is not filtered, it reaches the peritubular capillary network in a higher concentration compared to the filtrate.
  - *Tubular reabsorption/secretion and transcellular transport:* If the filtered drug is reabsorbed in the tubule, the concentration inside the cell becomes high. For example, gentamicin is filtered by the glomeruli and reabsorbed in the proximal tubular cell where it is stored as myeloid bodies best seen by electron microscopy. So, cumulative dosing may result in nephrotoxicity. If the drug is not subjected to tubular reabsorption, water reabsorption along the nephron causes increase in luminal concentration by nearly 100 fold. Some antibiotics exhibiting this type of pharmacokinetics are preferred for the treatment of urinary tract infections because of the high urinary concentration achieved (e.g. Nitrofurantoin). Some drugs which are not freely filtered are secreted into the tubule through transcellular transport. Drugs like furosemide are secreted into the proximal tubule through the organic anion transport system from where they travel through the tubular lumen to their site of action in the thick ascending limb of the loop of Henle.
  - *Enzymatic activity:* Many enzymes are involved in the normal functioning of the kidney. Drugs may damage or inactivate the enzyme systems thereby impairing renal function.
  - *Protein binding and uncoupling:* Some drugs which are protein bound remain inactive but when they are uncoupled from protein link, they become active. Since many drugs are handled by the kidney, uncoupling of protein bound drug may cause renal damage.

AGE-RELATED DECLINE IN RENAL FUNCTION AND IMPORTANCE OF GLOMERULAR FILTRATION RATE

The glomerular filtration rate (GFR) is a more reliable measure of kidney function compared to serum creatinine level. It is better to assess the GFR by the bedside using one of the commonly available formulas. Calculations based on Cockcroft-Gault formula, Chronic Kidney Disease Epidemiology Collaboration (CKD-EPI) formula and Modification of Diet in Renal Disease (MDRD) formulas are now easily available on line and offline and help to assess GFR by the bedside before prescribing. MDRD formulas are more reliable in children and the aged. Ideally, the GFR should be entered in the file together with vital signs, height, weight, body surface area and BMI. From the age of 30–35 onwards, even in normal persons, the GFR falls from the normal values of approximately 120 mL/min at the rate of 0.75–1 mL/minute/year steadily and gradually thereafter. Therefore, the normal GFR of a 60-year-old person may be in the range of 90 mL/min, a 90-year-old about 60 mL/min and so on. Since the symptoms of uremia manifest only in stage 3 of CKD (< 30 mL/min), an old person does not develop uremic symptoms during normal life span. The serum creatinine may not increase corresponding to low GFR because of the reduced muscle mass in old age. The 'normal' creatinine level may tempt the clinician to order an adult dose of drugs for an older patient as well **(Box 14.1)**.

The drug handling capacity of the kidney decreases as the GFR declines and care should be taken while deciding the dose of drugs in renal failure. Dosing in renal failure should therefore take into consideration the GFR and not the age or serum creatinine alone. The importance of low GFR in old age is often overlooked in clinical practice.

Although individual drugs may not have exhibited nephrotoxicity in short term trials, long-term studies with the use of multiple drugs or combinations are not available. These combinations could potentially harm the kidney over a long time. Long-term use of NSAIDs like even aspirin may manifest as renal failure only when combined with a hypotensive episode or concurrent administration of other potentially nephrotoxic drugs. Cumulative dosing and unsupervised, long term 'polypharmacy' may lead to renal damage.

GLOMERULAR FILTRATION RATE IN RENAL DISEASES

Changes in GFR in acute kidney injury and chronic kidney disease (CKD) have been explained in respective chapters. GFR below 60 mL/min even in the absence of structural or other functional abnormalities is an independent

Box 14.1 Examples of eGFR calculation by 3 methods in 2 different case scenarios

1. Case 1→ Male	Age—40 years,	Weight—80 kg, Serum creatinine—1 mg%	
2. Case 2→ Female	Age—70 years,	Weight—50 kg, Serum creatinine—1 mg%	
GFR calculated by:	CG formula	CKD-EPI (off. line)	MDRD (off. line)
1. Case 1	111 mL/min	93.73 mL/min/1.73 m^2	82.8 mL/min/1.73 m^2
2. Case 2	48.6 mL/min	57.03 mL/min/1.73 m^2	54.8 mL/min/1.73 m^2

Note the marked decrease in eGFR for the same level of serum creatinine in the 2 cases. Note that the age, sex and body weight are different.

Abbreviations: eGFR, estimated glomerular filtration rate; CG, cockcroft-Gault; CKD-EPI, chronic kidney disease-epidemiology; MDRD, modification of diet in renal disease

criterion for the diagnosis of CKD (stage 3). The recent classification has further subdivided stage 3 into 3a (45–59 mL/min) and 3b (30–44 mL/min). [Please see the chapter on CKD for more details].

MECHANISMS OF DRUG-INDUCED RENAL DAMAGE

Drugs can cause renal damage in many ways. As with all diseases, the mechanisms of damage can be approached as pre-renal, intrinsic renal and post-renal. The pre-renal mechanisms are applicable mainly to drugs causing:

- Hyper-catabolism/anti-anabolism, e.g. steroids, tetracyclines
- Reduction of blood volume, e.g. diuretics, aquaretics.
- Reduction of blood pressure, e.g. hypotensive agents
- Vascular thrombosis, e.g. oral contraceptives
- Hemodynamic changes: Hemodynamic injury can be caused by imbalance between the vasoconstrictive and vasodilatory autocoids which are synthesized and metabolized in the kidney. They are mainly the prostaglandins and Thromboxane A2 (TxA2). The cyclo-oxygenase isoenzymes COX 1 and COX 2 are involved in prostaglandin production. Drugs inhibiting this system can lead to impaired autoregulation of renal circulation and hemodynamically mediated injury, e.g. nonsteroidal anti-inflammatory drugs (NSAIDs), angiotensin-converting enzyme inhibitors (ACEIs).

Among the mechanisms affecting the intrarenal systems, the following are important (only a few examples are given in each).

- Immune-mediated damage to blood vessels—vasculitis, e.g. microscopic polyarteritis
- Immune-mediated damage to glomeruli, e.g. penicillamine.
- Hemoglobinuria/myoglobinuria causing acute tubular necrosis, e.g. antimalarials
- Acute damage to tubulointerstitium, e.g. gold, penicillamine
- Chronic damage to tubulointerstitium, e.g. analgesic abuse
- Direct tubular toxicity, e.g. aminoglycosides, amphotericin, cisplatin, mercuric chloride)
- Patchy/cortical necrosis, e.g. arsenic, high dose gentamicin
- Renal papillary necrosis, e.g. analgesics

The postrenal causes are mainly those causing obstruction to the urinary flow. The important ones are:

- Intratubular obstruction due to crystals, e.g. indinavir, acyclovir, triamterene, sulfonamides.
- Stones causing obstructive uropathy, e.g. triamterene, chemotherapeutic agents (causing tumor lysis and urate sludge blocking ureters)
- Retroperitoneal fibrosis, e.g. hydralazine, methysergide
- Ureteric block due to sloughed papilla, e.g. analgesics
- Bleeding and blood clots, e.g. anticoagulants, cyclophosphamide (hemorrhagic cystitis).

Principles and Methods of Drug Dosing in Renal Failure

Drugs which are primarily excreted by the kidneys need modification of doses depending on the kidney function. The decrease in the dose depends on the severity or renal failure as assessed by estimated GFR. Elderly individuals and females require much lower doses as compared to the standard adult dose. The dose modifications may be made by many methods and formulas. It is necessary for the clinician to be familiar with one set of calculations or formulas and use them judiciously. In the case of most drugs, the drug information pamphlet available in the packing may be used to decide dose modifications based on eGFR.

The first dose of most drugs even in patients who are in renal failure is the same as the dose for those with normal renal function of the same age, sex and body weight. This is called the loading dose and is independent of the degree of renal dysfunction. It helps to achieve therapeutic blood level early. The subsequent doses are based on the degree of renal dysfunction, extrarenal elimination, pharmacodynamic and pharmacokinetic properties of the drug. The dose modification is to maintain the blood level of the drug in the therapeutic range. If the drug has a narrow therapeutic window, the gap between the minimum therapeutic dose and minimum toxic dose is narrow and very careful monitoring is necessary.

Assuming that the nonrenal clearance is unchanged, the dose of drugs excreted by the kidney should be reduced in proportion to the degree of renal dysfunction. The main principle is highlighted with two examples.

1. If the kidney function is 25% of normal (eGFR around 25 mL/min) and the drug is excreted 100% by the kidneys, the maintenance dose will be 25% of the loading dose.
2. If the kidney function is 25% of normal (eGFR around 25 mL/min), and the drug is excreted 50% by the kidneys, and 50% extrarenally, the maintenance dose will be 50% (representing full dose for nonrenal excretion) + 25% of 50% (modified dose for renal excretion) = 50 +12.5 = 62.5%—rounded off to 60% of the dose.

Therapeutic drug monitoring (TDM) to periodically assess the drug level in blood is ideal but not practical. It is used when a drug with narrow therapeutic window is used. TDM is usually used while using drugs like immunosuppressive drugs, aminoglycosides, digoxin, lithium and antiepileptic drugs. The timing of blood sampling is important while monitoring TDM. For most drugs, the trough level has to be maintained and in those cases, the sample is drawn just before the next dose of the drug becomes due. To assess the peak level, the sample is to be taken at the prescribed time after drug administration.

Most drug studies have assessed only the short and medium term toxicities of the drugs before marketing. The prolonged use for many years has not been fully evaluated in them. Therefore, delayed toxicity may occur and clinicians should be aware of the same. Similarly, combination of drugs, which may not be highly nephrotoxic independently or dose has been modified appropriately may eventually be nephrotoxic because of the combination. This can be highlighted by a few common examples of combinations in clinical practice—aminoglycosides with second-generation cephalosporins, acyclovir with aminoglycosides/vancomycin, NSAIDs with ACE inhibitors, NSAIDs with radiocontrast agents. The 4 important groups of drugs, which are commonly used and cause nephrotoxicity are aminoglycosides, NSAIDs, ACE inhibitors/A2RBs, and radiocontrast agents—together called the 'Nephrotoxic Quartet'.

Table 14.1 shows the dose modifications for the different commonly used groups of drugs acting on different systems and at different levels of renal dysfunction. The table gives a simplified view. For accurate calculation of individual drugs, please refer to the drug information pamphlet accompanying the packing.

Table 14.1 Drug dosing of antihypertensive drugs

Group of drugs	*Pharmacological name*	*Percentage of dose for glomerular filtration rate (GFR)*			*Remarks*
Subgroup		*>50 mL/min*	*10–50 mL/min*	*<10 mL/ min*	
Antihypertensive drugs					
ACE inhibitors	Captopril Enalapril Ramipril Lisinopril Perindopril	100	75	50/avoid	
	Fosinopril	100	100	75	
A2 RB	Losartan Telmisartan Valsartan Irbesartan Candesartan	100	100	100	Monitor response and potassium level
	Olmesartan	100	100	50	
Direct renin inhibitors	Aliskiren	50	25	Avoid	
Beta blockers	Carvedilol Esmolol Labetalol Metoprolol Propranolol Timolol Pindolol	100	100	100	No modification
	Bisoprolol Atenolol and other beta blockers	100 100	75 50	50 25	Atenolol accumulates in ESRD
Adrenergic modulators	Clonidine Guanabenz Doxazosin Prazosin Terazosin	100	100	100	No modification
	Methyldopa	100	50	25	Increase dosing interval
Vasodialators	Diazoxide (IV) Sodium nitroprusside	100	100	Avoid	
	Minoxidil	50	50	25	To regulae dose by assessing response
Calcium channel blockers		100	100	100	No dose modification

Contd...

Contd...

Group of drugs	*Pharmacological name*	*Percentage of dose for glomerular filtration rate (GFR)*			*Remarks*
Subgroup		*>50 mL/min*	*10–50 mL/min*	*<10 mL/min*	
Diuretics	Furosemide Torsemide Indapamide Metolazone Bumetanide	100	100	100	Loop diuretics like furosemide has to compete with organic anion transport system to be secreted into proximal tubule and reach its site of action. Higher doses are often required in renal failure.
	Thiazides Spironolactone Amiloride Triamterene Acetazolamide and others	100	50	Avoid	Thiazides—ineffective Spironolactone—hyperkalemia Acetazolamide—weak
Antiarrhythmic drugs	Amiodarone Propafenone	100	100	100	No change except hypothyroidism
Nitrates	Isosorbide Nitroglycerine	100	100	100	No modification
Inotropic agents	Dopamine Dobutamine	100	100	100	No modification
Antidiabetic drugs	Insulins	100	75	50	Dose depends on response. Action of endogenous and exogenous insulins are prolonged because of impaired renal degradation of insulin in the kidneys

Contd...

Contd...

Group of drugs	*Pharmacological name*	*Percentage of dose for glomerular filtration rate (GFR)*			*Remarks*
Subgroup		*>50 mL/min*	*10–50 mL/min*	*<10 mL/ min*	
Oral	Voglibose Glipizide Glimepiride Gliclazide Metformin Miglitol Acarbose	 100 100	 100 50 25	 50 Avoid Avoid Avoid Avoid Avoid	Use with caution Glimepiride— Start low-dose and titrate
	Chlorpropamide Acetohexamide Glyburide Tolbutamide	Avoid 50–75 100	Avoid Avoid Avoid 100	Avoid Avoid Avoid 100	
Lipid lowering drugs	Simvastatin Lovastatin Pravastatin Gemfibrozil Cholestyramine Probucol	100	100	100	No modification
	Benzafibrate Nicotinic acid	100	50	25	Flushing with nicotinic acid
	Clofibrate Fenofibrate	100	50	Avoid	
Antineoplastic drugs	Busulfan Cytarabine Daunorubicin Doxorubicin Fluorouracil Paclitaxel Tamoxifen Vincristine Vinblastin	100	100	75	
	Mitomycin C	100	75	50	
	Cyclophosphamide	100	100	75	
	Bleomycin Cisplatin Etopiside Melphalan Nitrosuria Idarubicin	100	50	25	
	Streptozocin	100	50	Avoid	
	Hydroxyurea	100	50	50	
	Carboplatin	100	75	50	
	Methotrexate	100	50	Avoid	

Contd...

Contd...

Group of drugs	*Pharmacological name*	*Percentage of dose for glomerular filtration rate (GFR)*			*Remarks*
Subgroup		*>50 mL/min*	*10–50 mL/min*	*<10 mL/min*	
Common antibiotics					For most antibiotics, initial dose is the regular dose. Maintenance dose is modified for the remaining course after initial loading dose
Penicillin group					
Oral penicillins	Penicillin V Ampicillin Amoxycillin Dicloxacillin	100 100 100 100	100 100 100 100	75 75 75 75	
Parenteral penicillins	Penicillin G Piperacillin/ Tazobactam Ticarcillin/ clavulunate	100 100 100	75 75 66	50 50 33	
Cephalosporins					
Oral cephalosporins	Cephalexin Cefpodoxime Cefuroxime Cefadroxil Cefradine Cefixime	100 100 100 100 100 100	100 100 100 100 100 100	100 100 100 50 50 50	
Parenteral	Cefoperazone Cefazolin Ceftazidime Cephaotaxine Cefuroxime	100 100 100 100 100	100 66 66 66 66	100 33 33 33 33	
Carbapenems	Imipenem/ cilastatin Ertapenem Doripenem Meropenem	75 100 100 100	33 50 50 66	25 Avoid 25 33	
Monobactam	Aztreonam	100	50	25	
Quinolones	Moxifloxacin Ciprofloxacin (oral) Ciprofloxacin (intravenous) Ofloxacin Norfloxacin	100 100 100 100 100	100 50 66 66 66	100 50 33 33 33	

Contd...

Contd...

Group of drugs	*Pharmacological name*	*Percentage of dose for glomerular filtration rate (GFR)*			*Remarks*
Subgroup		*>50 mL/min*	*10–50 mL/min*	*<10 mL/ min*	
Macrolides	Erythromycin Clarithromycin Azithromycin	100 100 100	100 100 100	100 100 100	
Lincosamides	Clindamycin	100	100	100	
Aminoglyco-sides	Gentamicin Kanamycin	75 75	50 50	25 25	Monitor dose with therapeutic dose monitoring (TDM)
	Amikacin Tobramycin Streptomycin Netilmicin	75 75 75 75	50 50 50 50	25 25 25 25	Half of full dose after hemodialysis Additional dose reduction in old age
Oxazolidi-nones	Linezolid	100	100	100	Myelosuppres-sion
Cationic polypeptides	Polymyxin E (colistin) Polymyxin B	100 100	100 75	100 25	Oral
Glycopep-tides	Vancomycin (oral)	100	100	100	Only for oral GFR < 10 half
	Vancomycin (intravenous)	100	25	12	On hemodialy-sis—1/2 dose af-ter hemodialysis only dose every week. GFR < 10 half dose every week.
Other antibiotics	Chloramphenicol Minocycline Tigecycline Tetracycline Doxycycline Nitrofurantoin Metronidazol Tinidazole Ornidazole	100 100 100 Aviod 100 100 100 100 100	100 100 100 Avoid 100 Avoid 100 100 100	100 100 100 Avoid Avoid Avoid 100 100 100	Hypercatabolic Ineffective in renal failure.
	TMP/ SMZ	100	50	50	Trimethoprim/ Sulphameth-oxazol

Contd...

Contd...

Group of drugs	*Pharmacological name*	*Percentage of dose for glomerular filtration rate (GFR)*			*Remarks*
Subgroup		*>50 mL/min*	*10–50 mL/min*	*<10 mL/min*	
Antiviral drugs					
Oral	Indinavir	100	100	100	Crystalluria,
	Zidovudine	100	100	100	nephrolithiasis,
	Acyclovir	100	100	50	AKI
	Ribavirin	100	100	50	Oral only for
	Ganciclovir	100	66	33	prophylaxis
	Lamivudine	100	50	25	
	Valaganciclovir	100	50	25	TTP, HUS
	Cidofovir	Avoid	Avoid	Avoid	
Intravenous	Ganciclovir	100	50	25	Intravenous for treatment
Antifungal drugs					
Oral	Griseofulvin	100	100	100	Hepatotoxic
	Ketoconazole	100	100	100	
	Miconazole	100	100	100	
	Itraconazole	100	100	50	
	Fluconazole	100	75	50	
Intravenous	Amphotericin B	100	100	100	Nephrotoxic. Lipid formulations prefered
	Itraconazole	100	Avoid	Avoid	
	Voriconazole	100	Avoid	Avoid	
	Posaconazole	100	Avoid	Avoid	
	Echinocandins	100	100	100	Caspofungin, Micafungin and Anidulafungin—Avoid rapid infusion
Antiparasitic drugs					
	Albendazole	100	100	100	
	Mebendazole	100	100	100	
	Pyrantel pamoate	100	100	100	Intestinal nematodes
	Praziquantel	100	100	100	Schistosomal infections
	Diethylcarbamazine				
	Ivermectin	100	100	100	Lymphatic filariasis
	Chloroquine	100	100	50	Lymphatic filariasis Malaria
	Quinine	75	50	25	Falciparum malaria
	Mefloquine	100	100	100	
	Primaquine	100	200	100	Cure from relapses of *P. vivax* (malaria)
	Artemesinin	100	100	100	

Contd...

Contd...

Group of drugs	*Pharmacological name*	*Percentage of dose for glomerular filtration rate (GFR)*			*Remarks*
Subgroup		*>50 mL/min*	*10–50 mL/min*	*<10 mL/min*	
Neuromuscular agents					
	Vecuronium	100	100	100	No modification
	Atracurium				
	Ketamine				
	Propofol				
	Succinylcholine				
Anesthetics					
	Halothane	100	100	100	
	Desflurane	100	100	75	
	Sevoflurane	100	75	50	
	Etomidate	100	75	50	
	Sufentanil				
	Thiopental				
	Morphine				
	Meperidine				
Other drugs					
	Neostigmine				
	Pyridostigmine	100	50	Avoid	
	Pancuronium				
	Tubocurarine				
Anticonvulsants					
	Phenytoin				No dose change
	Carbamazepine				
	Valproate	100	100	100	
	Ethosuximide				
	Tiagabine				
	Gabapentin	75	50	25	
	Levetiracetam	100	75	50	
Anti-Parkinson drugs					
	Amantadine	75	37.5	17.25	
	Levodopa				
	Carbidopa				
	Bromocriptine	100	100	100	No dose modification
	Rasagiline				
	Anticholinergics				

Contd...

Contd...

Group of drugs	*Pharmacological name*	*Percentage of dose for glomerular filtration rate (GFR)*			*Remarks*
Subgroup		*>50 mL/min*	*10–50 mL/min*	*<10 mL/min*	
Antidepressant/antipsychotic					
	Imipramine Amitriptyline Nortriptyline Protriptyline Isocarboxazid Doxepin Sertraline Fluoxetine Citalopram	100	100	100	No dose modification
Sedatives/hypnotics					
	Midazolam Chlordiazepoxide Lorazepam Alprazolam Nitrazepam diazepam clonazepam Zolpidem Clobazam	100 100 100	100 100 100	50 50 100	No dose modification
Gastrointestinal agents					
	Domperidone Dolasetron Granisetron Ondansetron Palonosetron Cimetidine Famotidine Ranitidine Nizatidine	100 100 100 100 100	100 100 100 100 100	100 50 50 50 50	
Pulmonary system					
	Methylxanthine group Beta-2 agonists Anticholinergics Montelukast	100 100 100 100	100 100 100 100	100 100 100 100	No dosage change

SUMMARY

- Most drug trials have assessed only the short and medium term toxicities of the drugs before marketing. The use of drugs for many years has not been fully evaluated in most of them. Therefore, delayed toxicity may occur and clinicians should be aware of the same.
- Combination of drugs, which may not be highly nephrotoxic individually when given in modified doses, may eventually be nephrotoxic when combined with other drugs. This can be highlighted by a few common examples of combinations in clinical practice—aminoglycosides with second-generation cephalosporins, acyclovir with aminoglycosides/vancomycin, NSAIDs with ACE inhibitors, NSAIDs with radiocontrast agents.
- The 4 important groups of drugs, which are commonly used and cause nephrotoxicity are aminoglycosides, NSAIDs, ACE inhibitors/A2RBs, and radiocontrast agents—together called the '*Nephrotoxic Quartet*'.
- The clinician should remember that the new drug might not be always the 'best drug'. It is prudent to be familiar with some common drugs and use them judiciously since drug-induced AKI is a very common cause of iatrogenic problems.

Multiple Choice Questions

1. **The following factors are responsible for high vulnerability to renal damage except:**
   a. High metabolic activity of tubular cells
   b. High medullary osmolality
   c. Uncoupling of drugs in kidney
   d. Blood flow rate at 1 mL/gram/minute
   e. Glomerular filtration

2. **Stage 3b of CKD represents GFR of:**
   a. 50–60 mL/min
   b. 40–50 mL/min
   c. 30–45 mL/min
   d. 45–60 mL/min
   e. 25–35 mL/min

3. **Choose the correct set of answers from following.**
   The prerenal mechanisms causing drug-induced renal damage are:
   A. Diuretic-induced hypovolemia
   B. Uncoupling from protein binding
   C. Hypercatabolism
   D. Vascular thrombosis
   E. Hypotension
   F. Crystal formation
   a. A, B, D, F are correct
   b. A, C, E, F are correct
   c. A, C, D, E are correct
   d. B, D, E, F are correct

4. **A normal individual will have the highest GFR at the age of:**
   a. Neonatal period
   b. 5–10 years
   c. 20–25 years
   d. 30–35 years
   e. 40–45 years

5. **What will be the eGFR by Cockroft-Gault formula in a 40-year-old man weighing 72 kg and serum creatinine level of 4 mg%:**
   a. 75 mL/min
   b. 60 mL/min
   c. 45 mL/min
   d. 25 mL/min
   e. 15 mL/min

6. **The following drugs cause crystalluria:**
   a. Gentamicin
   b. Nitrofurantion
   c. Indinavir
   d. Sodium bicarbonate
   e. Lente insulin

7. **The following drug is incriminated as a cause of retroperitoneal fibrosis.**
   a. Hydralazine
   b. Hydrochlorothiazide
   c. Hydroxyuria
   d. Hydroxychloroquine

8. **The following ACE inhibitor drugs require dose modification in renal failure except:**
   a. Enalapril
   b. Ramipril
   c. Lisinopril
   d. Fosinopril
   e. Perindopril

9. **The following oral antidiabetic drugs are avoided in stage 3 of CKD, except:**
   a. Glyburide
   b. Gliclazide
   c. Glimepiride
   d. Acarbose
   e. Chlorpropamide

10. **Match the following:**

1. Pharmacodynamics	U. Low for protein bound drugs
2. Pharmacokinetics	V. High margin of safety
3. Bioavailability	W. Therapeutic drug monitoring preferred
4. Volume of distribution	X. What the drug does to the body
5. Narrow therapeutic window	Y. Percentage of drug reaching circulation
	Z. What the body does to the drug

Answers

1\. d 2. c 3 c 4. d 5. d 6. c 7. a 8. d
9\. c 10. 1 = X, 2 = Z, 3 = Y, 4 = U, 5 = W

SUGGESTED READING

1. Aronoff. G, Bennet WM (Eds), et al. Drug prescribing in renal failure. Dosing Guidelines for Adults and Children, 5th edition. American College of Physicians, Philadelphia. USA.
2. Brunton LL (Ed). Goodman and Gilman's Pharmacological basis of Therapeutics, 12 edition. McGraw-Hill companies, San Diego, California, USA.
3. Floge J, Johnson R, Feehally J. Comprehensive Clinical Nephrology, 5th edition, Elsevier.
4. Kasi Visweswaran R (Ed). Prescribing drugs in renal diseases. Tree Life media publishing for practice, Mumbai, India, 2004.

CHAPTER 15

Renal Replacement Therapy in Chronic Kidney Disease Patients

Georgi Abraham, Tarun K George

INTRODUCTION

Chronic kidney disease is defined as a structural or functional renal abnormality for more than three months, usually associated with reducing glomerular filtration rate (GFR). As the GFR continues to fall, there is an increase in the stage of chronic kidney disease (CKD) and the various functions of the kidney get compromised. End-stage renal disease (ESRD) or kidney failure is the term used when the GFR <15 mL/min/1.73 m^2, and this is associated with features of uremia.

India has a rising trend in the prevalence of diabetes and hypertension. Associated with this, there is an increasing prevalence of CKD. The CKD stage III and above (i.e. GFR < 60 mL/min/1.73 m^2) in the adult population ranges from 4-6% in different studies. Unfortunately, in India only 2-4% of patients with ESRD seek any of the following definitive therapy.

RENAL REPLACEMENT THERAPY

Renal replacement therapy (RRT) refers to the modalities available to carry out the core renal function of excretion during renal failure. They are dialysis and renal transplant. This may be carried out in an acute and chronic setting. In an acute setting continuous renal replacement therapy (CRRT), slow low-efficiency dialysis (SLED), and sometimes peritoneal dialysis are used. In the chronic situation—hemodialysis, peritoneal dialysis and renal transplant are the options for replacing the damaged renal function **(Fig. 15.1)**.

The important steps in the management of CKD are—confirm, rule out and treat. After confirming the presence of CKD and staging the disease, a systematic and thorough approach to rule out reversible causes must be sought. Factors that are over commonly looked are as follows:

Prerenal factors:
- Bilateral renal artery stenosis.
- Uncontrolled hypertension.

Renal causes factors:
- Active glomerular and tubulointerstitial diseases
- Nephrotoxic agents
- Recurrent pyelonephritis.

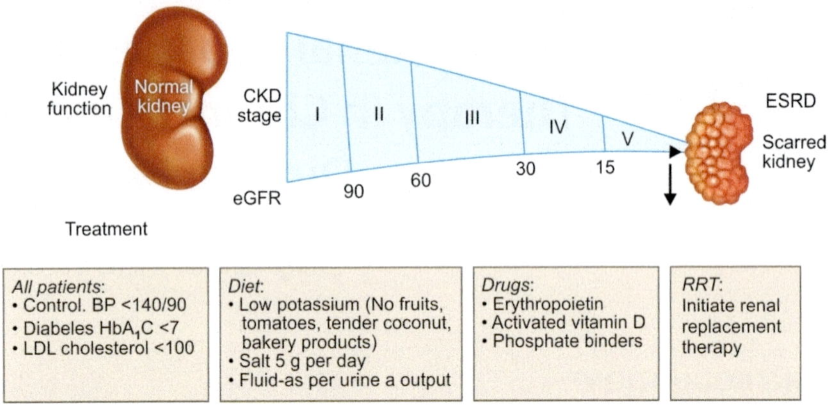

Figure 15.1 CKD treatment involves conservative management and renal replacement therapy. All patients must receive therapy appropriate for the current renal function prior to and even during RRT

Abbreviations: CKD, chronic kidney disease; GFR, glomerular filtration rate; ESRD, end stage renal disease; RRT, renal replacement therapy

Postrenal factors:
- Stone
- Stricture ureters
- Enlarged prostate
- Bladder neck obstruction.

As a person's renal function continues to deteriorate, the doctor must prepare the patient and family about the options of RRT. After reaching the stage of end-stage renal disease (ESRD) the options available are hemodialysis, peritoneal dialysis or transplantation.

The indications for dialysis are as follows:
- Persistence of uremic symptoms—nausea, vomiting, anorexia, fatigue, mental status changes, itching and muscle cramps
- Hyperkalemia unresponsive to medications
- Extracellular volume expansion not responding to diuretic therapy
- Refractory metabolic acidosis
- Bleeding diathesis due to platelet dysfunction
- Pleuritis or pericarditis due to uremia

Dialysis is usually initiated when the estimated GFR (eGFR) <10 mL/min per 1.73 m^2.

Hemodialysis

This is the process of removing excess water and clearing the blood of impurities, such as creatinine, urea, and anions. Here, the solute composition of blood is altered by exposing it to a physiological solution (dialysate) across a semipermeable dialysis membrane. The parts involved are the dialyzer, the dialysate and the blood. It involves a circuit, which removes the blood from the body, passes it through the dialyzer and removes electrolytes, urea and water through the dialysate, before returning it back into the body.

- *The principle of hemodialysis*: Underlying principle is the diffusion of solutes and ultrafiltration of water. In diffusion the solutes move from area of high to a low concentration. In ultrafiltration, the water in the blood compartment is driven out by a hydrostatic pressure through a semipermeable membrane. The semipermeable membrane is impermeable to cells and plasma proteins and allows the movement of solutes and water.
- *The access*: Here, the blood leaves the body and also returns through it. This is usually an arteriovenous fistula (AVF), arteriovenous graft (AVG) and even a catheter through which the blood can be obtained for the dialysis. The most convenient access is the fistula. The arteriovenous (most often an end to side anastomosis of the cephalic vein to the radial artery) channel creates an arterialization of the vein through which large needles can access the blood, which is at a high pressure. The blood is drawn from the arterial end into the hemodialysis machine and returned to venous part. The fistula has a mean patency of five to seven years. The drawback is that after the surgery it takes 2–4 months for the fistula to mature before it can be used and there can be issues of improper maturation or early thrombosis **(Fig. 15.2)**.
  - AVGs are synthetic, usually PTFE (Poly tetra fluro ethylene). Tubings that connect an artery to a vein. They take less time to mature, but they are more prone to infections and clots. These can be used when the veins are of a smaller caliber or when there has been repeated venipuncture **(Fig. 15.3)**. The catheters are used when dialysis has to be suddenly initiated in an unplanned setting. It is usually placed in the internal jugular **(Fig. 15.4)** or femoral vein. It can be a temporary bridge until a fistula becomes functional. The femoral vein catheter predisposes to high risk of infection. The subclavian vein is usually avoided since, if stenosis occurs, the opportunity of a permanent fistula in that forearm is lost. A tunneled catheter is also placed in femoral or internal jugular vein but it is tunneled under the skin, thereby reducing the chances of line related infection.

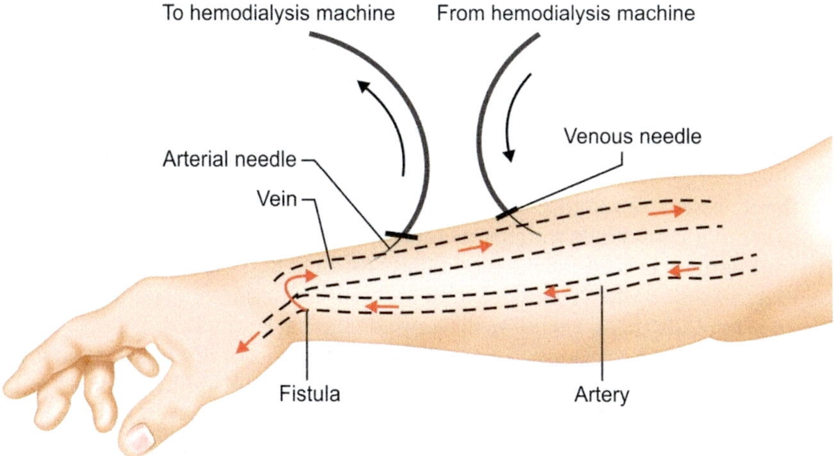

Figure 15.2 Fistula

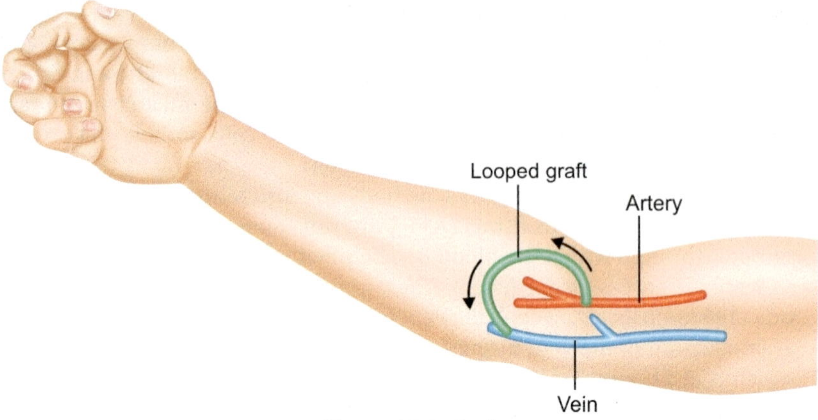

Figure 15.3 Graft

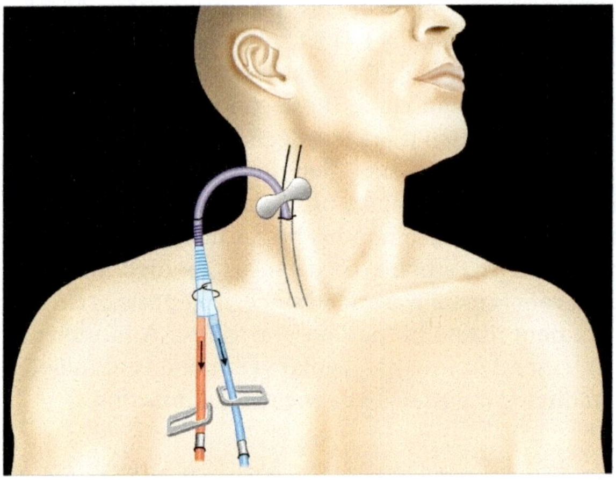

Figure 15.4 Catheter used in the internal jugular vein

- *The dialyzer*: This is a chamber where the blood and the dialysate flow in opposite directions. This is a plastic chamber with bundles of capillary tubes through which the blood circulates, while the dialysate flows through the outer side in opposite direction—the counter current principle. The membrane of the dialyzer can range from 1.5 to 2 m^2. The membranes are generally made of synthetic materials which are biocompatible and hence do not activate the complement cascade as the blood flows through it. In the Indian scenario the dialyzer unit is often rinsed, cleared and reused for the same patient
- *The dialysate*: This is a solution of components that is adjusted in concentration according to the patient's serum. The composition of the dialysate involves sodium, potassium, calcium and bicarbonate, which is individualized to the patients requirements. Patients can be exposed to up to 120 L of water during the dialysis, hence the water has to be subjected to thorough cleansing process of filtration, softening, deionization and reverse osmosis

- Comparing a standard hemodialysis solution and serum **(Table 15.1)**
- *The blood delivery system*: The blood is drawn from the patient, pumped through the dialysis machine where it equilibrates with the dialysate and is returned back to the patient. The blood is heparinized in the system to prevent it from clotting within the machine. The flow rate ranges from 250 to 500 mL/min. There are several checks and safety monitors to prevent air from entering, prevent leakage, etc.
  - Most patients require a hemodialysis sitting of 3 times a week (i.e. on alternate days). The end points are clinically attaining a euvolemic state without any evidence of fluid retention, uremia or electrolyte abnormalities.
  - **Figure 15.5** demonstrates a dialysis circuit.

Complications

- *Hypotension*: Due to fluid removal and poor compensatory autonomic responses
- *Muscle cramps*: Due to hypovolemia and low sodium dialysates
- *Anaphylactoid reactions*: From components in the dialyzer membrane
- *Dialysis disequilibrium syndrome*: This occurs when a rapid reduction in urea levels after dialysis causes an intravascular hypo-osmolar state and leads to cerebral edema. Patients develop neurological features of headache, nausea, restlessness and altered sensorium. It can be avoided by initiating dialysis at a low blood flow rate. Therapy involves reducing/stopping the dialysis and treating the symptoms
- *Cardiovascular diseases:* They are the major cause of death in patients with ESRD due to the previous comorbidities, chronic inflammation and changes in volume. They should be initiated on appropriate therapy, such as statins, aspirin and beta blockers.

Table 15.1 Comparing a standard hemodialysis solution and serum

Component	*Dialysate concentration (mEq/L)*	*Normal Serum Concentration (mEq/L)*
Sodium	135–145	135–145
Potassium	2–3	3.5– 5.0
Magnesium	0.5–0.75	1.5–2.0
Calcium	2.5–3.5	8.4–10.2
Chloride	98–124	95–105
Bicarbonate	25–35	22–28
pCO2	40–110 mm Hg	33–45 mm Hg
pH	7.1–7.3	7.35–7.45
Acetate	3–8 m M/L	0.025 mM/L
Citrate	0.8–1 mM/L	0.16 mM/L
Glucose	0–200 mg/dL	80–200 mg/dL

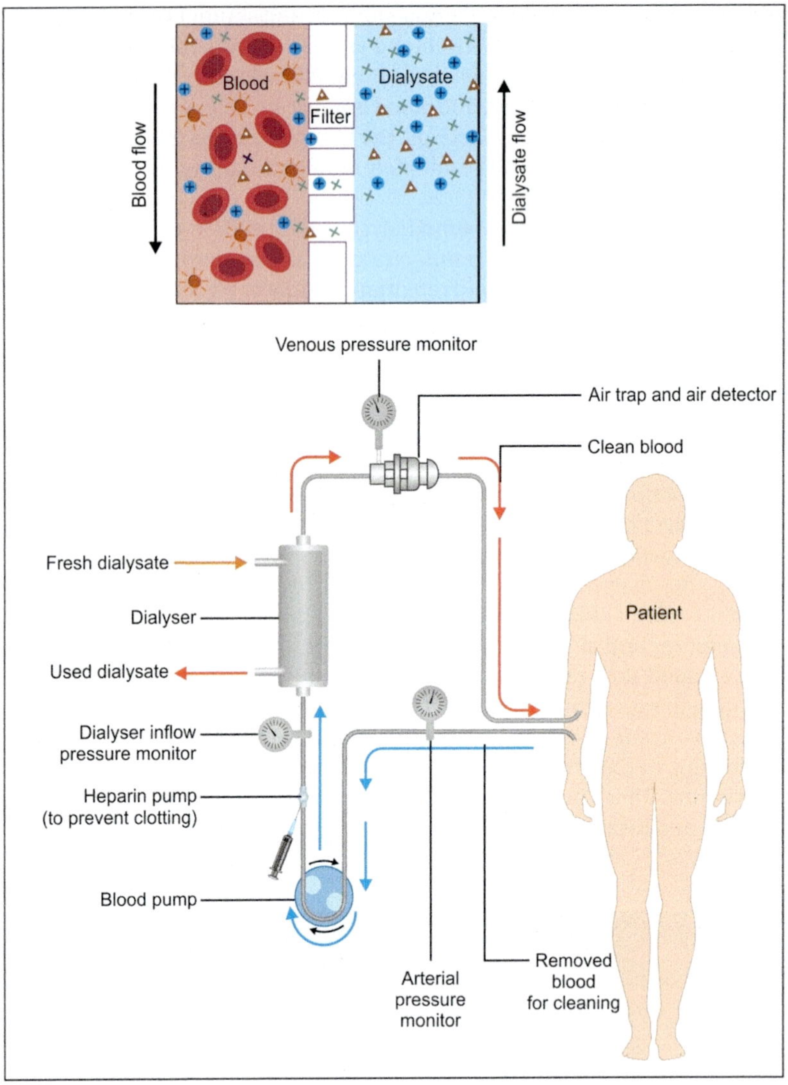

Figure 15.5 Dialysis circuit with cellular level exchange
Factoid: Dr Willem Kolff, a Dutch physician and the father of dialysis made the first dialysis machine in 1943 from sausage skins, orange juice cans and a washing machine

Peritoneal Dialysis

Principle of Peritoneal Dialysis

Here, the peritoneal membrane is used as a natural semipermeable membrane. The dialysate is infused into the peritoneal cavity and there is a diffusion of solutes and filtration of water between the blood in the capillaries and the dialysate solution. Usually, 1.5–3 liters of a dextrose containing fluid is used, and it is allowed to dwell for a period of 2–4 hours. After the rate of diffusion gradient between the two fluids diminishes and when equilibrium between the plasma and the dialysate is reached the spent dialysate is replaced with fresh one. Peritoneal dialysis may be carried out in two ways: as a continuous ambulatory PD (CAPD) where the patient manually changes the fluid 3–4 times in 24 hours and continuous cycling PD (CCPD) where an automated cycler performs the exchanges while the patient is in bed **(Fig. 15.6)**.

A peritoneal catheter is surgically inserted and used to access the cavity. The volume of the fluid ranges from 1.5 L to 3 L. The dialysate here is usually composed of Na 132, Cl 96, lactate 40, Mg 0.25 and Ca 1.75 (in mmol/L). The osmolality varies from 346 mmol/L upwards. A non-absorbable carbohydrate solution (icodextrin) was introduced as an osmotic agent and it demonstrates more efficient ultrafiltration than with dextrose solutions. Although rised stylet cathters are used for acute PD, flexible Tenckhoff catheters are preferred for both acute and chronic PD.

The patients undergo a peritoneal equilibrium test that assesses the peritoneal membranes characteristics of transferring glucose and creatinine across the membrane. Patients who are slow transporters do well with fewer exchanges and longer dwells while the opposite is true for high transporters.

Complications

Peritonitis: It usually occurs due to nonsterile techniques. Here the common organisms are of skin origin (such as the gram-positive *Staphylococcus*), sometimes gram-negative rods and rarely fungal and mycobacterial. The patient

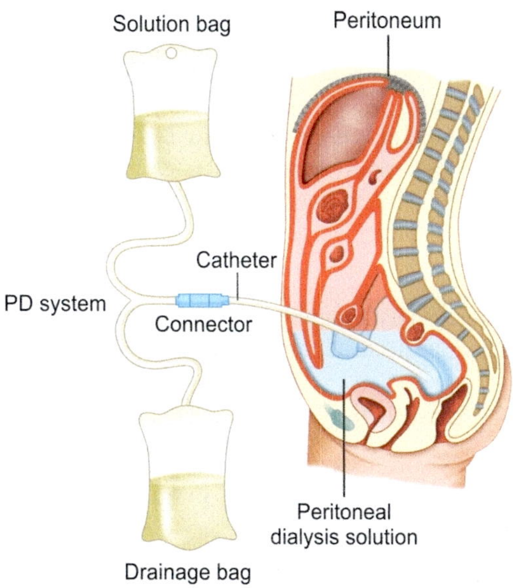

Figure 15.6 Illustration of peritoneal dialysis

Factoid: In 1946 the *first successful 'peritoneal irrigation' was carried out by Frank, Seligman and Fine. They used continuous lavage through surgically implanted rubber and stainless steel tubes. Peritonitis was a fatal complication in many of these patients*

develops pain, fever and a cloudy dialysate fluid associated with elevated peritoneal fluid leucocytes predominantly neutrophils. These have to be treated with appropriate antibiotics and even catheter removal if it is not resolving.

Tunnel infection: There can also be infection around the catheter, which is known as a *tunnel infection.*

Metabolic complications: Metabolic complications, particularly loss of albumin and protein require a higher intake of dietary protein. These patients also develop *hyperglycemia* from the dextrose in the solution and are prone to insulin resistance and *hypertriglyceridemia.*

Mechanical complications: *These* include pain during the inflow and outflow, blockage of the system, distressing abdominal distension, pulmonary atelectasis, pleural effusions and migration of intraperitoneal portion of catheter.

Renal Transplantation

This is the treatment of choice for patients with ESRD. However, the limiting factor is the cost and the availability of kidneys for transplant. In the early years, the major problem was graft (transplanted kidney) rejection. Since then there have been major progresses in immunosuppression so that now the mean graft survival rates are around 10–15 years. The Transplantation Human Organ Act (THO) was passed in 1994 in India to streamline donation and transplantation however there is a wide gap between the donation rate and the number of patients on the transplant list.

Indications

Patients with ESRD. The major causes of ESRD are diabetes, hypertension, chronic glomerulonephritis and cystic kidney diseases. In certain cases like hepatorenal syndrome, a combined liver and kidney transplant while in severe type I diabetes a kidney-pancreas transplant is done. There are few conditions that recur in the transplanted kidney—IgA nephropathy, some glomerulonephritides, oxalosis and diabetes. However the rate is low.

Contraindications

Metastatic cancer, severe HIV immunodeficiency, active or recurrent infections, advance cardiac failure and substance abuse.

Pretransplant Assessment

Most patients are either on dialysis or have an eGFR <20 mL/min/1.73 m^2. A preoperative work-up of assessing cardiac, pulmonary, bladder function and viral status is done for all patients.

Donor status: The donors can be living or deceased. The live donor could be a twin, related or unrelated one. The deceased donation can be from either brain dead or donation after cardiac death. It is required that the donor is in good health without any disease (such diabetes, cardiac illness, malignancy, etc.)

that can compromise their renal function in the future. Most centers require the donor to have a GFR of at least 80 mL/min/1.73 m^2.

Compatibility: The donor and the recipient should be ABO blood group and HLA antigen crossmatch compatible. Incompatibility increases activation of the immune system and graft rejection. Nowadays, desensitization protocols are available to reduce risk of rejection in incompatible transplants. Also in conditions where a pair of donor and recipient is incompatible, they can be exchanged for a compatible kidney from another pair, i.e. kidney paired donation.

Procedure

The kidneys are removed either from a living or a deceased donor. In the case of a living donor often both resection and implantation occurs in the adjacent surgical theatres. In a deceased donor transplant, if it is in another location, the resected kidney needs to be preserved in a hypothermic container with or without a continuous preservative perfusion. This reduces the metabolism and degradation reactions. The kidney can be stored up to 40 hours prior to implantation. The time that the organ is without blood supply is called ischemia time. The warm ischemia time is while the kidney is still in the body and when the vessels are clamped preventing perfusion. The cold ischemia time is the period while it is in transit from the donor to the recipient. However longer the ischemia time, the less viable the organ becomes.

- Most often the diseased kidneys are not removed. The transplanted kidney is often placed in the right iliac fossa because of the availability of space and more vessels available for reconstruction. The surgery usually takes around three hours. The donor the surgery is now often done by a laparoscopic assisted method. Usually the left kidney is removed as it has a longer renal vein and hence is easier to implant **(Fig. 15.7)**.
- In India if there is a deceased donor the operation is part of a multiorgan retrieval process where the heart, kidney, liver, pancreas and lung are removed and they are individually transported to centers where a predetermined matched recipient is earlier notified and awaiting.

Immunosuppressive Regimens

Drugs like cyclosporine (calcinuerin inhibitors), tacrolimus, mycophenolate, steroids and azathioprine are commonly used. These cause broad immunosuppression and hence the body is prone to various infections and even malignancies. Prior to transplant surgery patients receive an induction immunosuppression with antithymocyte globulin (ATG) or interleukin (IL) 2 receptor antibodies (such as basiliximab). These are followed by maintenance immunosuppression, such as tacrolimus/cyclosporine with mycophenolate and prednisolone. Therapeutic drug monitoring is required to ensure appropriate levels of drugs like tacrolimus and cyclosporine. After 6 months, the dose of these drugs are cautiously reduced but are never withdrawn as it may lead to rejection.

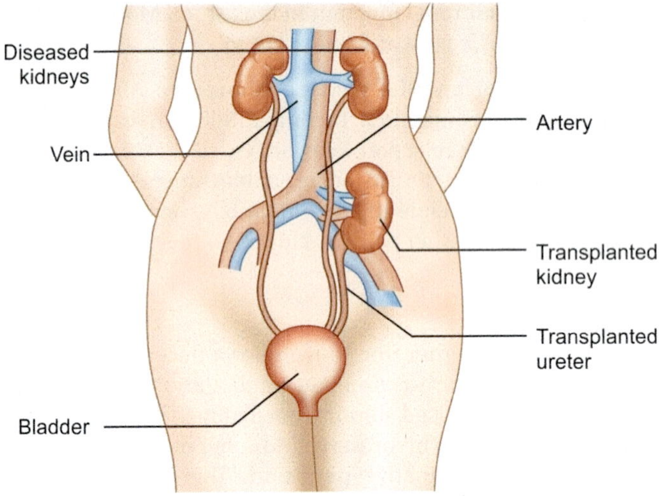

Figure 15.7 Deciding between different RRT options

Factoid: The first successful renal transplant was in 1954 where surgeons Joseph Murray and John Hartwell in collaboration with nephrologist John Merrill transplanted a kidney between identical twins in Bent Brigham Hospital, Boston.

Dr John Murray, was awarded the Nobel Prize for his work in organ transplantation

Complications

Hyperacute rejection: It occurs on the operating table due to ABO or HLA incompatibility. The kidney appears mottled, and it requires immediate nephrectomy.

Acute rejection: Is due to cellular or immune mediated injury. It presents within 6 months with features of fever, malaise, abdominal pain, oliguria and a rising creatinine. It can occur in up to 15% of transplants. It is crucial to rule out infections in such a scenario. An ultrasound and biopsy is done to confirm the diagnosis and it is treated with high dose steroids and immunosuppression like antithymocyte globulin or plasmapharesis.

Chronic allograft nephropathy: It occurs more than one year after transplant. There is a gradual decline in renal function with increasing proteinuria and hypertension. It is due to a combination of immune mediated and nonimmune factors like hypertension and dyslipidemia, which promote injury and poor functioning.

Infections: It occurs mostly in the first year after transplant and 40–80% experience an infection during this time. Patients in first 6 months receive the highest immunosuppression and have greatest risk of viral and opportunistic infections. **Table 15.2** shows a timeline of common post-transplant infections.

Anatomical complications: Renal artery and vein thrombosis, urine leaks from the anastomotic connection. Late complications are renal artery stenosis and ureteric strictures.

Table 15.2 Timeline of post-transplant infections

Within 1 month	*1–6 months*	*More than 6 months*
• Nosocomial infections: - MRSA, VRE, *Candida* species • Wound infections, anastomotic leaks • Donor derived infections - HSV, HIV, CMV	• If no prophylaxis given—PCP, HSV, CMV, EBV • Polyomavirus BK infection • *C. difficile* colitis, *Cryptococcus neoformans, Mycobacterium tuberculosis*	• Community acquired pneumonia • Urinary tract infections • *Nocardia* • Late viral infections—CMV of retina and colitis, hepatitis B and C, HSV skin cancers and lymphoma

Abbreviations: MRSA, Methicillin-resistant *Staphylococcus aureus*; VRE, vancomycin resistant organism; HSV, herpes simplex virus; HIV, human immunodeficiency virus; CMV, cytomegalovirus; PCP, *pneumocystis carinii* infection; EBV, Epstein-Barr virus

Table 15.3 Factors to decide between three RRT options

Factors	*Hemodialysis*	*Peritoneal dialysis*	*Transplant*
Expertise and infrastructure	Requires dedicated centers	After training can be done by self at home	Needs multidisciplinary team in tertiary level hospital
Availability	Most commonly used mode of RRT	Lack of trained personnel and poor patient education restricts usage	Available in select institutions. Permanent solution
Cost	Approx. ₹12,000–36,000 per month (varies as per center)	Almost same as hemodialysis	Approx. ₹4–5 lakh initial cost (center dependent) with up to ₹10,000 per month as maintenance cost

Malignancies: Higher risk of skin malignancies, late onset lymphoma, stomach and liver cancers.

Drug-related toxicities: Calcineurin inhibitors (such as cyclosporine) can cause renal ischemia and has multiple drug interactions. Steroids have many side effects specifically weight gain, dyslipidemia, diabetes and hypertension. Azathioprine causes bone marrow suppression.

Table 15.3 summarizes how should the doctor and patient decide between the three options.

SUMMARY

- All patients with declining renal function should be evaluated for reversible and treatable causes.
- All patients should have appropriate treatment for their risk factors.
- They should be educated on the progression of disease and the need for renal replacement therapy. The modality of choice should be individualized for the patient.
- Hemodialysis is carried out up to 3 times a week. It is widely available.

- Peritoneal dialysis can be done at home. It requires training and clean surroundings to perform.
- Renal transplant is a more permanent solution that is initially expensive and available in select centers.

Multiple Choice Questions

1. **Which of the following is not an indication to initiate dialysis in a patient with chronic kidney disease?**
   a. Hyperkalemia not correctible by medical management.
   b. Patient with pericarditis and uremia.
   c. Renal artery stenosis with shrunken kidneys asymptomatic patient.
   d. Fluid overload state with only 300 mL of urine output per day.

2. **The most common cause of death in patients with end-stage renal disease is:**
   a. Dialysis related complications
   b. Urinary tract infections and sepsis
   c. Cardiovascular causes, such as ACS, sudden cardiac death and stroke
   d. Acute uremic complications.

3. **The following is true about hemodialysis:**
   a. Can be offered for all age groups and even in ICUs
   b. Requires deionized water
   c. Blood volumes flows can be up to 500 mL/min in the system
   d. All of the above

4. **Which is false about dialysis disequilibrium syndrome?**
   a. Occurs in hemodialysis
   b. Is an anaphylactic response due to the components of the dialyzer membrane
   c. Patient complains of headache, nausea and restlessness
   d. The dialysis needs to be stopped or flow rate reduced.

5. **Which of the following is not given via a peritoneal dialysis solution?**
   a. Heparin
   b. Potassium
   c. Antibiotics
   d. Insulin

6. **Which of the following is a complication of peritoneal dialysis?**
   a. Tunnel site infection
   b. Hypoalbuminemia
   c. Dyslipidemia
   d. All of the above

7. **A patient on peritoneal dialysis presents with fever, abdominal pain and turbid dialysate fluid for 2 days. You suspect an infectious peritonitis. What is the most likely organism?**
   a. *E. coli* from the perineum
   b. *Staphylococcus epidermidis* from the skin
   c. *Mycobacterium tuberculosis* which is acquired
   d. Anaerobic bacteria from the gut

8. **Which of the following drugs are not used in immunosuppression in a patient with renal transplant?**
   a. Cyclophosphamide
   b. Mycophenolate
   c. Prednisolone
   d. Anti-thymocyte globulin

9. Which of these patients with ESRD is not a candidate for renal transplant?

a. 30-year-old type 1 diabetic with uncontrolled sugars and eGFR of 10 mL/min per 1.73 m^2

b. 50-year-old multivalvular rheumatic heart disease in severe heart failure, pulmonary artery hypertension with history of smoking and recent ACS with current ejection fraction of 25%.

c. 60-year-old lady with SLE, now controlled and cured breast cancer

d. 40-year-old man with family history of autosomal dominant polycystic kidney disease (ADPKD).

10. The most commonly employed mode of renal replacement therapy in India is:

a. Intermittent hemodialysis

b. Renal transplant

c. Continuous ambulatory peritoneal dialysis

d. Continuous cycling peritoneal dialysis.

Answers

1. c	2. c	3. d	4. b	5. b	6. d	7. b	8. a
9. b	10. a						

SUGGESTED READING

1. Abboud H, Henrich WL. Clinical practice. Stage IV chronic kidney disease. N Engl J Med. 2010;362(1):56.
2. Abraham G, George TJ, Shroff S, et al. Evolution of renal transplant in India over the last four decades. Clinical Kidney Journal. 2009;3(2):203-7.
3. As it was in the beginning: A history of Peritoneal Dialysis by Dr Russel A. Palmer *http://www.pdiconnect.com/content/2/1/16.full.pdf*
4. Current status of end-stage renal disease care in India and Pakistan. Vivekanand Jha-Kidney Intern Suppl. 2013;3:157-60.
5. Guidelines of the Renal Association—Planning, Initiating and Withdrawal of renal replacement therapy *http://www.renal.org/guidelines/modules/planning-initiating-and-withdrawal-of-renal-replacement-therapy#sthash.bCkH5Jsl.dpbs*
6. KDOQI. Clinical practice guideline for hemodialysis adequacy: Update. National Kidney Foundation. Am J Kidney Dis. 2015;66(5):884-930.
7. Khanna U. The economics of dialysis in India. Indian J Nephrol. 2009;19(1):1-4.

Index

Page numbers followed by *f* to figure, *fc* to flow chart, and *t* to table

D

E

F

G

H

I

J

K

L

Q

R

S

T

U

V

W